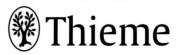

# Medical Thoracoscopy/Pleuroscopy: Manual and Atlas

Robert Loddenkemper, MD
Professor
Former Head of Department of Pneumology II
Lungenklinik Heckeshorn
HELIOS-Klinikum Emil von Behring
Berlin, Germany

Praveen N. Mathur, MD
Professor of Clinical Medicine
Indiana University School of Medicine
Indianapolis, IN, USA

Marc Noppen, MD, PhD
Associate Professor
Free University of Brussels, VUB
Chief Executive Officer and Head
Interventional Endoscopy Clinic
University Hospital UZ Brussels
Brussels, Belgium

Pyng Lee, MD
Associate Professor
Division of Respiratory and Critical Care
Department of Medicine
National University Hospital
Singapore

241 illustrations

Thieme
Stuttgart · New York

*Library of Congress Cataloging-in-Publication Data*
Medical thoracoscopy/pleuroscopy : manual and atlas /
Robert Loddenkemper ... [et al.].
    p. ; cm.
ISBN 978-3-13-108221-3 (hardback : alk. paper)
1. Thoracoscopy–Handbooks, manuals, etc.
2. Thoracoscopy–Atlases. I. Loddenkemper, Robert.
    [DNLM: 1. Thoracoscopy–methods. 2. Pleural Cavity–
surgery. 3. Thoracoscopy–Atlases. WF 980 M4896 2010]
    RC941.M43 2010
        617.5'4–dc22                                2010023078

**Important Note:** Medicine is an ever-changing science undergoing continual development. Research and clinical experience are continually expanding our knowledge, in particular our knowledge of proper treatment and drug therapy. Insofar as this book mentions any dosage or application, readers may rest assured that the authors, editors, and publishers have made every effort to ensure that such references are in accordance with **the state of knowledge at the time of production of the book.**

Nevertheless, this does not involve, imply, or express any guarantee or responsibility on the part of the publishers in respect to any dosage instructions and forms of applications stated in the book. **Every user is requested to examine carefully** the manufacturers' leaflets accompanying each drug and to check, if necessary in consultation with a physician or specialist, whether the dosage schedules mentioned therein or the contraindications stated by the manufacturers differ from the statements made in the present book. Such examination is particularly important with drugs that are either rarely used or have been newly released on the market. Every dosage schedule or every form of application used is entirely at the user's own risk and responsibility. The authors and publishers request every user to report to the publishers any discrepancies or inaccuracies noticed.

© 2011 Georg Thieme Verlag,
Rüdigerstrasse 14, 70469 Stuttgart, Germany
http://www.thieme.de
Thieme New York, 333 Seventh Avenue,
New York, NY 10001, USA
http://www.thieme.com

Cover design: Thieme Publishing Group
Typesetting by Ziegler + Müller, Kirchentellinsfurt,
Germany
Printed in Germany by Offizin Andersen Nexö
Leipzig GmbH, Zwenkau, Germany

ISBN 978-3-13-108221-3            1 2 3 4 5 6

# Foreword

The fact that my medical career started back in the first half of the last century means, of course, that I must be very old, which I am–well past 80–but it also means that for over 60 years I have been both witness to and participant in the spectacular advances that have revolutionized the understanding and practice of medicine in general and of pulmonary medicine in particular. Certainly, this experience provides an advantageous perspective from which to write a foreword to this edition of *Medical Thoracoscopy/ Pleuroscopy: Manual and Atlas*, a thoroughly revised and updated book about a resurgent procedure that is both underappreciated and underutilized in many countries, including the United States, and that is gaining importance in the diagnosis and treatment of a variety of pleuropulmonary diseases.

In the 1950s, at the beginning of my career as a pulmonologist, I cared for many patients with tuberculosis, the signature disease of the specialty. But during the ensuing decade, tuberculosis began to decrease in incidence and became mostly a curable instead of a chronic and often fatal condition; in addition, the focus of its care shifted from the hospital (or sanatorium) to the clinic (or office). Pulmonary physicians, however, became even busier than before as their responsibilities shifted from patients with tuberculosis to those with diseases that were by no means new but which we began to see in increasing numbers– asthma, chronic obstructive pulmonary disease, and cancer of the lung: a trend that to a large extent continues today.

By the mid-1960s, I took advantage of the steadily diminishing number of patients with tuberculosis that required hospitalization in my 158-bed "TB Building" at San Francisco General Hospital by converting one of the newly emptied wards into an intensive care unit for patients with respiratory disease. The burgeoning number of intensive care units at the time provided a welcome home to physicians trained in pulmonary medicine, not only because of the frequency with which serious lung conditions –such as community-acquired pneumonia, status asthmaticus, and exacerbations of COPD–were the cause of admission, but because of the recurring need for mechanically assisted ventilation in desperately ill patients. Pulmonary specialists were well-versed in respiratory physiology, including the mechanics of breathing, which was a subject of much research and academic activity, and which coincided with considerable corporate interest in the development and marketing of ventilators. Soon, my dedicated "respiratory" facility became a full-fledged "medical" intensive care unit, and I became more and more involved in critical care, becoming an expert in a subspecialty that did not even exist when I was certified in pulmonary medicine.

Today's clinicians–skilled in contemporary medical practices and in the use of life-saving pharmacology and technology–take for granted what older physicians appreciate and still marvel at. And this is true not just in the practice of intensive care or pulmonology, but in each one of the many branches of medicine. Everyone agrees: remarkable discoveries have improved the lives of both patients and their doctors. Consider only one example: the spectacular advances that have occurred in diagnostic methodology. Currently, not many diseases escape definitive diagnosis by available microbiological, biochemical, and pathological analyses of specimens obtained from all the usual sources and, when needed, from hard-to-reach, formerly inaccessible sites. Moreover, application of highly advanced diagnostic methods quickly identified previously unknown and important clinical scourges, such as Legionnaire's disease, hantavirus pulmonary infection, human immunodeficiency virus infection and its partner in death and disability the acquired immunodeficiency syndrome, mad cow disease, and, more recently, severe acute respiratory syndrome (SARS): all of which have come to light during my professional lifetime.

Modern practitioners are blessed with imaging techniques of exceptional clarity and precision, which have replaced older sometimes dangerous and always unpleasant diagnostic methods: my father nearly died from an air encephalogram; today he would have been easily diagnosed by magnetic resonance imaging. Not many practicing pulmonary specialists realize how difficult bronchography was for doctors to perform and for patients to endure; now, when we need to map the extent and severity of bronchiectasis, we simply write an order for high-resolution computed tomography of the lungs. All of us welcomed ultrasonography into our diagnostic armamentarium, a convenient and noninvasive way of looking–for the first time–deep inside the heart, blood vessels, abdomen, and pelvis to identify anatomical and functional abnormalities, including the presence and location of pleural fluid in the chest.

Within the last decade or so, we have witnessed the flourishing of a breed of subspecialists called interventionists, descendents of a group of intrepid pioneers who, as the authors of this *Manual and Atlas* tell us, started probing body cavities around a century ago. Now, however, endowed with ultra-modern high-tech instruments, interventionists not only examine the insides of various cavities and organs, but they are able to do something about the abnormalities they find there. Surgeons are, without doubt, the consummate interventionists, but the practice has broadened to other chiefly "medical" specialists. Currently, we have interventional radiologists, interventional cardiologists, and interventional gastroenterologists. Plus, there is a scattering of interventional pulmonologists but, as the authors of this *Manual and Atlas*, who come from Europe, North America, and Asia, persuasively state, there should be many more. After proper training and experience in medical thoracoscopy or pleuroscopy (interchangeable terms), pulmonary specialists have much to offer in the diagnosis and management of patients with lung disease, especially those with pleural effusions, but including those with pneumothorax, empyema, and other conditions as well.

A brief review of my 60-plus years of repeated frustrations trying to diagnose and manage patients who presented with pleural effusions of uncertain etiology underscores the valuable additions to pulmonary medicine now provided by medical thoracoscopy. Traditionally, in teaching hospitals, thoracenteses are performed by interns and residents, and I did my share, although I don't remember doing very many. I also carried out a few artificial pneumothoraces, including one induction, for collapse therapy of pulmonary tuberculosis, although pneumoperitoneum was the preferred treatment in both hospitals I trained in.

Back then, the fluid we aspirated was not of much diagnostic value; measurements of the numbers and types of white blood cells and the protein concentration seldom altered clinical thinking, and cultures were only occasionally positive. The availability of cytology helped considerably, and we were even more delighted when, practically simultaneously, the Cope and Abrams needles appeared: here at last was a chance of making a definitive diagnosis. But not always. The report of one of my first biopsies, which provoked a brisk hemorrhage, showed a "fragment of arterial wall." Later, we profited from the diagnostic orientation afforded by Light's criteria, greatly improved culture methods, including for anaerobic organisms, and the development of biochemical tests such as N-terminal pro-brain natriuretic peptide (NT-BNP), adenosine deaminase, and gamma-interferon.

Obviously, all these additions and refinements helped. Although it is hard to generalize because of differences in technical approaches and in clinical settings, the yield from analysis and culture of thoracentesis fluid plus histo-logical examination and culture of specimens obtained by closed pleural biopsy establish a diagnosis of tuberculous pleurisy with effusion in 70–80% of cases. (Even though finding a high level of adenosine deaminase or gamma-interferon in blood or discovering caseating granulomas in pleural tissue provides a satisfactory working diagnosis, it remains important—and increasingly so—in some settings to culture *Mycobacterium tuberculosis* and to identify drug-resistant strains.) Image-guided pleural biopsy undoubtedly raises the diagnostic yield above 80% in patients with tuberculous pleural effusion, but it is close to 100% with thoracoscopy and the result of culture of thoracoscopic specimens is higher than from any other source. Sadly, these more sensitive procedures are seldom available where they are needed most: in resource-poor countries where the incidence of tuberculosis is extremely high.

Studies in patients who turn out to have malignant pleural effusions typically show a low diagnostic return from closed pleural biopsy when pleural fluid cytology is negative. Here again, the yield is increased by image-guided pleural biopsy, but raised even higher by thoracoscopy, which is clearly the best way of diagnosing pleural malignancies when suspicion is high and simpler approaches are unrevealing; thoracoscopy also furnishes the opportunity for performing talc poudrage under direct vision for optimum pleurodesis: when the procedure is indicated.

So for more than half a century, the work-up of patients with pleural effusion of unknown etiology has steadily improved, always in the direction of more reliable and safer ways of making an accurate diagnosis, thus paving the way for effective treatment. The point is that diagnostic algorithms are constantly evolving and that they now include medical thoracoscopy.

The appearance of this *Manual and Atlas* is timely, and the book fills a pressing need: it details the latest methodology; it offers numerous photographs of the various abnormalities that may be encountered during medical thoracoscopy; and it discusses controversial issues regarding indications and provides evidence-based recommendations for when the procedure should be carried out. And there is more. As stated earlier, medical thoracoscopy has been used and is being tried in patients with conditions other than pleural effusion, and the book deals with what these conditions are and how the procedure may help. Here at last is an excellent way for pulmonary specialists to start taking advantage of the diagnostic and therapeutic benefits of medical thoracoscopy.

*John F. Murray, MD, FRCP*
Professor Emeritus of Medicine
University of California, San Francisco

# Preface

Exactly a hundred years ago, Hans-Christian Jacobaeus published his pioneering article on the use of the cystoscope for examination of serous cavities, which he called thoracoscopy and laparoscopy. Although he developed thoracoscopy primarily as a diagnostic method in pleural effusions, he soon used and propagated it for lysis of pleural adhesions, by means of thoracocautery, to accomplish an artificial pneumothorax. The technique became very popular in the preantibiotic era for collapse treatment of pulmonary tuberculosis.

Around 1950, with the advent of antibiotic treatment for tuberculosis, the era of pneumothorax therapy came to an end and other diseases became increasingly important to the chest physician. Consequently, a generation of physicians already familiar with therapeutic application of thoracoscopy, mainly in Europe, began to use this technique on a much broader basis for evaluation of many pleuropulmonary diseases. The *Atlas of Diagnostic Thoracoscopy*, published in 1985, summarized these experiences.

However, during the last 25 years, many new developments have had an enormous impact on the application of thoracoscopy. Imaging techniques such as CT and MRI very often deliver the diagnosis in localized chest lesions. Transbronchial lung biopsies and bronchoalveolar lavage (BAL) in combination with HRCT frequently allow the differentiation of diffuse lung diseases. In the early 1990s, tremendous advances in endoscopic technologies stimulated the development from thoracoscopy to minimally invasive thoracic surgery/video-assisted thoracic surgery (VATS). For better distinction from "surgical thoracoscopy," the term "medical thoracoscopy" was introduced. With the introduction of the semirigid (semiflexible) pleuroscope, the term "pleuroscopy" became popular. Talc poudrage, performed during thoracoscopy, has now become widely accepted as the preferred method for pleurodesis, and medical thoracoscopy/pleuroscopy (MT/P) is meanwhile considered to be one of the main areas of interventional pulmonology.

All these changes during the last 25 years gave us reason to edit this new *Manual and Atlas*, which describes in detail the different technical approaches as well as today's diagnostic and therapeutic indications. We hope that this update on the various techniques, described by editors from Europe, North America, and Asia, together with the endoscopic photographs and the accompanying DVD with videos of typical cases, will further promote the use of this easy-to-learn technique.

We thank Olympus Europa Holding GmbH for support in the production of this book and the permission to use the procedural video of medical thoracoscopy under local anesthesia. We would also like to thank Angelika Findgott, Anne Lampater, Elisabeth Kurz, and Clifford Bergman for careful handling and aid in editing the book.

We are especially grateful to John F. Murray, Professor Emeritus of Medicine, University of California, San Francisco, and one of today's most preeminent pulmonologists, for his foreword in which he puts the method into the context of the whole field of respiratory medicine.

*Robert Loddenkemper*
*Praveen Mathur*
*Marc Noppen*
*Pyng Lee*

# Table of Contents

## Section B: Atlas

# Abbreviations

| | |
|---|---|
| **A–a gradient** | alveolar–arterial gradient |
| **ACCP** | American College of Chest Physicians |
| **ACGME** | Accreditation Council for Graduate Medical Education |
| **ADA** | adenosine deaminase |
| **ARDS** | acute respiratory distress syndrome |
| **BAPE** | benign asbestos pleural effusion |
| **CEA** | carcinoembryogenic antigen |
| **cm H$_2$O** | centimeters of water [pressure] 1 cm H$_2$O = 98.0665 pascals (Pa) = 0.980665 millibar (mbar) ≈ 1 mbar |
| **CME** | Continuing Medical Education |
| **COPD** | chronic obstructive pulmonary disease |
| **ECG** | electrocardiography |
| **HRCT** | high-resolution computed tomography |
| **IPF** | idiopathic pulmonary fibrosis |
| **IGRAs** | interferon-gamma release assays |
| **INR** | International Normalized Ratio |
| **LVRS** | lung volume reduction surgery |
| **MDR** | multidrug resistance |
| **MT/P** | medical thoracoscopy/pleuroscopy |
| **NBI** | narrow band imaging |
| **NETT** | National Emphysema Treatment Trial |
| **PET** | positron emission tomography |
| **PPE** | parapneumonic effusions |
| **PSP** | primary spontaneous pneumothorax |
| **RBILD** | respiratory bronchiolitis associated interstitial lung disease |
| **SSP** | secondary spontaneous pneumothorax |
| **TB** | tuberculosis |
| **TLB** | thoracoscopic lung biopsy |
| **UIP** | usual interstitial pneumonia |
| **VATS** | video-assisted thoracic surgery |
| **WLT** | white-light thoracoscopy |
| **XDR** | extensive drug resistance |

# Section A: Manual

# 1 Introduction

## The Role of Medical Thoracoscopy/ Pleuroscopy in Respiratory Medicine

Endoscopic procedures play an essential role in the diagnostic evaluation of patients with respiratory diseases. These techniques were mainly developed and refined during the last century. The recent tremendous advances in endoscopic technology with sophisticated instruments and telescopes with extremely high optimal resolution and small diameters, as well as developments in anesthesiology, offer a wide range of diagnostic and therapeutic possibilities.

Thoracoscopy, introduced 100 years ago, is—after bronchoscopy—the second most important endoscopic technique in respiratory medicine. In the past, the vast majority of respiratory specialists (pulmonologists/pneumologists/chest physicians) performed only flexible bronchoscopy, thoracentesis, and chest tube placement. A growing number now perform medical thoracoscopy/ pleuroscopy as well. Just as the art and science of flexible bronchoscopy has evolved since its introduction in the 1960s, medical thoracoscopy/pleuroscopy (MT/P) will follow as more pulmonologists, already adept and comfortable with flexible endoscopic instruments, venture to explore the pleural space with the semirigid (semiflexible) pleuroscope ("Thoracoscopy: window to the pleural space" [Colt 1999], "Pleuroscopy: a window to the pleura" [Mathur 2004]. MT/P is meanwhile considered to be one of the main areas of interventional pulmonology (Beamis and Mathur 1999; Seijo and Sterman 2001; Beamis et al. 2004; Lee et al. 2010).

The definition of interventional pulmonology is the art and science of medicine related to the performance of invasive diagnostic and therapeutic procedures that require additional training and expertise beyond that required within a standard training program in respiratory medicine (Beamis and Mathur 1999).

In many European countries medical thoracoscopy has already been part of the training program in respiratory medicine for many years (Dijkman et al. 1994; UEMS 1995; Loddenkemper et al. 2006; Loddenkemper et al. 2008). It has also become more popular in the United States, where according to the national survey in 1994, medical thoracoscopy was applied frequently by 5% of all pulmonary physicians (Tape et al. 1995). Although newer data are not available, the interest in the technique seems to be increasing (Lee et al. 2003; Loddenkemper 2003). However, training is lagging; in an American College of Chest Physicians (ACCP) survey of US pulmonary/critical care fellowship programs in 2002/2003, only 12% of the directors stated that MT/P was offered in their programs (Pastis et al. 2005). In the United Kingdom, where medical thoracoscopy was underutilized compared with the rest of Europe, there is also growing interest (Burrows et al. 2006; Medford et al. 2010). Meanwhile, the technique has been introduced successfully in Australia as well as in many Asian, South American, and some African countries.

MT/P is an invasive technique that should be used to obtain a diagnosis only when other, simpler methods are nondiagnostic (mainly in case of pleural exudates). But, in addition to its several diagnostic advantages, it offers certain therapeutic possibilities, in particular talc poudrage, to achieve pleurodesis (in case of recurrent pleural effusion or pneumothorax) (Loddenkemper 1998; Tassi et al. 2006; Rodriguez-Panadero 2008).

As with all technical procedures requiring special skills, there is a learning curve before full competence is achieved (Boutin et al. 1981a; Rodriguez-Panadero 1995). Appropriate learning is therefore mandatory (Loddenkemper 1998; Ernst et al. 2003). The technique is actually very similar to chest tube insertion by means of a trocar, the difference being that the thoracoscope/pleuroscope is introduced before the insertion of the chest tube. Thus, the whole pleural cavity can be visualized, and biopsies can be taken from all areas of the pleural cavity, including the chest wall, diaphragm, lung, and even mediastinum (Loddenkemper 1998). In general, medical thoracoscopy/pleuroscopy is easier to learn than flexible bronchoscopy if sufficient expertise in thoracentesis and chest tube placement has already been gained. When indicated, talc poudrage can be performed prior to chest tube insertion, allowing a very homogeneous distribution of talc on the visceral and parietal pleural surface. Today, this is the gold standard for nonsurgical pleurodesis (Rodriguez-Panadero and Antony 1997; Antony et al. 2000).

Although medical thoracoscopy/pleuroscopy are invasive techniques, it is necessary to outline important differences in comparison with surgical thoracoscopy or video-assisted thoracic surgery, which are much more invasive and expensive, usually requiring selective double-lumen intubation under general anesthesia, multiple points of entry, disposable instruments, and an operating theater (Kaiser and Daniel 1993). Because the term is now used for both the medical and the surgical procedures, a degree of uncertainty has arisen, which may lead to unnecessary surgical interventions for what are in fact medical indications.

Thus, to distinguish it better from the surgical approach, the term "medical thoracoscopy" was introduced (Mathur et al. 1994). This method is actually performed under local anesthesia or conscious sedation, via only one or two points of entry, by the respiratory physician in an endoscopy suite, using nondisposable instruments. To further clarify the difference from the surgical procedure, and to avoid confusion in the future, it has been suggested that the old term "pleuroscopy," as used in the early French literature (Piguet and Giraud 1923), and as proposed by Weissberg (1991) for the sake of clarity, should be favored over "medical thoracoscopy." Today, both terms are used in parallel, but often the term "medical thoracoscopy" is preferred for the technique using rigid instruments, and the term "pleuroscopy" for the technique using semirigid (semiflexible) instruments. Another alternative has been proposed in the United Kingdom, with the term "thoracoscopy for physicians" (Buchanan and Neville 2004).

The added term "video-assisted" can be confusing, since this is very often associated with video-assisted thoracic surgery (VATS). However, here it actually means only that direct inspection through the thoracoscope is not used, but rather the inspection is performed indirectly by video-assisted observation, which can be employed both with the semirigid (semiflexible) pleuroscope and with the rigid thoracoscope for medical thoracoscopy.

The recent development of medical and surgical thoracoscopy coincided with several technical improvements, as well as with a renewed interest in this field of respiratory medicine. This is underlined by the enormous increase in literature. In PubMed, under the terms "thoracoscopy," "pleuroscopy," "thoracoscopy and pleuroscopy," and "VATS," enormous numbers of publications (more than 8300) are cited today, demonstrating on the one hand the lack of distinction between the medical and surgical approach, and on the other hand the great interest in the technique, which has grown exponentially since the first edition of the *Atlas of Diagnostic Thoracoscopy* was published in 1985. Until 1982, the total world literature consisted of only approximately 240 publications relating to the clinical applications of thoracoscopy in pleuropulmonary diagnosis (Brandt et al. 1985; Loddenkemper 2004a).

In conclusion, medical thoracoscopy/pleuroscopy, in our experience, is easier to learn than flexible bronchoscopy, provided that sufficient skills in thoracentesis and chest tube placement have already been acquired and the appropriate mandatory training has been accomplished.

This book aims to lay the basis for learning and teaching the technique with its *Manual* part, explaining in depth the techniques, indications, results, contraindications, complications, etc., together with the *Atlas* part, showing in color endoscopic examples of different pathologies.

The associated DVD demonstrates the diagnostic and therapeutic techniques of medical thoracoscopy/pleuroscopy, together with some typical case presentations.

# History and Development of Thoracoscopy/Pleuroscopy

Thoracoscopy is based on the development of the artificial pneumothorax, of endoscopes, and of pleural drainage. It was the combination of these three essentials that led to the introduction of the technique in 1910 by Hans-Christian Jacobaeus (**Fig. 1.1a, b**), who worked as an internist in Stockholm, Sweden (Jacobaeus 1910).

## Artificial Pneumothorax

The first publication describing artificial pneumothorax can be found in the Hippocratic writings. In Chapter 59 of the second book of diseases "Adhesion of the lung to the pleura," it is stated: "If this disease (pleuritis) is caused by injury or is present in a patient with empyema as a result of a penetrating wound, one should attach an air-filled bladder to a tube and insert it. One should then take a strong instrument of tin and push. With such therapy, one should have the most luck" (Hippocrates, cited in Kapferer and Sticker 1933). Introducing air seems to indicate the establishment of pneumothorax, the little tube suggests drainage, and the tin instrument perforation of the chest wall (although the sequence is not quite clear). The bladder might have been used to catch pus or exudate in a closed system after establishing the pneumothorax.

It was only in 1821 that the Scottish physiologist Carson presented the concept of an artificial pneumothorax to the Liverpool Medical Society (Carson, cited in Schmidt 1938). Based on his experiences in rabbits, Carson seems to have been the first to conceive the idea of minimizing lung scarring in tuberculosis by producing a pneumothorax in humans. Later, in 1882, Forlanini in Italy proposed a closed pneumothorax induced by means of fine, sterile needles (Forlanini 1882). He used this method for the first time in a human in 1888 in the presence of a pleural exudate, and in 1894 he produced a pneumothorax in a previously normal pleural space. For the latter, he used nitrogen because of its very slow reabsorption since he wanted to produce a prolonged therapeutic collapse of the affected lung in patients with pulmonary tuberculosis. Saugmann introduced the water manometer for the purpose of producing a controlled pneumothorax in 1902 (Saugmann 1902, cited in Schmidt 1938; Faurschou and Viskum 1997). All of these pneumothorax experiments were performed for therapeutic purposes.

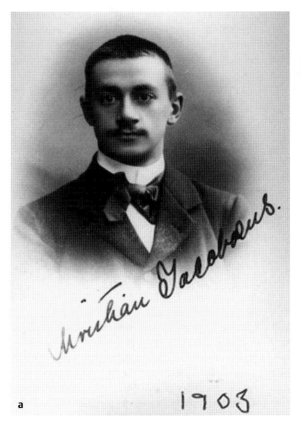
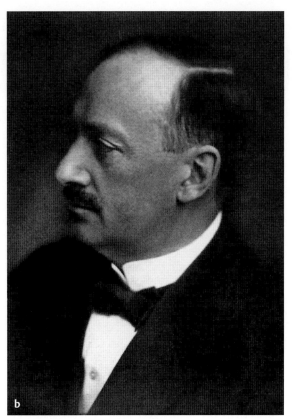

**Fig. 1.1**  Hans-Christian Jacobaeus (1879–1937). **a** In 1903 (courtesy of Gianpietro Marchetti). **b** In the 1930s.

## Pleural Drainage

The development of pleural suction drainage for the purpose of reexpanding the lung is closely connected to closed drainage of empyemas and to the therapy for pneumothorax. Some of this was even alluded to in the Hippocratic writings. It was probably Hewitt who, in the modern era, first developed the underwater seal for pleural drainage (Hewitt 1876, cited in Enerson and McIntyre 1966) and who, in 1876, provided instructions at the London Hospital concerning "the value of the pneumatic aspirator." The management of pleural empyema was the subject of a medical congress in Vienna in 1891, and in the same year Bülau wrote his famous article "On suction drainage in the treatment of empyema" (Bülau 1891). The large number of empyemas during the influenza epidemic in 1918 led to the recommendations of the Empyema Commission in Virginia (Empyema Commission 1918, cited in Enerson and McIntyre 1966).

According to Sattler, in 1940 "there were many opinions regarding the most useful and correct measures for the treatment of pneumothorax which were confusing, lacked uniformity or were completely contradictory" (Sattler 1940). Careful thoracoscopic evaluations and studies of pleurodesis, using continuous suction, together with the development of drainage procedures following lung resection, have resulted in the current, highly developed technique of continuous closed pleural suction drainage (Roe 1958; Munnell 1997).

## Introduction of Thoracoscopy as a Diagnostic Method

Hans-Christian Jacobaeus (1879–1937) primarily developed thoracoscopy as a diagnostic method. In 1910, he described the technique at the same time as laparoscopy in a paper entitled "On the possibility to use cystoscopy in the examination of serous cavities" (Jacobaeus 1910). At that time, as a result of the development of suitable optical systems in the nineteenth century, endoscopy was already being applied to all organs and hollow cavities with anatomical connections to the exterior (Moisiuc and Colt 2007).

Recently, it has been reported that Francis-Richard Cruise, born in Dublin/Ireland in 1834, was probably the first to perform thoracoscopy as early as 1866. This was brought to light in an article entitled "Thoracoscopy before Jacobaeus" (Hoksch et al. 2002). The authors also point out that the term "thoracoscopy" was well known in several French dictionaries before Jacobaeus defined it, as "exploration of the thoracic cavity" (Larousse 1878, cit-

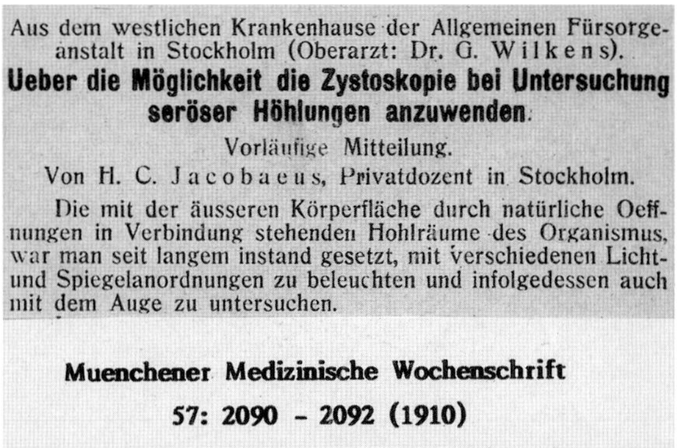

Aus dem westlichen Krankenhause der Allgemeinen Fürsorge-
anstalt in Stockholm (Oberarzt: Dr. G. Wilkens).

## Ueber die Möglichkeit die Zystoskopie bei Untersuchung seröser Höhlungen anzuwenden.

### Vorläufige Mitteilung.

Von H. C. Jacobaeus, Privatdozent in Stockholm.

Die mit der äusseren Körperfläche durch natürliche Oeff-
nungen in Verbindung stehenden Hohlräume des Organismus,
war man seit langem instand gesetzt, mit verschiedenen Licht-
und Spiegelanordnungen zu beleuchten und infolgedessen auch
mit dem Auge zu untersuchen.

### Muenchener Medizinische Wochenschrift
### 57: 2090 – 2092 (1910)

**Fig. 1.2**  Title page of the 1910 publication of Jacobaeus.

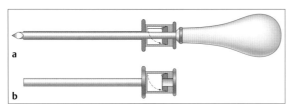

**Fig. 1.3**  Original trocar (**a**) and automatically closing valve (**b**) from Jacobaeus (1910).

ed by Hoksch et al. 2002). Cruise, who in 1865 had already published on an "Endoscope as an aid to the diagnosis and treatment of disease" (Cruise 1865), performed an "Examination of interior of pleura by endoscope" in an 11-year-old girl with empyema through a pleurocutaneous fistula that had developed after pleural drainage, and he used the technique for monitoring therapy. This was reported by Samuel Gordon, who cared for this patient for about 9 months but, because of a deteriorating course, asked Cruise to help him by using his endoscopic skills (Gordon 1866). Although it was published in the *Dublin Quarterly Journal of Medical Science*, the technique remained anecdotal.

Jacobaeus, in his pioneer paper (published in German in the *Münchener Medizinische Wochenschrift*, one of the leading journals at that time) (**Fig. 1.2**), mentioned two cases of tuberculous pleural effusion (pleuritis exsudativa) in which he studied the pleural surfaces after replacing fluid with air according to Holmgren's technique. Although not initially able to safely characterize the pleural changes, he expressed his confidence that the method would be successful with more training, and that it might even eventually yield prognostic information. Jacobaeus closed his publication by mentioning that he had no experience using the cystoscope in the pericardium, but that he believed that this might also eventually be possible (Jacobaeus 1910).

Jacobaeus began his "Preliminary Communication" by referring to endoscopy of organs with natural openings, such as the urinary tract, and referred to the work of Max Nitze, who, in 1877, developed the first cystoscope with a

telescopic lens and distal illumination (Nitze 1879). Jacobaeus then commented that closed cavities such as the peritoneum, pleura, and pericardium had not been examined endoscopically. For this kind of "cystoscopy," Jacobaeus defined three main prerequisites:

1.  The possibility to introduce a trocar (or puncture needle) into the relevant cavity without lacerating the inner organs and without causing too much pain.
2.  The introduction of a transparent medium into the cavity—Jacobaeus used filtered air for this purpose.
3.  A cystoscope of such small dimensions that it could be introduced through the trocar.

**Figure 1.3a, b** shows the trocar Jacobaeus used, which contained an automatically closing valve. It was built with the assistance of Dr. A. Ahlström, chief instrument maker at Stille-Werner in Stockholm. The whole apparatus had a diameter of only 17 Charrière (1 Charrière = 0.33 mm), with the cystoscope having a diameter of 14 Charrière.

Jacobaeus delineated the basic procedure as follows: The skin was disinfected and anesthetized with cocaine. Following a small skin incision, the trocar was introduced with or without prior insufflation of air into the cavity. Once the trocar was introduced, filtered air was insufflated by means of a simple Politzer air pump. The cystoscope was then introduced through the trocar, and the inspection was performed. Jacobaeus then described in detail how the peritoneum was examined. He called this "laparoscopy," and he initially practiced it in over 50 cadavers before successfully performing the procedure in three patients.

In the second, much smaller part of his discussion, Jacobaeus described in detail the examination of pleural cavities, which he called "thoracoscopy." He stated that in this procedure the three above-mentioned main prerequisites are fulfilled more closely than in laparoscopy, especially with regard to point (1) (introduction of the trocar), which he considered to be much less dangerous in the thorax. He referred to a technique developed by Dr. Israel Holmgren, who substituted the fluid with air ("exhalation of the exudate"). He also cited Forlanini's method, in which air or nitrogen was blown into the pleural space, and which under certain circumstances was used as a therapy for pulmonary tuberculosis. Jacobaeus mentioned that he planned to begin examination of the pleural cavity using Forlanini's treatment method (closed pneumothorax). This eventually led to the therapeutic application of thoracoscopy, which Jacobaeus himself initiated only a few years later in 1913 (Jacobaeus 1916), to facilitate pneumothorax treatment of tuberculosis by lysis of pleural adhesions by means of thoracocautery (Jacobaeus operation).

Jacobaeus therefore has to be regarded as the "father" of endoscopic procedures in serous cavities. Today, these techniques are widely used for diagnostic and therapeutic purposes by internists and surgeons. He was apparently aware neither of the above-mentioned publication in Ireland nor of the report by Georg Kelling, who worked in Dresden, Germany, which was published in 1902, also in the journal *Münchener Medizinische Wochenschrift* under the title "On Oesophagoscopy, Gastroscopy, and Coelioscopy" (Kelling 1902). Kelling described his experiences with laparoscopy (coelioscopy) in dogs using two ports of entry—one for a trocar through which air was insufflated and one for a trocar through which Nitze's cystoscope was introduced. Kelling definitely did not perform thoracoscopy, as incorrectly stated by Unverricht in 1923 and later by several other authors.

## Use of Thoracoscopy for Diagnostic Purposes

In the following years, Jacobaeus and several other European pulmonary specialists from Scandinavia, Germany, Italy, and several other European countries performed thoracoscopy for diagnostic purposes in pleural effusions, in spontaneous pneumothorax, in focal pulmonary disease, in diseases of the chest, in mediastinal tumors, as well as in anomalies of the heart and great vessels and in thoracic trauma (Brandt et al. 1985; Loddenkemper 2004b, Moisiuc and Colt 2007). Jacobaeus himself published in 1912 an extensive description of the technique and the results of (laparoscopy and) thoracoscopy, and finally in 1925 a comprehensive summary of his experiences, describing in detail his studies on the etiology and staging of tuberculous pleurisy, malignant effusion, rheumatoid effusion, empyema, parapneumonic effusion, and idiopathic pneumothorax. He divided tuberculous pleurisy into different stages, which are observations still valid to the present day. Additional insight into tuberculous pleurisy was provided by Unverricht (1931), who recognized that in many cases the spread of the disease was hematogenic. In malignant pleural effusion, Jacobaeus was often able to differentiate between primary and secondary tumors of the chest wall, pleura, lung, and mediastinum. He furthermore studied traumatic and nonspecific parapneumonic effusions. He thoracoscopically examined more than 100 cases of empyema, many of which were nontuberculous. He also appreciated that one frequently could not visualize the defect in idiopathic spontaneous pneumothorax.

**Figure 1.4a,b** shows some drawings of endoscopic situations made by Jacobaeus. Publications from different countries appeared sporadically, emphasizing the diagnostic value of thoracoscopy in pleural effusions (15 references in *Atlas of Diagnostic Thoracoscopy* edited by Brandt et al. 1985), in spontaneous pneumothorax (8 references), in focal pulmonary disease (8 references), in diseases of the chest wall (5 references), in mediastinal tumors (3 references), in anomalies of the heart and great vessels (3 references), and in thoracic trauma (2 references).

The highlight in the early history of diagnostic thoracoscopy was presented by Felix Cova from Italy in 1928 with his *Atlas thoracoscopicon*, in which most of the diseases that could be diagnosed by thoracoscopy were shown in the form of colored illustrations (**Fig. 1.5a,b**).

## Thoracoscopy as a Therapeutic Procedure in Tuberculosis (Jacobaeus Operation)

Although Jacobaeus developed thoracoscopy primarily as a diagnostic procedure, it was applied during the ensuing 40 years on a worldwide scale, almost exclusively for lysis of pleural adhesions by means of thoracocautery. As brief-

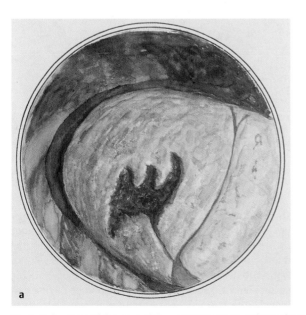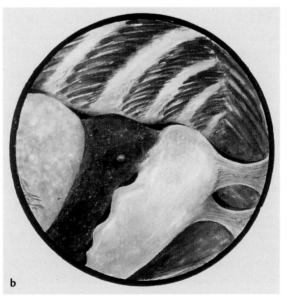

**Fig. 1.4a, b**  Original drawings of thoracoscopic situations by Jacobaeus. (Courtesy of Gunnar Hillerdal.)

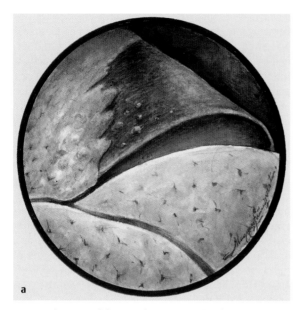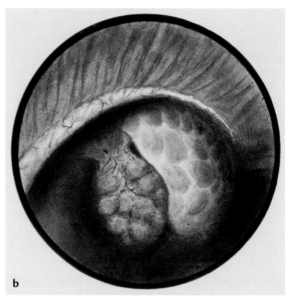

**Fig. 1.5a, b**   Original drawings from Cova's *Atlas Thoracoscopicon* (1928).

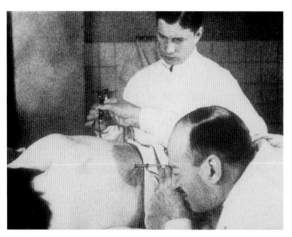

**Fig. 1.6**   Jacobaeus performing cauterization during therapeutic thoracoscopy. (Courtesy of Gunnar Martensson.)

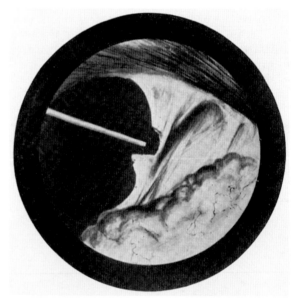

**Fig. 1.7**   Drawing showing the cauterization of membranous adhesions between the chest wall and the compressed lung. (From Jacobaeus 1922 b. Reprinted with permission from the Journal of the American College of Surgeons, formerly Surgery Gynecology & Obstetrics.)

ly mentioned above, in his first publication Jacobaeus anticipated the therapeutic value of thoracoscopy and developed the technique of cauterizing the adhesions between the parietal and visceral pleura, which prevented a complete artificial pneumothorax and was the basis of the collapse therapy for tuberculosis as developed in 1882 and introduced in 1888, both by Forlanini. Jacobaeus stated that during thoracoscopy he found stringlike or membranous adhesions within the artificial pneumothorax induced for pulmonary tuberculosis. This stimulated him to work out a method to remove these pleural adhesions, a process in which "thoracoscopy finds its real practical determination" (Jacobaeus 1916). Already in 1913 he had used the technique with two different points of entry under local anesthesia. He usually introduced the thoraco-

scope through the patient's back, either toward the apex or closer to the diaphragm, depending on the location of the adhesions on chest radiography performed after induction of an artificial pneumothorax (Jacobaeus 1922 a). **Figure 1.6** shows Jacobaeus performing therapeutic thoracoscopy and **Figure 1.7** shows the technique of thoracoscopic cauterization ("burning of membranous adhesions between the chest wall and the compressed lung"), which

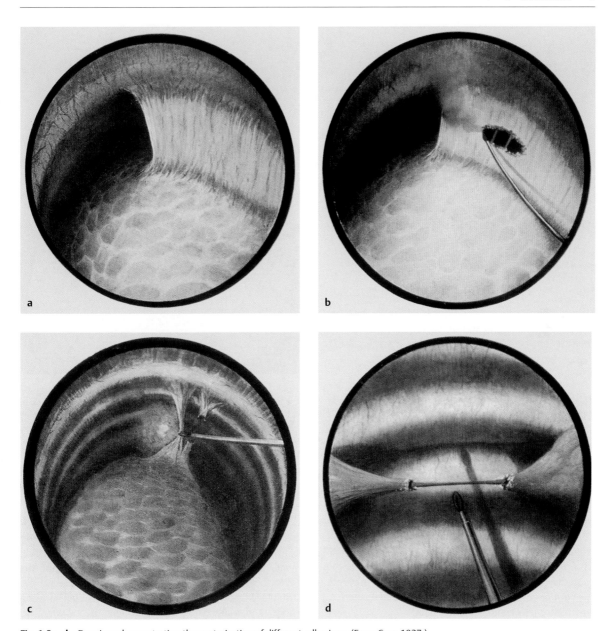

**Fig. 1.8a–d**  Drawings demonstrating the cauterization of different adhesions. (From Cova 1927.)

was the precursor of what we call today "minimally invasive surgery."

This technique became very popular in the pre-antibiotic era for treatment of pulmonary tuberculosis. Several textbooks were written on the subject, thorax models were mass-produced for students to practice on (Diehl and Kremer 1929; Unverricht 1931), and even an intrathoracic movie was produced to provide information about this method of treatment (Siebert 1930). The most comprehensive review during this period was written by O.M. Mistal from Montana in Switzerland in 1935 ("Endoscopy and pleurolysis"). With an introduction by Jacobaeus, it contained numerous illustrations of all the instruments and techniques used up to that time, as well as an extensive bibliography containing more than 500 references from Sweden, Denmark, Finland, Germany, Austria, Switzerland, Italy, France, Spain, Portugal, Great Britain, Canada, and the United States (Mistal 1935). Mistal called the technique "pleuroscopy" (or "pleural endoscopy"), a term first mentioned in 1923 (Piguet and Giraud 1923) and apparently preferred in the French-language literature.

The technique was called the "Jacobaeus operation," and this was also the title of Felix Cova's other book, published in Italian in Milan in 1927 (Cova 1927). **Figure 1.8** shows some drawings from this book. The publication by

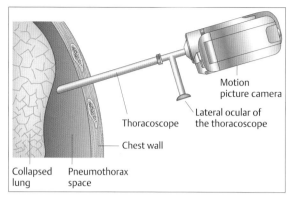

**Fig. 1.9** Schematic drawing of "Kinematography" during thoracoscopy. (From Siebert WW. Endothorakale Kinematographie. *Dtsch Med Wochenschr* 1930;1:1006.)

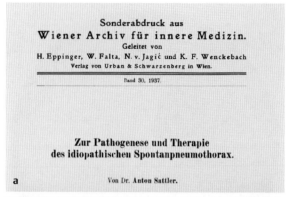

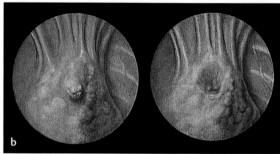

**Fig. 1.10** Title page of Anton Sattler's article on "Pathogenesis and therapy of idiopathic spontaneous pneumothorax" (Sattler 1937b) (**a**). The drawings demonstrate that a ruptured bleb is kept open by pleuropulmonary adhesions (**b**).

Siebert from Berlin on "Endothoracic Cinematography," which provided an illustration of how to make an intrathoracic film, could be considered to be a precursor of today's video endoscopy (Siebert 1930) (**Fig. 1.9**).

## Thoracoscopy as a Therapeutic Tool in Nontuberculous Disease

Anton Sattler, in Vienna, was probably the first to use thoracoscopy in the treatment of patients with idiopathic spontaneous pneumothorax (Sattler 1937a,b). **Figure 1.10** shows the title page of the reprint of this publication. Between 1937 and 1981 he published a large series of papers (cited in Brandt et al. 1985) on this subject (Sattler 1981). Many others, again mainly in Europe, used a similar technique for this indication. With thoracoscopy, bleeding from torn adhesions or bronchopleural fistulas could be cauterized by electrocoagulation. Adhesions preventing the closure of ruptured blebs could be divided, and localized pleurodesis could be undertaken.

In 1947, E. Kux, in Germany, used thoracoscopy in the treatment of hyperhidrosis. He published his experiences in 1954 in a book entitled *Thoracoscopic Interventions in the Nervous System* (Kux 1954). His main indication for sympathectomy was upper limb hyperhidrosis (Kux 1978). He also described vagotomy for other indications. R. Wittmoser later delineated similar procedures in several diseases that may be influenced by the autonomous nervous system (Wittmoser 1990, 1992).

Jacobaeus had already demonstrated in 1925 the use of thoracoscopy in patients with empyema (Jacobaeus 1925). Subsequently, this procedure has been used only rarely for empyema therapy (Weissberg 1981; Kaiser 1989; Boutin et al. 1991). Thoracoscopy can indeed be beneficial in empyema therapy, as it may help to break up loculations of pus and by removing fibrinopurulent membranes with forceps to create one large, unilocular cavity, thus facilitat-

ing drainage and irrigation. Even foreign bodies were removed thoracoscopically (Weissberg 1991).

Individual case reports have mentioned further therapeutic uses of thoracoscopy for drainage and obliteration of cysts (Swierenga et al. 1974), removal of a surgical swab following thoracic surgery and causing empyema (Weissberg 1981), removal of a small benign pleural fibroma (Mengeot and Gailly 1986), pericardial fenestration (Vogel and Mall 1990), and treatment of postoperative chylothorax (Janssen et al. 1994a).

In 1963, Roche and co-workers, in France, were probably the first to report on talc poudrage during thoracoscopy as a means of achieving pleurodesis in chronic, mainly malignant pleural effusions (Roche et al. 1963). The technique is now widely accepted and recommended because of its high success rate (Antony et al. 2000).

**Table 1.1** summarizes those therapeutic indications of medical thoracoscopy/pleuroscopy which are still used today in addition to talc poudrage (see below).

**Table 1.1** Therapeutic indications for medical thoracoscopy/pleuroscopy today

| Main indication | Talc poudrage for pleurodesis |
|---|---|
| | • In malignant (or other chronic) pleural effusions |
| | • In pneumothorax |
| Further indications | • Empyema (opening of loculations) |
| | • Hyperhidrosis (upper dorsal sympathicolysis) |
| | • Pericardial fenestration |
| | • Removal of foreign bodies |
| | • Removal of benign tumors (?) |

## Further Development of Thoracoscopy as an Important Diagnostic Tool

There are several reasons for the initial emphasis on thoracoscopy being primarily a therapeutic tool. For one, the diagnostic potential was certainly not fully appreciated. For another, the therapeutic challenges at that time were focused on tuberculosis despite the description by Jacobaeus and Key in 1921 of five thoracoscopically diagnosed intrathoracic tumors, some of which were subsequently treated by surgery.

In North America particularly, there appears to have been considerable skepticism about thoracoscopy on the part of thoracic surgeons. This was demonstrated in a "Letter to the Editor" by Dr. H. Lilienthal from New York in 1922 commenting on an article by Jacobaeus (1922 b) in the leading surgical journal *Surgery, Gynecology and Obstetrics* (Lilienthal 1922). Lilienthal, speaking on behalf of American thoracic surgeons, favored the use of open thoracotomy for diagnostic purposes while agreeing that thoracoscopy might be of some value in the therapeutic lysis of pleural adhesions. He stressed the relatively high complication rate of 20%, and suggested that thoracoscopy was not a minor surgical procedure. In this context, cases with chronic empyema, which resulted from therapeutic thoracoscopy in collapse treatment of tuberculosis and which in three cases caused death within 1 to 2 years, were incorrectly attributed to diagnostic thoracoscopy. Equally discouraging to internists must have been the pronouncement of one of the major American thoracic surgeons, J. Alexander from Michigan, who, in 1937, following severe intrathoracic hemorrhage resulting from thoracocautery, warned against the performance of this procedure "in a sanatorium by a physician who is not surgically trained to rapidly open the thorax and ligate the artery."

However, there were also internists in the United States who recommended the use of the thoracoscope in pulmonary diagnosis. As early as 1924, J. J. Singer from St. Louis stated:

*For some reason medical men, as distinguished from surgeons, are very prone to make every effort to prevent operation and most of us doing chest work will go a long way to escape the surgeon's knife … When one considers that in the use of thoracoscopy we have a means by which the pleural cavity can be explored through a relatively small instrument without rib resection … it is reasonable to expect medical men to make use of this method. (Singer 1924)*

Singer concluded from his early experience that "the use of the thoracoscope is a great aid in the diagnosis of chest conditions." Another internist, R. C. Matson from Portland, Oregon, who in 1936 used a forceps introduced through a second entry port to obtain biopsies from lung tumors, stated that "Thoracoscopy is undoubtedly one of the most neglected procedures in clinical medicine" (Matson 1936).

In the years between 1950 and 1960, with the advent of antibiotic therapy for tuberculosis, the era of pneumothorax therapy of pulmonary tuberculosis came to an end. **Figure 1.11** illustrates this decrease of "thoracocauteries" and the increase of "diagnostic thoracoscopies" together with the numbers of other diagnostic endoscopies (bronchoscopy and mediastinoscopy) and other biopsy techniques (perthoracic needle biopsy and open lung biopsy) in this transition period (1948–1981) at Lungenklinik Heckeshorn/Berlin (from *Atlas of Diagnostic Thoracoscopy*, Brandt et al. 1985).

As the number of tuberculosis patients in the industrialized countries gradually declined, other diseases became more important to the chest physician. Consequently, a generation of physicians already familiar with the therapeutic application of thoracoscopy began to use this technique on a much broader basis for the diagnostic evaluation of many pulmonary diseases. As has been mentioned, until 1966 the total world literature included only approximately 80 publications relating to diagnostic indications of thoracoscopy. However, by 1982, over 160 additional papers had been published describing the clinical applications of thoracoscopy in pleuropulmonary diseases (Brandt et al. 1985; Loddenkemper 2004 b).

The indications for thoracoscopy were greatly expanded by the use of various biopsy techniques for localized and diffuse lung diseases. Anton Sattler in Vienna (1956) and Hans-Jürgen Brandt and co-workers in Berlin (Brandt 1955; Brandt and Kund 1964; Brandt et al. 1985) were the first to apply thoracoscopy to the complete spectrum of pleuropulmonary diseases. They systematically studied large numbers of patients and published their data. Thus, the modern development of this technique and its dissemination throughout Europe can be attributed to these groups as well as to Swierenga et al. in the Netherlands (1974), Boutin et al. in France (1975), and Enk and Viskum in Denmark (1981), who also reported their experience in a large number of patients. Storey already in 1957 and Bloomburg in 1978, both in the US, used thoracoscopy in several indications, too.

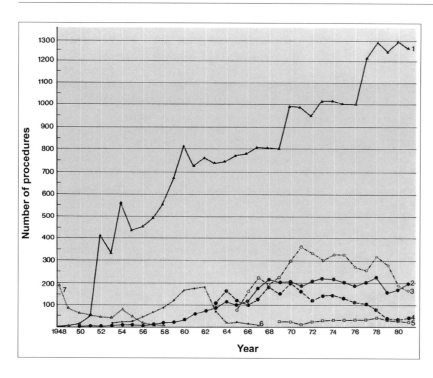

**Fig. 1.11**  Development of therapeutic and diagnostic thoracoscopy compared with other diagnostic endoscopic and biopsy techniques (Lungenklinik Heckeshorn/Berlin, 1948–1981). (From Brandt et al. 1985.)
**1** Brochoscopies
**2** Diagnostic thoracoscopies
**3** Perthoracic needle lung biopsies
**4** Mediastinoscopies
**5** Open lung biopsies
**6** Lymph node biopsies
**7** Thoracocauteries

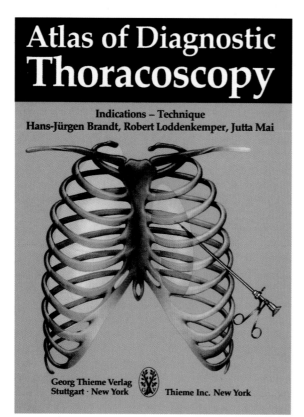

**Fig. 1.12**  Front cover of the *Atlas of Diagnostic Thoracoscopy* published in 1985.

Swierenga published the first atlas of color photographs of thoracoscopy. This monograph depicted spontaneous pneumothorax as well as mediastinal and chest wall tumors (Swierenga 1978). Brandt and co-workers at Lungenklinik Heckeshorn in Berlin summarized their experiences of over 3000 diagnostic thoracoscopies in the first edition of the *Atlas of Diagnostic Thoracoscopy*, published in German in 1983 (Brandt et al. 1983). In 1985, the English translation by Michael T. Newhouse from Hamilton, Canada, was published (Brandt et al. 1985) (**Fig. 1.12**). **Figure 1.13** shows Hans-Jürgen Brandt performing rigid thoracoscopy, while his co-worker and co-editor Jutta Mai is watching through the teaching optics.

It is also an example how this modern technique spread over the world. Michael Newhouse had learned the technique from Roland Keller (Keller et al. 1974; Oldenburg and Newhouse 1979; Newhouse 1989) during a visit to Basel, Switzerland. Keller, in turn, had been taught by Hans-Jürgen Brandt during a one-year visit to Berlin. Praveen Mathur, from Indianapolis, studied thoracoscopy under Michael Newhouse (Mathur 1994). Other US experts who have promoted thoracoscopy include Henri Colt in San Diego (1992) and Yossef Aelony et al. in Harbor City, California (1991). They had learned the technique from Christian Boutin in Marseille.

Boutin's group published their thoracoscopy experience in 1991 in a book entitled *Practical Thoracoscopy* (Boutin et al. 1991). Other books on diagnostic thoracoscopy were published in Italy (Alcozer and Dorigoni 1984), in Spain (Quetglas et al. 1985), and in Israel (Weissberg 1991). All of these publications made the technique more widely known.

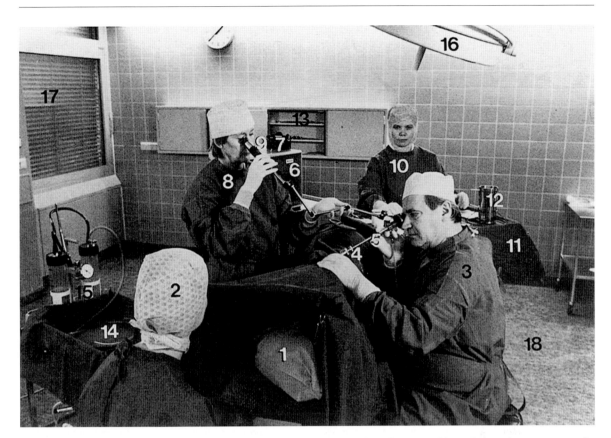

**Fig. 1.13** Historical photograph of Hans-Jürgen Brandt performing diagnostic thoracoscopy, assisted by Jutta Mai, who observes the procedure through a teaching optic. The figure also demonstrates the set-up for performing thoracoscopy. Sterile draped patient (**1**) in lateral decubitus position monitored by a nurse (**2**). Thoracoscopist in sterile outfit (**3**), holding the trocar shaft in his left hand (**4**), guiding the thoracoscope with his right hand (**5**). Combination light unit with cold light source and flash generator (**6**). Camera (**7**). Assistant (**8**) with teaching optics (**9**), to which a color TV camera can be attached. Nurse for sterile instruments (**10**) with instrument table (**11**) and hot water container (**12**) to warm and clean the optic. Formalin-tight sterile instrument cupboard (**13**) (for this photograph the door is open). Sterile suction drainage equipment (**15**), surgical light (**16**), blinds (**17**), conductive, washable floor (**18**). (From Brandt et al. 1985.)

Pulmonologists nowadays use two different techniques for the performance of diagnostic and therapeutic thoracoscopy (Loddenkemper 1998; Rodriguez-Panadero et al. 2006). One method recommends a single entry site, the use of a usually 9-mm rigid thoracoscope (or of a semirigid/semiflexible 7-mm pleuroscope) with a working channel for accessory instruments and an optical biopsy forceps, most often performed under local anesthesia. The other method requires two entry sites—one for a 7-mm trocar for the examination telescope and the other for a 5-mm trocar for accessory instruments—including the biopsy forceps, and is performed usually with conscious sedation or general anesthesia. The rigid instruments are developed, respectively, by Karl Storz GmbH and Richard Wolf GmbH, two German-based companies, and the semirigid (semiflexible) pleuroscope, which is very similar to a flexible bronchovideoscope, by the Japanese Olympus Corporation (Pleuravideoscope).

Flexible bronchoscopes had already been used for thoracoscopy, mainly by pulmonologists in North America.

Several case reports from 1975 describe this technique, which has been termed "pleuroscopy" (Ben-Isaac and Simmonds 1975; Brezler and Abeles 1975; Gwin et al. 1975). Presumably, these flexible bronchoscopes were used because more suitable instruments were not generally available. Miller and Hatcher (1978) and Oldenburg and Newhouse (1979) abandoned this method because of unsatisfactory results and were in favor of thoracoscopy with rigid instruments. Flexible bronchoscopes showed several disadvantages, mainly that they provide less adequate orientation within the pleural cavity, since a fixed anatomical guidance as in the tracheobronchial tree is not present, and that the biopsies are much smaller. Other publications on the use of flexible bronchoscopes appeared in 1988 (Davidson et al. 1988), 1990 (Edmondstone) and 1995 (Robinson and Gleeson 1995). Special semiflexible instruments with rigid shafts and flexible tip were developed in Japan as early as 1978 by Yoshihito Takeno, a surgeon, who used them in pneumothorax treatment (Takeno 1993). The first study in pleural effusions with a semirigid LTF thoracofiberscope, developed by the Japanese Olympus Corporation, was reported by MacLean and co-workers from the United Kingdom (McLean et al. 1998); the pleura was well visualized, but the working channel of 2 mm was felt to be somewhat too small. The next generation of semirigid pleuroscope was developed for the market by Olympus Corporation in 2002, with a working channel of 2.8 mm, and incorporated video imaging (Ernst et al. 2002). This model is now widely used (Lee and Colt 2005).

Another approach to simplifying thoracoscopy, published in the *New England Journal of Medicine* in 1974, was the proposal to use smaller (12- and 14-gauge) instruments 1974 (Ash and Manfredi 1974: this was done at the VA hospital before Praveen Mathur joined). However, this technique has not been proven to be successful. The image quality was very poor and biopsies were difficult to obtain. The same is true for the recently proposed "minithoracoscopy," which consists of a rigid 3-mm endoscope (Tassi and Marchetti 2003). A disadvantage is that a second entry is needed for forceps biopsy and for insertion of a chest tube. Janssen and co-workers compared minithoracoscopy using the 3-mm and the 2-mm sets with standard rigid thoracoscopy using the 7-mm set. The diagnostic yield of the 3-mm set was 100%, the same as for the 7-mm set. The yield of diagnostic biopsies using the 2-mm set was only 40% (Janssen et al. 2003).

A more surgically oriented modification of the thoracoscopic technique was introduced by W. Maassen in Essen, Germany, and called "direct thoracoscopy." This procedure uses a mediastinoscope and general anesthesia with double-lumen intubation (Maassen 1972). The technique which resembles an open-lung or pleural biopsy by a minithoracotomy, has the advantage that it can be performed in circumstances where a pneumothorax cannot be induced (Lewis et al. 1976). An alternative technique, termed "extended thoracoscopy," has been described for cases with pleuropulmonary adhesions (Janssen and Boutin 1992; see the section "Access to the Pleural Space," Chapter 11. p. 78 ff.).

In 1980, many of the leading European experts gathered in Marseille at the First International Symposium on Thoracoscopy, which was organized by Christian Boutin (Boutin 1981). The congress was attended by participants from 16 countries and addressed mainly diagnostic aspects of thoracoscopy. Another international symposium was held in Berlin in 1987 (Loddenkemper 1989). These conferences summarized the current state of the art of diagnostic thoracoscopy as performed by pulmonologists, and highlighted the widespread use of the procedure in many European countries.

## Development of Thoracoscopy for Minimally Invasive Thoracic Surgery ("Surgical Thoracoscopy")

In 1978, K. Semm, a gynecologist in Kiel, Germany, pioneered laparoscopic surgery for various gynecological indications (Semm 1978). In 1982, he was also the first to perform a laparoscopic appendectomy (Semm 1993). In the following years, laparoscopic techniques were introduced for cholecystectomy and for many other abdominal surgeries (Cuschieri 1990, Cuschieri et al. 1992). This development was also made possible by the tremendous advances in endoscopic technology: Newer endoscopic telescopes provided extremely high optical resolution with very small-diameter instrumentation. In addition, new endoscopic instruments, such as forceps, scalpels, staplers, laser fibers, and video cameras were developed (Kaiser and Daniel 1993).

These advances in abdominal surgery, along with a trend toward minimally invasive surgery, stimulated thoracic surgeons to try this technique in surgery for pleuropulmonary disorders. In the early 1990s, many reports were published almost simultaneously in Europe (Inderbitzi and Molnar 1990; Inderbitzi and Althaus 1991; Donelly et al. 1993), the United States (Miller 1991; Wakabayashi 1991; Landreneau et al. 1992; Lewis et al. 1992; Bensard et al. 1993; McKenna 1994; Landreneau et al. 1995), and other parts of the world. The technique was called "therapeutic" or "surgical thoracoscopy," as well as "video-controlled" or "video-thoracoscopic surgery" or "minimally invasive" or "video-assisted thoracic surgery" (VATS) (LoCicero 1992).

VATS requires general anesthesia with selective endobronchial intubation and usually at least three points of entry. Indeed, it is a surgical procedure for which an operating theater and disposable, often expensive, instruments are needed. Textbooks describing the technique and its multiple indications were published (Kaiser and Daniel 1993), and in 1994 "Practice Guidelines" for video-assisted thoracic surgery were proposed by the Society of Thoracic Surgeons (Council of Society of Thoracic Surgeons 1994).

In the United States, where only a few pulmonary physicians performed thoracoscopy, a heated debate ensued about whether thoracoscopy should be performed by pulmonologists or be limited to the domain of the thoracic surgeon (Lewis 1994; Faber 1994; Harris et al. 1995). Praveen Mathur, at that time, visualized this conflict in a cartoon (**Fig. 1.14**).

In most parts of Europe, this was not a controversial issue (Loddenkemper and Boutin 1993; Brandt 1997; Maiwand 1997), as many pneumologists had been performing thoracoscopies well before the introduction of VATS. However, in any debate on this issue, it is of most importance to differentiate "surgical thoracoscopy" from the (medical) thoracoscopic technique introduced originally by Jacobaeus and currently performed by pulmonologists (see a more detailed description in the following chapter). Today,

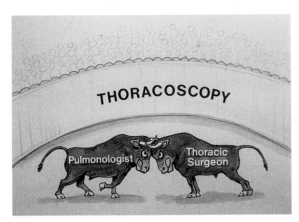

**Fig. 1.14** Cartoon illustrating the conflict between pulmonologists and thoracic surgeons as a bull fight (Praveen Mathur).

American surgeons agree that medical thoracoscopy/pleuroscopy is in the domain of pulmonologists, but correctly insist that adequate training is essential (Lewis 1994). There is no doubt that a strong professional relationship between the pulmonologist and the thoracic surgeon must be maintained (Hartman and Antony 1995).

For better distinction, the term "medical thoracoscopy" was introduced (Mathur et al. 1994). However, since the term "thoracoscopy" is still used to describe both the medical and the surgical procedures, a certain amount of confusion has arisen and persists. This possibly has led and still leads to some unnecessary surgical interventions for what are or should be, in fact, medical indications. To avoid continuing confusion, it has been proposed "for the sake of clarity" (Weissberg 1991) to return to the old term "pleuroscopy", already introduced in France in 1923 (Piguet and Giraud 1923). However, there is no uniform opinion among respiratory physicians (Rodriguez-Panadero et al. 2006). Some feel that the term "medical" is not appropriate since thoracoscopy will always be an invasive procedure. But this does not solve the dilemma that the approach of physicians should be distinguished from the very different surgical approach, which would best be defined as video-assisted thoracic surgery (VATS). However, the term "pleuroscopy" has now become quite popular with the introduction of the semirigid (semiflexible, flexrigid) pleuroscope by Olympus Corporation. Both terms—*medical thoracoscopy* and *pleuroscopy*—are therefore used in this book as equivalent (MT/P).

# 2 Differences between Medical Thoracoscopy/Pleuroscopy and Surgical Thoracoscopy/Video-assisted Thoracic Surgery

As already explained in Chapter 1, two different techniques have emerged, video-assisted thoracoscopic surgery (VATS) and medical thoracoscopy/pleuroscopy (MT/P). VATS is performed in an operating room under general anesthesia with selective intubation. For MT/P the patient does not need to be intubated and usually breathes spontaneously with moderate sedation and local anesthesia. The main differences between the two techniques are listed in **Table 2.1**. However, we feel that it is appropriate to explain the differences in the techniques as well as in the indications of MT/P and VATS in more detail because appreciation of the precise distinction between the two procedures is sometimes lacking.

A variety of definitions for MT/P have now emerged. In a paper in the *New England Journal of Medicine* it is given as follows:

*Pleuroscopy as performed by interventional pulmonologists differs from video-assisted thoracic surgery, in that local anesthesia and conscious sedation are most often used in lieu of general anesthesia, a single thoracic puncture is made rather than multiple incisions, and the procedure can be safely performed in an ambulatory care setting. Although pleuroscopy is primarily used for the diagnosis and management of pleural disorders, it can also be used to perform lung biopsy and manage spontaneous pneumothorax. Mortality rates associated with pleuroscopy are extremely low, ranging from 0.01–0.24%. Complications of the procedure include bleeding, persistent pneumothorax, and intercostal nerve or vessel injury. (Seijo and Sterman 2001)*

Another definition is mentioned in the ACCP Guidelines on "Interventional Pulmonary Procedures":

*Medical thoracoscopy/pleuroscopy is a minimally invasive procedure that allows access to the pleural space using a combination of viewing and working instruments. It also allows for basic diagnostic (undiagnosed pleural fluid or pleural thickening) and therapeutic procedures (pleurodesis) to be performed safely. This procedure is distinct from video-assisted thoracoscopic surgery, an invasive procedure that uses a sophisticated access platform and multiple ports for separate viewing and working instruments to access pleural space. It requires one-lung ventilation for adequate creation of a working space in the hemithorax. Complete visualization of the entire hemithorax, multiple angles of attack to pleural, pulmonary (parenchymal), and mediastinal pathology with the ability to introduce multiple instruments into the operative field allow for both basic and advanced procedures to be performed safely. (Ernst et al. 2003)*

## Video-assisted Thoracic Surgery (VATS)

The indications for VATS are different from those for MT/P, although there are some gray zones with overlapping indications for both techniques (**Table 2.2**).

Surgeons can be more ambitious since they are able to perform thoracotomy promptly if needed. Many operations traditionally performed via thoracotomy can now be done using VATS (LoCicero 1992; Miller et al. 1992; McKenna 2000; Yim et al. 2001; Loddenkemper and McKenna 2005). VATS involves the use of small incisions to perform therapeutic interventions in the chest without spreading the ribs. The surgeon generally needs at least three entry sites (**Fig. 2.1**). However, it often may become necessary to perform an additional minithoracotomy, 5–7 cm long, to remove large specimens. VATS, which takes its roots from MT/P, has now been technically developed so far that it can replace thoracotomy in almost all indications, if certain limitations such as dense pleural symphysis are not present. VATS requires an operating room, general anesthesia with single-lung ventilation, more than two—usually three—entry sites, and complex instruments.

**Table 2.1** Main differences between medical thoracoscopy/pleuroscopy versus surgical thoracoscopy/video-assisted thoracic surgery (VATS)

| Feature | Medical thoracoscopy/pleuroscopy | VATS |
| --- | --- | --- |
| Purpose | Diagnosis Pleurodesis | Minimally invasive thoracic surgery |
| Location | Endoscope suite Operating room | Operating room |
| Anesthesia | Local with moderate sedation | Single-lung ventilation |
| Technique | Single puncture Double puncture | Multiple punctures |
| Instruments | Nondisposable Simple | Disposable Complex |

**Table 2.2**  Indications for medical thoracoscopy/pleuroscopy (MT/P) versus surgical thoracoscopy (VATS) versus the middle column where both methods can be used

| MT/P | MT/P or VATS | VATS |
|---|---|---|
| Pleural effusions | Spontaneous pneumothorax | Lung procedures |
| Pleural effusions of unknown etiology | Staging | Lung biopsy |
| Staging of lung cancer | Pleurodesis by talc poudrage | Lobectomy |
| Staging of diffuse malignant mesothelioma | Empyema (stage I/II) | Pneumonectomy |
| Pleurodesis by talc poudrage or any other agent | Drainage | Decortication |
| | Diffuse pulmonary diseases | Lung volume reduction surgery |
| | Localized lesions | Pleura procedures |
| | Chest wall, diaphragm | Pleurectomy (pneumothorax) |
| | Sympathectomy, splanchnicectomy | Drainage/decortication (empyema stage III) |
| | | Esophageal procedures |
| | | Excision of cyst, benign tumors, esophagectomy, anti-reflux procedures, mediastinal procedures |
| | | Resection of mediastinal mass |
| | | Thoracic duct ligation |
| | | Pericardial window |
| | | Sympathectomy |

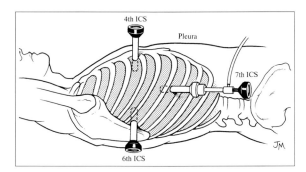

**Fig. 2.1**  Schematic drawing of the VATS access through three entry sites. (From Beamis JF Jr, Mathur PN, eds. Interventional Pulmonology. New York: McGraw-Hill; 1999. Reprinted with kind permission of McGraw Hill.)

It is a more invasive and expensive technique with a higher risk.

The procedures that can be performed by VATS are on the lung, esophagus, heart, pleural space, and mediastinum. This would include resection of lung mass; bullectomy, pleurectomy, pleural abrasion; collection of biopsy samples from thoracic lymph nodes from the mediastinum and hilus; resection of mediastinal cysts; drainage of vertebral abscess; treatment of bronchopleural fistula, lobectomy, pneumonectomy and esophagectomy, and some further procedures. The scope of indications is gradually being extended to include almost all the surgical in-

dications. In most cases the benefits for the patient are obvious in terms of postoperative pain, hospital stay, and recovery. However, it has a higher initial cost than open thoracotomy (Van Schil 2003). It has also been performed as an outpatient procedure (Molins et al. 2006; McKenna et al. 2007). Chronic pain after VATS is not uncommon. Persistant pain was observed 3–18 months after VATS (36%) as often as after thoracotomy (33%) in patients undergoing lung resections (Furrer et al. 1997). A similar incidence of chronic pain (32%) was seen after VATS performed for spontaneous pneumothorax (Passlick et al. 2001).

MT/P, on the other hand, is used mainly for diagnostic purposes in pleural diseases. The most common indications for pleuroscopy are diagnosis of pleural effusion with inspection of the pleural cavity, combined with biopsies from the parietal and visceral pleura, as well as treatment of malignant or other therapy-refractory effusions by talc pleurodesis (poudrage). There are also some further indications as shown in the following chapters.

## General Approach to VATS Procedures

VATS procedures, compared with a thoracotomy, allow a minimally invasive approach that will reduce the morbidity and mortality for patients and will allow a quicker return to normal activities. Increasing evidence suggests that this is true. VATS should be a standard complete operation done for the standard indications and is not a compromised operation. VATS lobectomy does allow a standard complete anatomical resection of the lobe with lymph node sampling or dissection (McKenna 1994; Howington 2007). A variety of equipment is available for VATS. Instruments used may be instruments designed for laparoscopy, instruments designed for thoracoscopy, or standard instruments that are used for open procedures. There are many disposable endoscopic instruments that are used, but some may prefer to use standard instruments for open thoracic procedures (Rocco et al. 2008). Even robotic systems have been applied in VATS (Al-Muffarej et al. 2010).

### Anesthesia

VATS is performed under general anesthesia with one-lung ventilation and collapse of the other lung, which gives good exposure. Single-lung ventilation is performed by the use of a double-lumen tube or more commonly with the use of bronchial blockers. Unlike with a laparotomy, there is no need for carbon dioxide insufflation into the pleural space. It is important that the pleural space is not insufflated under positive pressure, so as not to create a tension pneumothorax. Most thoracic surgeons have their own variation along with their anesthetist. Most important is that this unit has to work as a team and its members must understand each other's needs.

### Indications and Contraindications

Most thoracic surgery can now be performed with VATS, provided the necessary training is completed and the practice guidelines for VATS are observed, such as those proposed by the Society of Thoracic Surgeons (McKneally et al. 1992; Society of Thoracic Surgeons 1994; Kaiser 1994b).

For example, a large number of lobectomies are performed by VATS. The surgeon has to determine when a thoracotomy or VATS is appropriate. Basically, the choice of procedure is based on the goal of the operation. Certain situations may require a thoracotomy: a mass attached to the chest wall that requires resection of the mass and the ribs, or a mass that is too large for removal through a small incision; suturing requirements beyond the skills of the surgeon; and pleural adhesions from chemotherapy, radiation therapy, or infection that make dissection more difficult.

Certain procedures can be performed either way, such as an open lung biopsy. However, if the patient is unable to tolerate single-lung ventilation it may be more appropriate to perform a thoracotomy. Surgeons should understand their own limitations; these may include skills in operating with video assistance, though these skills will improve with time. The ability of general surgeons (nonthoracic surgeons) with their abdominal surgery video skills has brought several nonthoracic surgeons into dabbling in thoracic surgery.

## Lung Procedures Performed with VATS

Almost all pulmonary procedures can be performed with VATS and currently it is a common skill for thoracic surgeons. They should understand their own technical limitations, however.

### Lung Biopsy

Lung biopsy is the most common procedure performed by VATS (Ayed 2003; Qureshi et al. 2007). This usually involves three standard incisions, which generally do not vary except that the incision in the mid-axillary line may be in the fourth intercostal space or the fifth intercostal space for interstitial lung diseases or parenchymal infections. An endoscopic stapler is used to resect the appropriate area of lung parenchyma.

### Wedge Resection

Careful inspection of the preoperative chest CT scan is extremely important to allow the surgeon to know where the mass is located. All masses can be palpated because the lung is a very mobile organ. The mass can then be manipulated by forceps and grasper. When resected, the mass should be placed into a bag for removal through the utility incision to prevent tumor seeding.

A variety of new techniques have emerged for preoperative localization of a mass, such as wire localization, or use of dye or of radioisotopes under certain circumstances (Mack et al. 1993). If the mass is small (< 1 cm), more than 1 cm below the pleural surface, or a ground-glass opacity that would be soft and difficult to palpate, the radiologist can place a hook wire under CT guidance. The wire should then be cut at skin level. The patient then goes to the operating room for the VATS procedure. The surgeon resects the area of lung within the hook wire. An endoscopic stapler is used to resect the appropriate area of lung parenchyma. VATS wedge resection is a procedure very commonly performed by surgeons. The morbidity and mortality are extremely low.

### Pulmonary Metastases

VATS can be used for either the diagnosis or the treatment of pulmonary metastases (Mack et al. 1993; Lenglinger et al. 1994; Burdine et al. 2002; Mutsaerts et al. 2002; Pittet et al. 2007; Gonfiotti et al. 2007; Treasure et al. 2008). The procedure is performed with the standard technique for a wedge resection. If the intent of the procedure is therapeutic, careful, complete palpation is imperative because additional lesions, not identified on CT scan, are found in approximately 30% of patients. This indication for VATS is controversial because some surgeons question how well the entire lung can be examined during a VATS procedure. The advent of thin-cut CT scans, allows much better visualization of pulmonary lesions that otherwise could only be palpated.

## Lobectomy

Although most surgeons perform lobectomies via a thoracotomy incision, there is now a large and growing worldwide experience with VATS lobectomy to suggest that the VATS approach may have advantages over an open lobectomy (McKenna 1998; Nakajima et al. 2000; Hoksch et al. 2003; Li et al. 2003; Nomori et al. 2003; Shigemura et al. 2006; Shigemura and Yim 2007; Swanson et al. 2007; Whitson et al. 2007; Balderson and D'Amico 2008; Congregado et al. 2008; Solaini et al. 2008; Iwasaki et al. 2008; Mahtabifard et al. 2008; Park and Flores 2008; Reed et al. 2008).

This standard procedure should involve a complete anatomical dissection and removal of lymph nodes. Generally an 8-mm trocar and thoracoscope are placed in the mid-axillary line of the eighth intercostal space. This is followed by a 2-cm incision which is placed in the mid-clavicular line of the sixth intercostal space. The utility incision is an incision of approximately 4–5 cm in the fourth or fifth intercostal space in the mid-axillary line. Standard instruments are used to dissect and transect the artery, vein, and bronchus for the lobe to be removed. The mortality rate with VATS is less than 1% (Mack et al. 1993; Qureshi et al. 2007), it has a lower complication rate (Qureshi et al. 2007), lower costs (Li et al. 2003), less impairment of shoulder function (Nomori et al. 2003), no significant impact on the vital capacity and 6-minute walk (Fishman et al. 2003), and less use of postoperative analgesics. Long-term survival of either VATS lobectomy or an open procedure is the same; thus, when appropriate, if the surgeon is familiar with VATS lobectomy it may be the preferred operation (McKenna 1998; Fishman et al. 2003; Shigemura et al. 2006; Iwasaki et al. 2008; Park and Flores 2008). The important issue is that proper mediastinal dissection has to be performed. Thoracic surgeons with good skills have little difficulty with dissection of pulmonary vessels and controlling bleeding. To reduce tumor seeding at the site of the incisions, the mass has to be placed in a bag prior to removal.

## Lung Volume Reduction Surgery

Lung volume reduction surgery (LVRS) is an effective treatment for selected patients with emphysema (Fishman et al. 2003). It has been successful in patients who have failed medical management and have an upper-lobe heterogeneous pattern of emphysema. LVRS carries a hospital mortality and morbidity rate of approximately 5% (Fishman et al. 2003). In a selected group of patients when compared with medical management, LVRS provides better exercise tolerance, pulmonary function, and quality of life. LVRS provides increased survival for patients with upper lobe emphysema and low exercise tolerance. LVRS involves resection of approximately 30% of the parenchyma of each lung. The National Emphysema Treatment Trial (NETT) showed that LVRS can be performed with equal efficacy by VATS and by thoracotomy via median sternotomy, but the VATS approach provided easier recovery with less expense.

LVRS can also be performed by VATS, with the patient in the lateral decubitus position. The standard three incisions are used. The lung is held with a forceps through the incision in the fourth intercostal space and the stapler enters the chest through the incision in the sixth intercostal space in the mid-clavicular line. As the emphysematous parenchyma does not hold staples well, some form of buttress is needed to prevent air leaks. The thoracic surgeon has to determine the location and amount of lung tissue to be resected. The preoperative CT scan and ventilation and perfusion scans can be helpful in the determination.

# Pleural Procedures Performed with VATS

## Treatment of Pneumothorax

VATS has proved a good approach for the treatment of spontaneous pneumothorax. It is performed when there is persistent leak, bilateral pneumothorax, or recurrent spontaneous pneumothorax. The standard incisions are used and the lungs are carefully inspected to identify the bleb that has caused the pneumothorax. The bleb and a margin of normal lung tissue are excised with staples. A mechanical pleurodesis is performed with a ring forceps that holds a gauze pad or the scratch pad used for the electrocautery. Long-term success for this procedure is 90–95%. However, there is controversy attached to this approach as the blebs seem not to be responsible for the pneumothorax.

Another pleural procedure may be indicated for catamenial pneumothorax, recurrent pneumothorax after surgical treatment, or when a bleb is not found. Then, a more aggressive pleural procedure, either a talc pleurodesis or a parietal pleurectomy, is performed (Boutin et al. 1995a; Schramel et al. 1997; Ayed et al. 2006; Noppen et al. 2006; Tschopp et al. 2006; Amjadi et al. 2007; Barker et al. 2007; Cardillo et al. 2007; Vohra et al. 2008).

However, the management of pneumothorax is also an excellent indication for MT/P, which is outlined in the section "The Place of Medical Thoracoscopy/Pleuroscopy in the Management of Pneumothorax," Chapter 3, p. 41 ff.

Pleural effusions are the domain of MT/P, for diagnostic purposes as well as for talc pleurodesis. It can also be successfully used in early empyema cases. The latter use is described in detail in Chapter 3 on indications for medical thoracoscopy/pleuroscopy ("Parapneumonic Effusions and Pleural Empyema," Chapter 3, p. 31 f.).

## Decortication

VATS has been used successfully in the treatment of empyema, especially in the later stages (Angelillo-Mackinlay et al. 1999; Cameron 2002; Chen et al. 2002; Hampson et al. 2008; Luh et al. 2008; Medford et al. 2008). Generally, the effusion is drained by either large-bore or small-bore chest tubes. If the purulent effusion (empyema) cannot be drained due to multiple loculations, the patient remains febrile, and more conservative therapies including antibiotics are failing, VATS should be considered, in particular when decortication is needed (empyema stage III) and the patient does not have a high surgical risk. The thickened visceral pleura (peel) is incised and a blunt dissection is made by which the peel can be removed from the lung. Gentle ventilation and partial expansion of the lung facilitate this dissection. The process continues until there is a minimal amount of pleural debris and the lung fully reexpands to fill the entire pleural space. However, there are thoracic surgeons who find VATS a tedious operation and find a muscle-sparing thoracotomy to be an efficient way to complete the decortication.

## Esophageal Procedures Performed with VATS

### Excision of Cysts and Benign Tumors

VATS has also been used for masses in the middle mediastinum (esophageal leiomyomas (Li et al. 2009 b), esophageal duplication cysts, bronchogenic cysts, or pericardial cysts) or the posterior mediastinum (benign neurogenic tumors). For these procedures, the standard incisions are used, and the lung is retracted anteriorly. For an esophageal mass, the longitudinal muscles of the esophagus are separated and retracted laterally. The cyst or tumor is mobilized with a combination of blunt and sharp dissection. Retraction by placement of a suture into the tumor may help separate the tumor from the esophagus.

### Anti-reflux Procedures

A significant number of Nissen fundoplications as an anti-reflux procedure are primarily performed with minimally invasive surgery (Grant et al. 2008; Chen et al. 2009; Hartmann et al. 2009; Vlug et al. 2009).

## Esophagectomy

VATS can used for mobilization of the esophagus and an open trans-hiatal esophagectomy, or can be a totally minimally invasive procedure utilizing laparoscopy for gastric mobilization and feeding jejunostomy, VATS for esophageal mobilization, and a cervical incision for the esophagogastrostomy. The technique for a minimally invasive esophagectomy has been well described (Perry et al. 2002). One randomized trial showed that the same operation and same node dissection can be achieved with equal survival. The ultimate role for the minimally invasive esophagectomy has yet to be defined. There is a significant learning curve for surgeons trying to master this technique (Perry et al. 2002; Osugi et al. 2003; Shichinohe et al. 2008).

## Mediastinal Procedures

### Thymectomy

Minimally invasive thymectomy has been performed for thymomas (Savcenko et al. 2002; Wright et al. 2002). Concern about spreading the tumor has led some surgeons to recommend a median sternotomy, rather than VATS, when a thymoma is present. However, VATS thymectomy for myasthenia gravis appears to offer results comparable with those of an open or transcervical thymectomy (Savcenko et al. 2002; Wright et al. 2002). The mean length of hospital stay for the VATS approach was 1.64 days (range 0–8 days) with a median stay of 1 day. The mean length of follow-up is 53 months (range 4–126 months). Overall, clinical improvement at follow-up was observed in 30 of 36 patients (83.0%), with 5 of 36 patients (14.0%) in complete stable remission (Savcenko et al. 2002).

### Thoracic Duct Ligation

Patients with a chylothorax due to thoracic duct leakage can undergo ligation of the thoracic duct via VATS. The duct can then be identified as it crosses through the diaphragm by the right anterior surface of the aorta. Several clips are placed on the duct (Terashima et al. 2003).

### Pericardial Window

A large pericardial window may be achieved through either the right or the left chest (O'Brien et al. 2005; Georghiou et al. 2005; Rocco et al. 2006). If there is a concomitant pleural effusion, the side of the pleural effusion should be chosen for the VATS so that a talc pleurodesis may be performed to control the pleural effusion.

## Sympathectomy

Sympathectomy is the treatment of choice for the treatment of palmar hyperhidrosis (Noppen et al. 1995; Noppen and Vincken 1996). Affecting 1–2% of the population, palmar hyperhidrosis can be a severely debilitating and socially embarrassing disease. The procedure can be performed by both VATS or MT/P (see Chapter 3, p. 48–50). The procedure is performed under general anesthesia and can be done on an outpatient basis. As the patient is in the supine position with the arms extended, a bilateral procedure can be performed without repositioning the patient. A 1-cm incision is made in the anterior axillary line at the inferior margin of the hair line. A trocar and the thoracoscope are passed through the incision. There are several approaches for the procedure. Some surgeons resect part of the nerve or burn the ganglion, while others transect or clip the nerve. The results appear to be similar after all procedures. Many patients have accessory nerves, and an attempt is made to identify and transect these nerves. The lung is then reexpanded, and the procedure is performed on the opposite side. Complications after sympathectomy are infrequent. These include Horner syndrome (<1%) and bleeding (Boley et al. 2007; Krasna 2008; Marhold et al. 2008; Li et al. 2009a; Martins Rua et al. 2009).

## Thoracic Lymphadenectomy

A complete lymphadenectomy, usually done as part of a lung cancer operation, can be performed by VATS (Congregado et al. 2008). The incisions are, therefore, usually the same incisions that are used for lobectomy.

Paratracheal node dissection starts with inferior retraction of the lung. Blunt dissection along the trachea, the pericardium over the ascending aorta, and the superior vena cava mobilizes all of the level 2, 3, and 4 lymph nodes. Subcarinal node dissection starts with anterior retraction of the lung through the incision in the sixth intercostal space in the mid-clavicular line. Blunt dissection along the pericardium, esophagus, and both main-stem bronchi mobilizes the subcarinal nodes.

## Cervical Mediastinoscopy versus VATS

Accurate staging is critical for determining the appropriate treatment for lung cancer. Cervical mediastinoscopy provides access for removal of paratracheal (level 2 and 4 nodes), pretracheal nodes (level 3), tracheobronchial angle/hilar nodes (level 10), and subcarinal nodes (level 7). The middle mediastinum is accessible to mediastinoscopy, but not the anterior mediastinal space. This procedure is performed through a 2-cm incision in the base of the neck. It is generally an outpatient procedure, done under general anesthesia (Karfis et al. 2008; Molins et al. 2008).

VATS has not replaced mediastinoscopy because the latter is a simpler procedure that does not require either hospitalization or a double-lumen tube. Therefore, if the goal of the procedure is biopsy of level 2, 3, 4, 7, and 10 nodes, mediastinoscopy is preferred over VATS.

## Anterior Mediastinotomy versus VATS

Biopsy of an anterior mediastinal mass or level 5 and 6 nodes is often accomplished with an anterior mediastinotomy (Chamberlain procedure) (Landreneau et al. 1993). Removal of the cartilaginous portion of the left second rib provides excellent exposure for these areas.

VATS has not replaced anterior mediastinotomy because the latter is a simpler procedure that does not require either hospitalization or a double-lumen tube. Therefore, if the goal of the procedure is biopsy of level 5 and 6 nodes, anterior mediastinotomy is preferred over VATS.

## Summary

MT/P compared with video-assisted thoracic surgery (VATS)/surgical thoracoscopy has the advantage that it can be performed under local anesthesia or conscious sedation, in an endoscopy suite, using nondisposable rigid instruments. Thus, it is considerably less expensive and, for the patient, less cumbersome.

MT/P procedures are safe procedures and are even easier to learn than flexible bronchoscopy, provided sufficient experience with chest tube placement has been gained. However, as with all technical procedures, there is a learning curve before full competence is achieved.

The main indications for MT/P are pleural effusions, in particular exudates of unknown etiology, or for staging in diffuse malignant mesothelioma or lung cancer, and for talc poudrage. But there are additional indications, which are outlined in the corresponding chapters.

VATS has made tremendous progress during the last decade. The advances in endoscopic technology, with sophisticated endoscopic instruments and endoscopic telescopes, allow the replacement of thoracotomy in many indications. Although it necessitates selective double-lumen intubation under general anesthesia, it is much less invasive, and increasing evidence suggests that it reduces the morbidity and mortality compared with thoracotomy. However, just as there is an overlap between MT/P and VATS procedures, there is also an overlap between VATS and open surgical procedures, and the decision between these procedures depends on the performance status and prognosis of the patient, as well as on the expertise of the thoracic surgeon.

# 3 Indications for and Results of Medical Thoracoscopy/Pleuroscopy

Medical thoracoscopy/pleuroscopy (MT/P) is today primarily a diagnostic procedure, but it can also be applied for therapeutic purposes (Mathur et al. 1994; Harris et al. 1995; Medford et al. 2010). Pleural effusions are by far the leading indication for MT/P both for diagnosis, mainly in exudates of unknown etiology, and for staging in diffuse malignant mesothelioma or lung cancer, and for treatment by talc pleurodesis in malignant or other recurrent effusions (Rodriguez-Panadero et al. 2006) or in cases of empyema (Brutsche et al. 2005). Staging of spontaneous pneumothorax combined with local treatment, in stages I and II, is also an excellent indication for MT/P (Boutin et al. 1995 a). Those who are familiar with the technique can use it, for example, for biopsies from the diaphragm, the lung, the mediastinum, and the pericardium, or for sympathectomy (Tassi et al. 2006). In addition, MT/P offers a remarkable tool for research as a "gold standard" in the study of pleural effusion and pneumothorax (Loddenkemper 1998) (see Chapter 6, p. 56). A survey performed in the then West Germany in 1984 gives an impression of the indications that were used by pneumologist at that time (**Fig. 3.1**).

At the Lungenklinik Heckeshorn in Berlin, during the last three decades there has been a definite trend toward an increase in the application of MT/P in pleural effusions, both in absolute and in relative numbers, as shown in

**Table 3.1** Reasons for the change in indications for medical thoracoscopy/pleuroscopy

- Introduction of transbronchial lung biopsy, bronchoalveolar lavage and HR-CT (diffuse lung diseases)
- New imaging techniques (CT, MRI) in localized lesions (lung, chest wall, diaphragm, mediastinum)
- Introduction of surgical thoracoscopy (VATS)

**Figure 3.2**. Correspondingly, there has been a decline in the other indications. This decrease in all indications other than pleural effusions is explained by several factors (**Table 3.1**). That the absolute number of MT/P in pleural effusions has risen so much is due to the fact that more and more medical thoracoscopies/pleuroscopies are performed in pleural effusions for diagnostic and therapeutic purposes. However, the absolute number of medical thoracoscopies in all indications has slightly decreased, since other hospitals have also introduced the thoracoscopic technique in the meantime and since VATS is performed in some of the other indications.

The indications for diagnosis in localized and chest-wall lesions have diminished considerably because imaging techniques such as computed tomography (CT) or

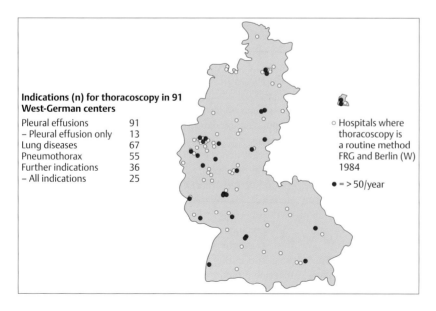

**Indications (n) for thoracoscopy in 91 West-German centers**

| | |
|---|---|
| Pleural effusions | 91 |
| – Pleural effusion only | 13 |
| Lung diseases | 67 |
| Pneumothorax | 55 |
| Further indications | 36 |
| – All indications | 25 |

○ Hospitals where thoracoscopy is a routine method FRG and Berlin (W) 1984

● = > 50/year

**Fig. 3.1** Survey of the indications for thoracoscopy in the then West Germany (FRG) 1984. Hospitals with more than 50 thoracoscopies per year are marked in red on the map.

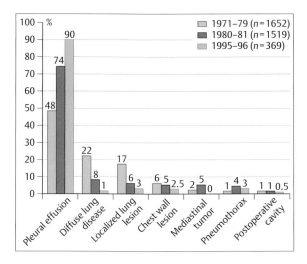

**Fig. 3.2** Change in indications for medical thoracoscopy at the Lungenklinik Heckeshorn, Berlin during the last three decades of the twentieth century.

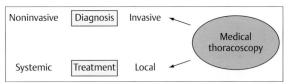

**Fig. 3.3** The role of medical thoracoscopy/pleuroscopy in the management of pleural effusions: invasive diagnosis and local treatment.

MT/P has its main role in the invasive diagnosis of otherwise undetermined pleural effusions and in local treatment (Fig. 3.3). In the following, a general overview of the different diagnostic and therapeutic possibilities is given and, in particular, the potential role of MT/P in the management of pleural effusions of different origins is described.

## Diagnostic Approach

Pleural effusions are common problems in pulmonary practice. It is estimated that approximately 25% of all consultations in the pulmonary service in the United States concern pleural diseases (Collins and Sahn 1987; Light 1997). The incidence of pleural effusions is calculated as being 300 per 100 000 in the United States (Light 2007) and 320 per 100 000 for Central Bohemia (Marel et al. 1993; Marel 2002). Pleural effusions may have many origins. They can be either the consequence of disease localized in the chest or the manifestation of extrathoracic or systemic diseases (Light 2007). The main cause (36%) is cardiac failure with unilateral or bilateral effusions. Among noncardiac effusions, parapneumonic effusions are the most common at 34%. Malignant pleural effusions follow, with 23% of cases. Pleural effusion is secondary to pulmonary embolism in 17%, to viral etiology in 11%, to liver cirrhosis in 6%, and to gastrointestinal diseases in 3% of cases.

Many other possible causes, albeit rare or extremely rare, play an important role in differential diagnosis. The discrepancy between the estimated incidence and the frequency distribution in the respiratory literature, in which the malignant causes are the most common—followed by infectious causes and idiopathic effusions—most probably results from patient selection (Loddenkemper 2004a).

Conversely, it may be concluded that, apart from cardiac effusions, effusions as sequelae of pneumonia, pulmonary embolism, liver cirrhosis, gastrointestinal disease, and autoimmune disease are usually easy to diagnose and, therefore, less frequently referred to the pulmonary specialist.

Thus, in the majority of cases, the etiology can be established by case history, clinical presentation, and imaging techniques. The next diagnostic step in a pleural effusion of still indeterminate origin is thoracentesis and direct examination of the pleural fluid (**Fig. 3.4**). Thoracentesis is

magnetic resonance imaging (MRI) very often deliver the diagnosis or allow the differentiation between malignant and benign disease. In addition, VATS or "surgical thoracoscopy" can be performed by preference in these indications for diagnosis and for the simultaneous removal of the lesion. Furthermore, the indications for thoracoscopic/pleuroscopic lung biopsies in diffuse lung diseases have decreased. This decrease is due to the improved diagnostic results of bronchoscopy using transbronchial lung biopsies and bronchoalveolar lavage as well as to the development of high-resolution CT (HRCT), which improves the definition of structural changes (e.g., the degree of fibrosis) and sometimes even gives the diagnosis (e.g., in pulmonary Langerhans cell histiocytosis).

The low number of pneumothorax patients in this series is explained by the policy at Lungenklinik Heckeshorn whereby the Department of Thoracic Surgery takes care of almost all patients admitted with spontaneous pneumothorax (Kaiser 2000; Kaiser et al. 2000). However, the surgeons include the routine application of a thoracoscope in nearly all cases for the inspection of the pleural cavity, prior to the insertion of the chest tube through the cannula. This is done under local anesthesia, which actually means that they perform a "medical thoracoscopy." The same approach is frequently used by the thoracic surgeons in cases of parapneumonic effusions and empyema, which are traditionally treated at this institution almost exclusively in the Thoracic Surgery Department (Kaiser 1989).

## Management of Pleural Effusions

Besides diagnosis, patients with pleural disorders may require evacuation of pleural fluid, guided parietal pleural biopsy, lung biopsy, or pleurodesis (Lee and Colt 2005).

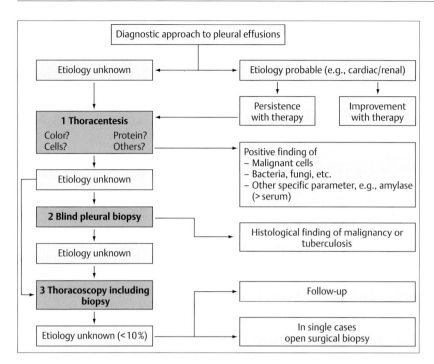

**Fig. 3.4** Algorithm for the diagnostic approach to pleural effusions.

indicated in all cases of pleural effusion of unknown origin, and in those effusions where the diagnosis was assumed on the basis of clinical criteria but which do not resolve under appropriate treatment (Light 2007).

In many cases, evaluation of the pleural fluid yields valuable diagnostic information or even permits a clear diagnosis. The most important criteria are appearance (color), protein content, and cellular components. Additional laboratory values as well as microbiological tests may also be helpful. However, even after extensive diagnostic work-up of the pleural fluid, the origin of several pleural effusions remains unclear (Storey et al. 1976; Hirsch et al. 1979; Lamy et al. 1980; Ferrer et al. 1996); additional biopsy techniques may therefore be indicated, but these can provide the final diagnosis only in cases with a distinct pathology of the pleural cavity, almost exclusively in malignancy and tuberculosis (Mathur and Loddenkemper 2002). Boutin and co-workers found that after extensive work-up, out of 1000 consecutive patients with pleural effusions, MT/P was indicated in 215 with chronic effusions, in whom it established the diagnosis in up to 97% (Boutin et al. 1981a).

Blind needle biopsies of the chest-wall pleura may establish the diagnosis in a few cases, particularly in tuberculous pleurisy (Valdés et al. 1998). The additional diagnostic yield in malignant pleural effusions is usually small, and it can be debated whether blind needle biopsy should routinely be performed in cases where a strong suspicion of malignancy is given (Antony et al. 2000). The next step for obtaining pleural biopsies, which offer a high diagnostic sensitivity in malignant pleural effusions together with a very high specificity to exclude these diagnoses, is MT/P or VATS (Rodriguez-Panadero et al. 2006). The choice between these two procedures is mainly determined by the facilities and preference of the diagnosing institution. In our view, MT/P should be preferred since it can be performed under local anesthesia or conscious sedation, without the need for general anesthesia, double-lumen intubation, and single-lung ventilation (Boutin et al. 1993), and thus is less cumbersome for the patient. Since it can be performed in an endoscopy suite with fewer personnel and using nondisposable instruments, it is also less expensive. Besides its diagnostic role, MT/P is useful in certain therapeutic circumstances, in particular to prevent recurrent pleural effusion by talc poudrage (Rodriguez-Panadero et al. 2006; Froudarakis 2008). The main indication is recurrent malignant pleural effusion (Antony et al. 2000).

In their concluding chapter on future directions in their *Textbook of Pleural Disease*, the editors Light and Lee (2008) discuss the potential role of medical thoracoscopy in the diagnosis and treatment of pleural diseases: Gary Lee predicts that thoracoscopy will be used more frequently in the diagnosis, while Richard Light predicts that thoracoscopy will be used less frequently in the diagnosis of pleural disease, as better noninvasive diagnostic tests will be developed. Both predict that thoracoscopy will be used early in the treatment of parapneumonic effusions and Richard Light predicts that more thoracic surgeons will become proficient at thoracoscopy and chest physicians will only perform the procedure where there are no thoracic surgeons trained for and interested in doing thoracoscopy. In contrast, Gary Lee states that there is already an increasing number of chest physicians performing tho-

**Table 3.2**  Advantages of medical thoracoscopy/pleuroscopy in the diagnosis of pleural effusions

- Fast and definite biopsy diagnosis including TB culture and hormone receptor assay
- Biopsies not only from chest wall pleura but also from diaphragm, lung, and mediastinum
- Staging in lung cancer and diffuse mesothelioma
- Exclusion of malignancy and tuberculosis with high probability
- Gold standard for scientific studies

**Table 3.3**  Advantages of medical thoracoscopy in the treatment of pleural effusions

- Complete and immediate fluid removal
- Evaluation of loculations (TB, empyema)
- Evaluation of the reexpansion potential of the lung
- Talc poudrage for pleurodesis with uniform distribution of talc (6–10 mL) under visual control (= nonsurgical gold standard)
- Early start to drug treatment, e.g., TB
- In addition better diagnosis + staging

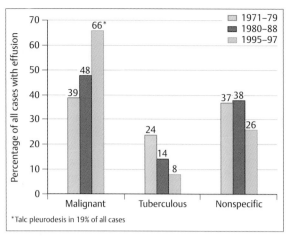

**Fig. 3.5**  Change in the etiology of pleural effusions that were examined thoracoscopically at the Lungenklinik Heckeshorn, Berlin during the last three decades of the twentieth century.

racoscopy worldwide and predicts that increasingly surgeons will only be involved in complicated cases. Richard Light believes that the demand for thoracoscopy will be relatively low (e.g., compared with bronchoscopy). As such, only a small percentage, not the majority of chest physicians will become proficient at thoracoscopy (Lee and Light 2008).

In the same textbook, the surgeons David A. Waller and Antonio E. Martin-Ucar from the United Kingdom predict in their chapter on "Surgery for Pleural Diseases" that medical thoracoscopy will be increasingly applied as initial diagnostic procedure, together with pleurodesis, when considering a malignant etiology of the pleural effusion (Waller and Martin-Ucar 2008).

Some authors feel that it is not necessary to perform MT/P in persistent pleural effusions to obtain a correct diagnosis, because the disease is incurable anyway and the prognosis is therefore poor. However, Harris and colleagues found that the clinical management was influenced by thoracoscopy in 155 out of 182 (85%) patients, of whom 98 (54%) had a malignant disease (Harris et al. 1995). Thoracoscopic findings resulted in important changes in treatment. Further surgical or therapeutic procedures were performed or deferred in 133 patients (72%), and subsequent medical treatment was directly affected by thoracoscopy in 66 patients (36%), of whom 36 underwent subsequent chemotherapy and 10 underwent radiotherapy.

The current policy of most thoracoscopists is therefore to use MT/P directly in almost all pleural exudates of un-

determined origin, and to perform closed needle biopsies of the pleura only in young patients (in whom tuberculous pleurisy is more likely, at least in countries with relatively high prevalence of tuberculosis), and in those patients who reject thoracoscopy or are too sick to tolerate it, or in whom, due to adhesions, a pneumothorax of adequate size most probably cannot be induced (here closed needle biopsies can be attempted) (Antony et al. 2000; Rodriguez-Panadero et al. 2006). **Tables 3.2** and **3.3** summarize the diagnostic and therapeutic advantages of MT/P.

**Figure 3.5** shows the changes in the etiology of pleural effusions in which MT/P was performed at Lungenklinik Heckeshorn during the previous three decades. Malignant effusions have now taken the lead and tuberculous effusions have decreased substantially, whereas the number of other pleural effusions has remained quite constant.

## Malignant Pleural Effusions

Malignant pleural effusions are a common clinical problem in patients with neoplastic disease (Antony et al. 2000). They are one of the leading causes of exudative effusions; some studies have demonstrated that 42–77% of exudative effusions are secondary to malignancy (Marel et al. 1993; Valdés et al. 1996), but this may be due to patient selection. In one postmortem series, malignant effusions were found in 15% of patients who died with malignancies (Rodriguez-Panadero et al. 1989a).

Nearly all neoplasms have been reported to involve the pleura. In most studies, however, lung cancer has been the most common neoplasm, accounting for approximately one-third of all malignant effusions. Breast carcinoma is the second most common. Lymphomas, including both Hodgkin disease and non-Hodgkin lymphoma, are also an important cause of malignant pleural effusions. Tumors less commonly associated with malignant pleural effusions include ovarian and gastrointestinal carcinomas. In 5–10% of malignant effusions, no primary tumor is identified (Chernow and Sahn 1977; Johnston 1985; Antony et al. 2000). The incidence of mesothelioma varies according to the geographical location (Greillier and Astoul 2008).

Autopsy studies suggest that most pleural metastases arise from tumor emboli, seeding to the visceral pleural surface, with secondary seeding to the parietal pleura (Rodriguez-Panadero et al. 1989 a). Other possible mechanisms include direct tumor invasion (in lung cancers, chest-wall neoplasms, and breast carcinoma), hematogenous spread to the parietal pleura, or lymphatic involvement (Antony et al. 2000). A malignant tumor can cause a pleural effusion both directly and indirectly. Interference with the integrity of the lymphatic system anywhere between the parietal pleural and mediastinal lymph nodes can result in pleural fluid formation. Direct tumor involvement with the pleura may also contribute to the formation of pleural effusions. Local inflammatory changes in response to tumor invasion may cause increased capillary permeability, with resulting effusions.

The term "paramalignant effusions" is reserved for those effusions that are not the direct result of neoplastic involvement of the pleura but are still related to the primary tumor (Antony et al. 2000). Important examples include: postobstructive pneumonia with a subsequent parapneumonic effusion; obstruction of the thoracic duct, with the development of a chylothorax; pulmonary embolism; and transudative effusions secondary to postobstruction atelectasis and/or low plasma oncotic pressures secondary to cachexia. Treatment of the primary tumor can also result in pleural effusions. Important causes in this category include radiation therapy and such drugs as methotrexate, procarbazine, cyclophosphamide, and bleomycin. Finally, concurrent nonmalignant diseases such as congestive heart failure may account for an effusion seen in a patient with cancer. MT/P offers the best

chances for differentiation between malignant and paramalignant effusions in lung cancer patients compared with pleural fluid cytology and pleural carcinoembryogenic antigen (CEA) (**Fig. 3.6**).

Most patients presenting with malignant pleural effusions have some degree of dyspnea on exertion, and their chest radiographs show moderate-to-large pleural effusions, ranging from approximately 500–2000 mL in volume (Antony et al. 2000). While only 10% of patients have massive pleural effusions on presentation, malignancy is the most common cause of massive pleural effusion, which is defined as occupying the entire hemithorax. About 15% of patients, however, will have pleural effusions < 500 mL in volume and will be relatively asymptomatic. The absence of contralateral mediastinal shift in these large effusions implies fixation of the mediastinum, main-stem bronchus occlusion by tumor (usually squamous-cell lung cancer), or extensive pleural involvement (as seen with malignant mesothelioma).

Computed tomography (CT) of patients with malignancies may identify previously unrecognized small effusions (Antony et al. 2000). It may also aid in the evaluation of patients with malignant effusions from mediastinal lymph node involvement and underlying parenchymal disease, as well as in demonstrating pleural, pulmonary, or distant metastasis. Identification of pleural plaques suggests asbestos exposure. Ultrasonography may aid in identifying pleural lesions in patients with malignant effusions and can be helpful in directing thoracentesis in patients with small effusions and avoiding thoracentesis complications.

Malignancy should be considered and a diagnostic thoracentesis performed in any individual with unilateral effusion or bilateral effusion and a normal heart size on the chest radiograph (Antony et al. 2000). It is reasonable to order the following pleural fluid tests when considering malignancy: cytology, nucleated cell count and differential, total protein, lactate dehydrogenase, glucose, pH, amylase, and tumor markers (optional).

Pleural fluid cytology is the simplest definitive method for obtaining a diagnosis of malignant pleural effusion (Antony et al. 2000). The diagnostic yield depends on such factors as extent of disease and the nature of primary malignancy. Studies have shown a large variation in diagnostic yields ranging from 22% to 94% (Heffner and Klein 2008). In some cases, differentiating between reactive mesothelial cells, mesothelioma, and adenocarcinoma can be problematic. Tumor markers such as carcinoembryonic antigen (CEA), Leu-1, and mucin may be helpful in establishing the diagnosis, as they are frequently positive in adenocarcinoma (50–90%) but rarely seen with mesothelial cells or mesothelioma (0–10%). Flow cytometry can complement cytology in some cases, particularly in lymphocytic effusions where lymphoma is suspected (Das 2006).

If the etiology remains unclear, invasive techniques are necessary to confirm the diagnosis. Closed needle biopsy of the chest wall pleura may establish the diagnosis in

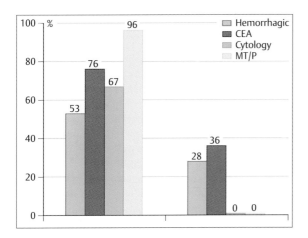

**Fig. 3.6**  Sensitivity (%) of different diagnostic criteria (hemorrhagic, CEA, cytology, MT/P) for differentiation between malignant (*n* = 67) and paramalignant (*n* = 25) pleural effusions in lung cancer patients at the Lungenklinik Heckeshorn, Berlin.

some additional cases, but usually adds little to the cytological diagnosis in most cases (Antony et al. 2000). This is related to the scars and irregular distribution of the tumor lesions in the pleural cavity when cytology is negative (Loddenkemper and Boutin 1993; Bielsa et al. 2008). In the series of 1000 consecutive patients with pleural effusions reported by Boutin and co-workers, 215 cases remained undiagnosed after repeated pleural fluid analysis and performance of pleural biopsies (Boutin et al. 1981a). This is in agreement with the results of several other authors, who, with or without the use of thoracoscopy, report that at least 20–25% of effusions remain undiagnosed (Storey et al. 1976; Hirsch et al. 1979; Lamy et al. 1980), although this certainly depends also on the selection of patient populations.

Most of the current guidelines recommend addition of a biopsy procedure when a first cytology is negative in effusions of unknown origin (Antony et al. 2000). Closed needle pleural biopsy of the costal (parietal) pleura is frequently advised in those cases. Closed needle biopsies have reported diagnostic yield of 40–75% in malignant pleural effusions. However, studies have shown that only 7–12% of patients with malignant pleural effusion may be diagnosed by pleural biopsy when fluid cytology is negative (Antony et al. 2000).

The relatively low yield of blind needle biopsy of the pleura is due to several factors, including early stage of disease with minimal pleural involvement, distribution of tumor in areas not sampled during blind biopsy, and operator inexperience. However, with the recent advances of imaging techniques some authors prefer CT-guided (Beauchamp et al. 1992; Metintas et al. 2010) or ultrasound (US)-guided (Chang et al. 1991) needle biopsies, which could replace blind needle biopsy in more than two-thirds of cases (Maskell et al. 2003), if abnormalities of the pleura can be identified with CT or US, as in mesothelioma. Cantó et al. studied the topography of pleural malignancies by medical thoracoscopy, and found that in 94% of their 203 cases the lower half of the pleural cavity was affected (**Fig. 3.7**). In 28% of cases, only the visceral pleura was involved and hence closed needle biopsy could not succeed (Cantó et al. 1983). Similar findings were seen in lung cancer (Cantó et al. 1985).

MT/P has a much higher diagnostic sensitivity and specificity than closed needle biopsy in malignant pleural effusions. Therefore, in cases of undiagnosed exudative effusions with a high clinical suspicion for malignancy, some clinicians may proceed directly to MT/P if cytology is negative and if the facilities for MT/P are available (Antony et al. 2000; Fletcher and Clark 2006). A theoretical cost analysis in the UK showed that MT/P saves considerable costs in unexplained pleural effusions compared with image-guided pleural biopsy (Medford 2010).

In a prospective intrapatient comparison, the diagnostic yield of the nonsurgical biopsy methods in malignant pleural effusions was studied simultaneously in 208 patients (Loddenkemper et al. 1983a). These included: 58

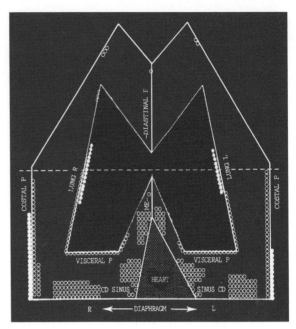

**Fig. 3.7** Location of pleural metastases at thoracoscopy. (Reproduced with permission from Canto et al., Chest 1983;84:176–9.)

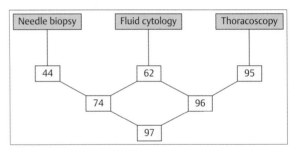

**Fig. 3.8** Sensitivity (%) of different biopsy methods in malignant pleural effusions (prospective simultaneous comparison, *n* = 206) (Loddenkemper et al. 1983b.)

diffuse malignant mesotheliomas; 29 cancers of the lung; 116 metastatic pleural effusions with 38 breast cancers; 30 cancers of various other origins; 58 of undetermined origin; and five malignant lymphomas. The overall diagnostic yield with cytological results from effusion was 62%, with needle biopsy (Tru-Cut) 44%, and with MT/P 95%, the latter showing a significantly higher sensitivity (*p* < 0.001) than needle biopsy with cytological results from effusions combined, which were positive in 74% of cases. All methods taken together were diagnostic in 97% of cases for malignant pleural effusion (**Fig. 3.8**). In six cases an underlying neoplasm was suspected at thoracoscopy but confirmed only by thoracotomy or autopsy in three cases each. Similar results were reported by several other investigators. In a study on 287 cases with malignant pleural effusion, there was virtually no difference in the yield of medical thoracoscopy for the different types of malignant effusions (Antony et al. 2000). The overall yield was

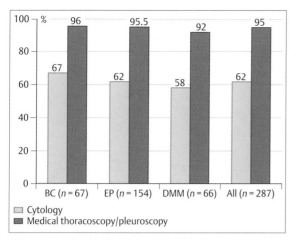

**Fig. 3.9** Diagnostic yield (%) of cytology and medical thoracoscopy/pleuroscopy in malignant pleural effusions of different origin at the Lungenklinik Heckeshorn, Berlin 1980–1986. BC, bronchial carcinoma; EP, extrathoracic primary; DMM, diffuse malignant mesothelioma. (From Antony et al. 2001, reprinted with permission from ERS Journals Ltd.)

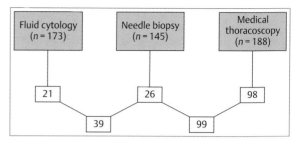

**Fig. 3.10** Sensitivity (%) of different biopsy methods in diffuse malignant pleural mesothelioma. (Modified from Boutin and Rey 1993).

62% for cytology and 95% for MT/P; the yield for cytology and in particular thoracoscopy did not vary much between lung carcinomas (67% versus 96%, n = 67), extrathoracic primaries (62% versus 95.5%, n = 154), or diffuse malignant mesotheliomas (58% versus 92%, n = 66) (**Fig. 3.9**).

A further advantage of MT/P in malignant pleural disease is that biopsies can be taken under direct visual control not only of the costal pleura but also of the visceral and diaphragmatic pleura (Loddenkemper 1998). Since the thoracoscopic biopsies provide larger tissue specimens, this provides an easier histological/immunohistological identification of the primary tumor, including determination of hormone receptors in breast cancer (Levine et al. 1986; Schwarz et al. 2004), and a better morphological classification in lymphomas (Viallat et al. 1986; Celikoglu et al. 1992; Kawahara et al. 2008; Steiropoulos et al. 2009) and in their differential diagnosis (Schwarz et al. 2009). An additional advantage is that the diagnostic procedure can easily be combined with the therapeutic procedure of talc poudrage for pleurodesis (see "Thoracoscopic Talc Pleurodesis," pp. 38–41, and Chapter 11, p. 93–94).

In addition, MT/P is helpful in staging of lung cancer, diffuse malignant mesothelioma, and metastatic cancers (Colt 1995 b). In lung cancer patients MT/P can determine whether the tumor has spread to the pleura, is secondary to venous or lymphatic obstruction, or is parapneumonic (Antony et al. 2000; Yoneda et al. 2007). As a result, it may be possible to avoid exploratory thoracotomy or to determine operability. Weissberg et al. (1981) performed thoracoscopy in 45 patients with lung cancer and pleural effusion. In 37 patients they found pleural invasion; three had mediastinal disease; the remaining five had no evident metastatic disease and, therefore, no contraindication to resection. Cantó and co-workers found similar re-

sults (Cantó et al. 1985). Of 44 patients, eight (18%) had no thoracoscopic evidence of pleural involvement, and six went to resection, where no tumor was found. A further study by Cantó et al. demonstrated that diagnostic sensitivity of malignancy was associated with the size of the effusion (Cantó et al. 1996). In conclusion, MT/P is the procedure of choice to differentiate between resectable and unresectable lung cancer if there is a pleural effusion present. In case of pleural metastasis, the stage of disease migrated previously to IIIB with a prognosis of stage IV (in the new staging system, malignant pleural effusion is classified as M1a and stage IV [Goldstraw et al. 2007]). In addition, the development of dedicated chemotherapy, even for metastatic non–small-cell lung cancer, warrants a specific diagnosis (Rodriguez-Panadero et al. 2006).

In diffuse malignant mesothelioma, the diagnostic yield of cytology is approximately 58%. MT/P can more often (**Fig. 3.10**) and more precisely provide a histological classification than closed pleural biopsy because of larger and more representative biopsies, along with more accurate staging (Boutin and Rey 1993; Boutin et al. 1993 b; Rusch 1995; Greillier and Astoul 2008; Scherpereel et al. 2010). This may have important therapeutic implications either for surgery or for local immunotherapy or local chemotherapy, since better results have been observed in the early stages (I and II) (Boutin et al. 1991; Astoul et al. 1993; Boutin et al. 1994; Nowak et al. 2002; Vogelzang et al. 2003; Stewart et al. 2004; Sugarbaker et al. 2004). However, recent studies have shown that thoracoscopy may be less efficient in diagnosing the histological subtype (Bueno et al. 2004; Greillier et al. 2007). In histologically proven mesothelioma, the patient has a right to claim financial compensation from the former employer in several countries (Rodriguez-Panadero et al. 2006). In addition, fibrohyaline or calcified, thick, pearly-white pleural plaques may be found. MT/P helps in diagnosing benign asbestos pleural effusion (BAPE) by excluding mesothelioma or other malignancies with high accuracy (Boutin et al. 1998; Greillier and Astoul 2008). Thoracoscopic lung biopsies as well as biopsies from lesions on the parietal pleura may demonstrate high concentrations of asbestos fibers, providing further support for diagnosis of asbestos-induced disease (Boutin et al. 1996).

Reasons for false-negative MT/P include insufficient and nonrepresentative biopsies, which depend largely on the experience of the thoracoscopist, and the presence of adhesions that deny access to neoplastic tissue (Loddenkemper and Boutin 1993).

Autofluorescence videothoracoscopy with rigid instruments, developed by Richard Wolf GmbH in Germany, may help in the future to avoid some of the false-negative results (Chrysanthidis and Janssen 2005) (see **Fig. 16.14 a, b** in the *Atlas* section).

Narrow-band imaging during semirigid pleuroscopy, developed by Olympus Corporation, Japan, may also detect earlier discrete pathologic changes (Schönfeld et al. 2009) (see Fig. **14.9a, b** in the *Atlas* section).

Another study, although under double-lumen intubation in general anesthesia, used fluorescence with 5-aminolevulinic acid in the diagnostic work-up for various pleural malignancies (D-LIGHT Auto Fluorescent System; Karl Storz, Germany). This method improved visualization of abnormal lesions and led to upstaging in four of 15 mesothelioma patients (Baas et al. 2006).

In a review of 4301 cases of diagnostic MT/P using rigid instruments in cases of chronic pleural effusion from 21 different studies, Boutin and co-workers reported that out of 1472 cancer cases a correct pathological diagnosis was achieved from thoracoscopic specimens in 1333 (92.5%). Conversely, 7.5% of thoracoscopic biopsies were false-negative (Boutin et al. 1991). Several explanations have been proposed:

1. In some cases of patients with cancer, pleural effusion is due not to malignant pleural effusion but to malignant obstruction of mediastinal or pulmonary lymphatics, which are not biopsied. This has been described both in lung cancer and cancer of the breast.
2. Rarely, an effusion is the late consequence of lymphatic obstruction due to mediastinal radiotherapy, which occurs in approximately 1% of cases (paramalignant pleural effusion).
3. The thoracoscopist learns with experience and has a suboptimal yield initially before full competence is achieved (a learning curve as experienced with all technical procedures).
4. Multiple biopsies must be taken systematically. There is no such thing as "too many." The costovertebral gutter and the diaphragm must be routinely sampled. Metastases sometimes cannot be recognized endoscopically.
5. If the biopsy is reported as negative in suspected malignancy, the pathologist should be asked to section all tissue, including "deepest," and to completely review all slides. This makes it possible to obtain additional diagnoses in some cases.
6. Sometimes the pleurae are covered with a fibrinous, necrotic layer, which requires removal to biopsy the parietal pleura behind it.
7. The major stumbling blocks for MT/P in cancer patients are cases of adherent pleura. The ability to obtain a biopsy depends on the practitioner's skill in dividing and cutting adhesions, and there are some cases in which biopsy is impossible.

**Table 3.4** Grading of intrapleural tumor spread in malignant pleural effusions by medical thoracoscopy/pleuroscopy ("lesion-size score", or tumor score [see Fig. 3.18b, p. 41])

| Pleural involvement | Isolated (1) | Diffuse (2) | Massive (3) |
|---|---|---|---|
| Parietal–chest wall | | | |
| Parietal–diaphragm | | | |
| Visceral | | | |
| Sum of points (maximum 9) | | | |

Modified from Sanchez-Armengol and Rodriguez-Panadero (1993).

In their routine experience, they achieved 95–97% sensitivity in cancerous effusions, and false-negative findings were almost always due to adhesions that denied access to the neoplastic tissue.

The main additional advantage in using MT/P to diagnose malignancy is that talc poudrage can be performed in the same procedure, which is probably the most often used conservative option today for pleurodesis, with high success rates of more than 80% (Rodriguez-Panadero and Antony 1997; Tan et al. 2006a). An even distribution of the talc powder to all parts of the pleura can be achieved by poudrage under visual control. The extent of the carcinomatous involvement of the pleural cavity can be determined macroscopically, which allows some prediction of the success of pleurodesis: the intrapleural tumor spread can be semiquantitated using a scoring system (Table 3.**4**) that has been shown to correlate quite closely with survival and with the success of talc pleurodesis (Sanchez-Armengol and Rodriguez-Panadero 1993; Antony et al. 2004). Furthermore, by visual inspection it can be judged whether the lung will reexpand, which is an important prerequisite for a successful pleurodesis.

## Tuberculous Pleural Effusions

In his pioneering publication in 1910 Jacobaeus reported that he performed his first thoracoscopies in two patients with tuberculous pleural effusion (pleuritis exudativa) (Jacobaeus 1910). At that time, tuberculous pleurisy was one of the main causes of pleural effusion. Since then this has changed considerably in industrialized countries with low TB incidence. However, in some countries with a high TB prevalence, tuberculous pleurisy is still the leading cause of pleural effusions (Light 2010).

In Germany, for example, tuberculous pleural effusion now occurs in less than 5% of patients with TB (Forssbohm et al. 2008), but is more frequent (15–90%) in AIDS patients, with an effusion being more common in patients with higher CD4+ counts (Gopi et al. 2007). The diagnosis

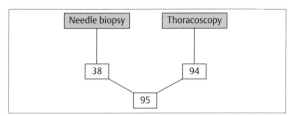

**Fig. 3.11** Histological yield (%) of blind needle biopsy and medical thoracoscopy/pleuroscopy in tuberculous pleural effusions (prospective simultaneous comparison, $n = 100$). (Modified from Loddenkemper et al. 1983 b.)

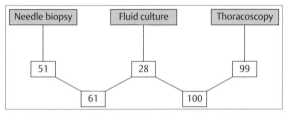

**Fig. 3.12** Combined histological and bacteriological yield (%) of different biopsy methods in tuberculous pleural effusions. (Modified from Loddenkemper et al. 1983 b.)

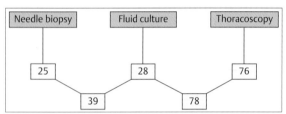

**Fig. 3.13** Cultural yield (%) of different biopsy methods in tuberculous pleural effusions. (Modified from Loddenkemper et al. 1983 b.)

of pleural tuberculosis is hampered by its paucibacillary nature (Chegou et al. 2008). Less than 10% of pleural fluids are smear-positive and culture is positive in only approximately 30% (20–50%) of cases. The diagnostic yield of closed needle pleural biopsies is much better than in malignant pleural effusions due to the usually more disseminated involvement of the whole pleural surface. In a review of the literature on 1225 cases, the yield averaged 69% with a range of 28–88%, including results for multiple biopsies and TB cultures (Loddenkemper et al. 1983b). A study from South Africa showed that ultrasound-assisted needle biopsies were diagnostic for TB in 81.8% with the Abrams needles and in 65.2% with the Tru-Cut needles (Koegelenberg et al. 2009).

However, the diagnostic accuracy of MT/P is even better, because the pathologist is provided with multiple biopsies selected under visual control, and because the cultural proof of growth of TB bacilli is more often positive (Loddenkemper et al. 1978). MT/P therefore still has its value in the diagnosis of tuberculous pleurisy since it offers a high diagnostic sensitivity and specificity, and, in addition, a higher chance to determine drug resistance (Zarić et al. 2008).

In a prospective intrapatient comparison, an immediate diagnosis in 100 TB cases could be established histologically by MT/P in 94%, compared with needle biopsy (Tru-Cut) with only 38% positive results (**Fig. 3.11**) (Loddenkemper et al. 1983b). In individual cases, this may be of clinical importance because antituberculous chemotherapy can be started without delay. The combined yield of histology and bacteriological culture was positive for MT/P in 99% and for needle biopsy in 51%, and when culture results from effusions were added, in 61% of cases (**Fig. 3.12**). The percentage of positive TB cultures was twice as high from thoracoscopic biopsies, including cultures from fibrinous membranes (78%), which are always worth examining, as the percentage of cultures from pleural effusions and needle biopsies combined (39%) (**Fig. 3.13**).

Thus, MT/P much more often provides a bacteriological confirmation of the diagnosis of TB and, furthermore, the possibility of performing susceptibility tests. In five of the 78 positive cases (6.4%), resistance to one or more antituberculous drugs was found that had an impact on treatment and prognosis. It is of interest that the chance for a positive TB culture was much higher (87%) in cases were fibrin production in the pleural cavity was present. The typical changes with diffusely thickened pleura, multiple adhesions, and sometimes formation of encapsulating membranes with fluid loculations, were present in 76% of cases. By comparison, the pathognomonic picture of so-called "sagolike" pleuritis with miliary tuberculous granulomas and without fibrin layers was seen in only 24% of cases. In these cases, a positive TB culture was obtained from all biopsied specimens in only 50%, giving a highly significant difference ($p < 0.0005$).

Interestingly, the study also showed that the chance of positive TB cultures from pleural effusion alone was statistically much better in cases with a low pleural glucose level (< 50 mg/dL), indicating an increased metabolism of TB bacilli and/or a higher degree of inflammation (59% positive versus 25% with glucose levels above 50 mg/dL, $p < 0.005$). But the first group comprised only 17% of the patients, suggesting that they were diagnosed at quite an early stage. Cell count differentiation showed mainly lymphocytes in 71%, neutrophils in 9%, predominating in the early stages of growth without fibrin production, and in 20% in no characteristic cells at all.

In another prospective study on 40 cases from South Africa, MT/P had a diagnostic yield of 98% in comparison with an 80% diagnostic yield of Abrams needle biopsies (Walzl et al. 1996). This led to the conclusion that in areas with high prevalence of TB, closed needle biopsy alone—in this study three biopsies were obtained and each was examined histologically and microbiologically—can contribute significantly to the diagnosis of tuberculous pleurisy.

In a further study from the same institution in Stellenbosch, South Africa, 51 patients with undiagnosed exudative pleural effusion were recruited for a prospective, direct comparison between bronchial wash, pleural fluid microbiology, biochemistry (adenosine deaminase

[ADA]), cell count, closed needle biopsy, and MT/P (Diacon et al. 2003). The final diagnosis was TB in 41 patients (82%). The sensitivities of histology, culture, and combined histology/culture were 66%, 48%, and 79%, respectively, for closed needle biopsy, and 100%, 76%, and 100%, respectively, for MT/P. Since the combination of ADA, lymphocyte/neutrophil ratio ≥ 0.75 plus closed needle biopsy reached 93% sensitivity and 100% specificity, the authors concluded that this high diagnostic accuracy is sufficient in an area with a high incidence of tuberculosis. However, if this combination of tests is negative despite a high clinical suspicion of tuberculous pleurisy, if antibiotic resistance is of concern, or if other possible diagnoses are considered, they recommend MT/P as the method of choice for the final diagnosis.

A retrospective study from Japan achieved similar results in 32 patients with tuberculous pleurisy. Semirigid pleuroscopic biopsies were positive in 93.8% with histological and bacteriological examination and in 65.6% with pathological examination alone (Sakuraba et al. 2006a).

Several laboratory and microbiological tests have been developed during recent years, including nucleic acid amplification and detection, markers of specific and nonspecific immune response such as ADA, and T cell-based interferon-gamma release assays (IGRAs), which may allow the diagnosis of TB as the cause of pleural effusion with high sensitivity and specificity (Trajman et al. 2008; Light 2010). However, at least in countries with low prevalence of TB, the accuracy may not be sufficient in individual cases (Hooper et al. 2009). This is underlined by a further study from Japan in which 138 patients underwent MT/P for unexplained pleural effusion (Sakuraba et al. 2009). Of 50 patients who had effusions with ADA levels of less than 50 IU/L, a tuberculous pleurisy was diagnosed in six patients (12%) by thoracoscopic biopsy. These patients would have been diagnosed with nonspecific pleurisy otherwise. It is questionable whether patients should undergo treatment with antituberculous drugs merely on the suspicion of a tuberculous etiology of the pleurisy. In our opinion, in these cases MT/P should be performed to prove or exclude TB.

A further important argument in favor of MT/P is provided by the fact that thoracoscopic biopsies much more often yield positive TB cultures (see above, Loddenkemper et al. 1983b), which give rise to the possibility of obtaining susceptibility tests that, in particular in patients born in countries with high resistance rates, especially of multidrug resistance (MDR) or extensive drug resistance (XDR) (World Health Organization 2009), may have a considerable impact on the correct treatment and the final outcome after therapy (Baumann et al. 2007; Gopi et al. 2007).

In addition, the immediate and complete drainage of the pleural fluid, achieved during and after MT/P, is associated with greater and direct symptomatic improvement than is any subsequent therapy. This was demonstrated in a further study from Stellenbosch on the effect of corticosteroids on the treatment of TB pleurisy (Wyser et al. 1996). Up to now, no studies have been done that compare the impact of MT/P with its fast diagnosis, complete drainage, and subsequent early drug treatment to a group of patients with drug treatment alone.

Although some authors are not much concerned with long-term complications of tuberculous effusions (Sahn 2002), the positive role of early removal of the pleural fluid has been shown recently in a double-blind, randomized, placebo-controlled trial from Taiwan (Chung et al. 2008). In this study, it was demonstrated that early effective drainage, combined with complete antituberculous treatment, may hasten clearance of pleural effusion, reduce residual pleural thickening occurrence, and accelerate pulmonary function recovery in patients with symptomatic loculated tuberculous pleural effusion who were irrigated in addition with streptokinase instead of saline alone. This is in accordance with the experience at Lungenklinik Heckeshorn where, after early MT/P with complete evacuation of the pleural fluid—if necessary combined with mechanical opening of loculations—and subsequent pleural drainage, no single case of tuberculous pleurisy was observed in 20 years that needed surgical decortication for fibrothorax.

## Parapneumonic Effusions and Pleural Empyema

The optimal management of parapneumonic effusions (PPE) and empyema in the fibrinopurulent state (stage II) is still controversial, with a lack of controlled studies, whereas the organizational stage (stage III) is reserved almost exclusively for surgical interventions, since this stage shows continued fibroblast migration and the production of pleural fibrosis with lung trapping (Colice et al. 2000). The initial evaluation should focus on three critical questions: (1) Should the pleural space be drained? (2) How should the pleural space be drained? (3) Should fibrinolytics be instilled? (Koegelenberg et al. 2008).

Treatment goals in stage II, besides eradication of the causative pathogen, include evacuation of all (infected) pleural fluid, prevention or breakdown of (multi-)loculations, and prevention of lung trapping by fibrin deposition on the visceral and parietal pleura. This is rarely achieved by antibiotic treatment alone, but needs pleural space drainage in almost all cases. Local pleural treatment options can be separated into medical (conservative) and surgical (Loddenkemper et al. 2004). The medical options include (serial) therapeutic thoracentesis, small-bore tubes, or standard chest tubes, often combined with instillation of fibrinolytic agents and/or irrigation of the pleural cavity. This can be combined with MT/P. Arguments in favor of conservative treatment are that (1) it is less invasive and (2) it can be applied even in severely sick patients (with sepsis, on ventilator, in the intensive care unit, on immunosuppressive disease/treatment, or in other severe concomitant diseases).

There are only few publications on the use of MT/P in the diagnosis and treatment of PPE and empyema. As early

**Table 3.5** Role of medical thoracoscopy/pleuroscopy in the management of complicated parapneumonic effusion/empyema

- Technique similar to chest tube insertion
- Direct visualization of loculations
- Inspection and characterization of the pleural surface
- Breakdown of fibrinous septae and creation of one single pleural space

Brutsche et al. (2005).

**Table 3.6** Outcome (%) in parapneumonic pleural effusions in the management of complicated treatment

| Outcome | D. Kaiser[a] (n = 376) | W. Frank[b] (n = 66) | Total (n = 442) |
|---|---|---|---|
| Complete remission | 82 | 64 | 79 |
| Partial remission | 10 | 25 | 12 |
| Failure | 8 | 11 | 9 |
| Surgery necessary | 6 | 6.5 | 6 |
| 30 days mortality | 3 | 10 | 4 |

From Loddenkemper et al. (2004) with permission from ERS Journals Ltd.
[a] Department of Thoracic Surgery, Lungenklinik Heckeshorn (1985–2000).
[b] Department of Pneumology, Treuenbrietzen (1995–2002).

as 1925, Jacobaeus reported on 100 cases of empyema in which he performed thoracoscopy (Jacobaeus 1925). Boutin et al. recommend the use of MT/P for breaking up loculations of pus, thereby creating one large, unilocular space, and for insertion of a large drainage tube under direct vision (Boutin et al. 1991). Karmy-Jones and co-workers recommend this approach for patients who are unable to tolerate one-lung anesthesia (Karmy-Jones et al. 1997). Weissberg (1981) as well as Kaiser (1989), both thoracic surgeons, used the technique successfully in many cases of empyema as well as the respiratory physician Wolfgang Frank (Loddenkemper et al. 2004). Solèr and co-workers have described the successful use of MT/P in the treatment of early parapneumonic empyema (Solèr et al. 1997). Tassi and co-authors recommend choosing the trocar point of entry by ultrasonography to identify the point where the pus collection is largest and the position of the diaphragm, which is often elevated. They also outline the steps that should be taken including the thoracoscopic/pleuroscopic exploration of the thoracic cavity to identify additional loculations and, very rarely, foreign bodies (Tassi et al. 2006).

In cases with multiple loculations, it is possible to open these spaces by removing fibrinopurulent membranes with the forceps and, thus, create one single cavity that can be drained and irrigated with high efficiency. This was demonstrated in a retrospective study of 127 patients of whom 94% were treated successfully for multiloculated empyema (Brutsche et al. 2005). Only 6% of the patients required a surgical approach. The treatment should be performed early in the course of parapneumonic effusion/empyema, before the adhesions become too fibrinous and adherent. Thus, if the indication for placement of a chest tube is present and if the facilities are available, MT/P should be performed at the time of chest tube insertion. Overall, medical thoracoscopy is a procedure technically similar to chest tube placement but it enables the creation of a single pleural cavity by mechanical opening of loculations and removal of fibrinous material, allowing successful local treatment (**Table 3.5**).

Henry Colt reported successful thoracoscopic drainage in six of seven patients. In three, thoracoscopy was performed because of loculated, complicated parapneumonic effusions. In each case an empyema was ultimately diagnosed and the multiloculated pleural space effectively drained. Four other patients with empyema were referred after failure of chest tube drainage. Treatment was suc-

cessful in three and in one surgical decortication was indicated because it was evident that thoracoscopic debridement alone would not be satisfactory (Colt 1995 a).

It has been shown that for patients with complicated parapneumonic effusions morbidity is lower in those who are treated with thoracoscopy or VATS than in those who receive tube thoracotomy alone (Colice et al. 2000).

At Lungenklinik Heckeshorn, by far the majority of fibrinopurulent effusions/empyemas could be managed successfully by nonsurgical treatment including antibiotics, pleural drainage (± medical thoracoscopy), intrapleural fibrinolytics, and irrigation (Kaiser 1989; Loddenkemper et al. 2004). A surgical approach became necessary only when medical treatment failed or in the later organizational stages of empyema. In 442 cases, complete remission was achieved in 79%, partial remission in 12%, and failure occurred in 9%. Surgery was necessary in 6% and the 30-day mortality was 4% (**Table 3.6**).

Thus, in our opinion, if the indication for placement of a chest tube is present and if the facilities are available, medical thoracoscopy should be performed at the time of chest tube insertion, since it allows staging and additional therapeutic measures. However, prospective studies on the use of medical thoracoscopy in the treatment of early empyema have not yet been performed. Successful thoracoscopic treatment has also been reported in children (Kern and Rodgers 1993; Stovroff et al. 1995).

VATS is definitely a more invasive procedure because general anesthesia and selective double-lumen intubation are necessary. If possible, this should be avoided in these often very sick patients. The advantages of MT/P compared with VATS include lower costs and better tolerance by frail patients who may not tolerate lung deflation, which is required for VATS (Heffner et al. 2009). However, surgery is certainly indicated in the later, organizational stage with dense and extensive adhesions (Colice et al. 2000).

**Figure 3.14** shows the proposed therapeutic approach (algorithm) in the different stages of parapneumonic effusion/empyema (Loddenkemper et al. 2004). Local expertise and availability are likely to dictate the initial treatment choice (Koegelenberg et al. 2008).

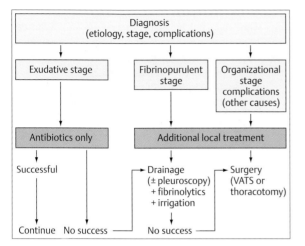

**Fig. 3.14** Algorithm for the management of parapneumonic effusions/empyema. (From Loddenkemper et al. 2004, reprinted with permission from ERS Journals Ltd.)

## Effusions of Other Origin

In other pleural effusions, when the origin remains indeterminate, the main diagnostic value of MT/P lies in its ability to exclude, with high probability, malignant or tuberculous disease (Loddenkemper 1998; Light 2006). In cases of pleural effusions that are neither malignant nor tuberculous, MT/P may occasionally give macroscopic clues to their etiology.

In rheumatoid effusions, in which tuberculosis often has to be excluded, typically white fibrin deposits on the visceral or parietal pleura can be demonstrated (Ferguson 1966; Faurschou 1974, 1989; Faurschou et al. 1985). Histologically, marked fibrosis can often be found in the subpleural tissue, rarely rheumatoid granulomas. In advanced cases, the walls of the pleural cavity are covered with extremely dense fibrin so that neither the lung nor the parietal pleura can be recognized. In pleural effusions due to systemic lupus erythematosus, MT/P may reveal nodules on the visceral pleura, and immunofluorescence of biopsy samples of these nodules demonstrates immunoglobulin deposits (Bouros et al. 2008).

Pleural effusions due to liver cirrhosis may show characteristically greatly distended, tortuous veins on the diaphragm, sometimes even bearing venous varices plus marked capillary hyperemia.

In pleural effusions following pancreatitis, the parietal pleura can be thickened by whitish fibrin, sometimes with disseminated small calcified areas. Henry Colt and a coworker describe a case with right chest pain and enlarging exudative pleural effusion four months after laparoscopic cholecystectomy in which only MT/P revealed bilious concretions in the parietal pleura and essentially contributed to a successful treatment (Brazinsky and Colt 1993).

When pleural effusions are secondary to underlying primary pulmonary problems, such as pneumonia or pulmonary infarct, the diagnosis can frequently be made by macroscopic examination during MT/P, and then confirmed microscopically from a biopsy of the lung. A few studies report on the successful thoracoscopic diagnosis of rare pleural effusions due to amyloidosis (Astoul et al. 1992) or sarcoidosis (Akçay et al. 2008).

As already mentioned, MT/P is helpful in differentiating between malignant and paramalignant pleural effusions in lung cancer (Antony et al. 2000), and it is well suited for the diagnosis of a benign, asbestos-related pleural effusion, which, by definition, presents a diagnosis of exclusion. Usually, this diagnosis is confirmed only by long-term observation (Greillier and Astoul 2008). Occasionally MT/P has to be repeated, which is easily performed (Breen et al. 2009). However, MT/P allows an immediate confirmation by excluding malignant pleural mesothelioma with a high specificity (Boutin et al. 1998).

In some selected cases of recurrent pleural effusions of nonmalignant etiology, including chylothorax, hepatic effusions, and refractory effusions due to cardiac etiology or in systemic lupus erythematosus, talc poudrage during MT/P may be successfully applied (Audier et al. 1967; Sudduth and Sahn 1992; Vargas et al. 1994; Rodriguez-Panadero and Antony 1997; Mares and Mathur 1998; Breuer et al. 2005).

Occasionally it is impossible to perform MT/P because of dense pleuropulmonary adhesions, often observed after repeated aspirations of larger volumes of pleural fluid. Here an extended medical thoracoscopy with the blunt dissection technique, which needs sufficient experience (Janssen and Boutin 1992), or a closed needle biopsy can be tried (see "Access to the Pleural Space," Chapter 11, p. 78 ff.). Only in selected cases may it be worthwhile to consider as a further diagnostic step "surgical thoracoscopy" (VATS) or exploratory thoracotomy, eventually combined with decortication (Ryan et al. 1981; Loddenkemper and McKenna 2005).

## "Idiopathic" Pleural Effusions

When MT/P is used in the diagnostic work-up of pleural effusions, the proportion of so-called idiopathic pleural effusions usually falls markedly below 10% (Cantó et al. 1977; Boutin et al. 1981a; Loddenkemper 1981; Martensson et al. 1985), whereas studies in which MT/P does not belong to the diagnostic armamentarium mostly report failure to obtain a diagnosis in over 20% (Storey et al. 1976; Hirsch et al. 1979; Lamy et al. 1980; Ozkara et al. 2007). No doubt the failure rate depends on the selection of patients and on the definition of "idiopathic" (Janssen et al. 2004; Venekamp et al. 2005). Sometimes, the number of eosinophils in the pleural effusion may be elevated, pointing, for example, to a viral etiology (Loddenkemper 1981).

Several studies have tried to determine the diagnostic accuracy of MT/P in the setting of undiagnosed pleural effusion, but the results vary widely, with a range of 69–90%. Closer evaluation of the study designs reveals that the duration of follow-up was occasionally short and frequently not mentioned at all. One well-designed Canadian study with follow-up periods between 1 and 2 years found a sensitivity of 91%, specificity of 100%, accuracy of 96%, and negative predictive value of 93% (Menzies and Charbonneau 1991). A study from Denmark reported a diagnostic accuracy of only 69% with a 5-year follow-up (Enk and Viskum 1981).

In a retrospective study from The Netherlands, a long-term follow-up was undertaken in 709 patients who underwent MT/P for unexplained exudative pleural effusion after (repeated) thoracentesis (Janssen et al. 2004). Of the 709 patients, 391 (55%) had nonmalignant pleuritis. Of these, 183 (26% of the total group) had pleuritis resulting from a true benign disease. In 208 patients (29% of the total group), the cause of pleuritis remained inconclusive. After long-term follow-up, the cause of pleural effusion in this last group appeared in 31 patients (4.3% of the total group); all finally developed a malignancy, most often a mesothelioma (10 patients), five an adenocarcinoma of an unknown primary, four non–small-cell and one small-cell lung cancer, four non-Hodgkin lymphoma, three breast cancer, and four other cancers. This means that in this study 31 (15%) of 208 MT/P with an inconclusive result appeared to be false-negative after a mean follow-up of 4.4 months. Thus, after long-term follow-up of all patients who underwent MT/P, the sensitivity of the examination was 91% and the specificity 100%; the positive predictive value being 100% and the negative predictive value 92%.

In a further retrospective study, from Belgium, the evolution of 75 patients who underwent diagnostic MT/P because of an unexplained exudative pleural effusion, and in whom the histological diagnosis of nonspecific pleuritis was made (Venekamp et al. 2005), was examined. Of the 75 patients, 8.3% eventually developed a malignancy during the mean follow-up period of 32.9 (±27.4) months (range 3–110 months). In the remaining patients (91.7%), the clinical evolution followed a benign course. Ultimately, a probable cause was established on clinical grounds in 40 patients. True idiopathic pleuritis was finally observed in 25% of patients with the histological diagnosis of nonspecific pleuritis. Recurrence of the effusion occurred in 10 out of 60 patients (16.7%) after a mean period of 26.2 months. The authors concluded that the majority of nonspecific pleuritis patients (91.7%) followed a benign course, with spontaneous resolution of the effusion in 81.8% of cases. In the majority of patients, a probable cause of the pleuritis could be identified. True "idiopathic benign pleuritis" hence occurs in only a minority (25%) of highly selected patients. The total number of patients in whom MT/P was performed during the study period was not given; thus the true percentage of idiopathic pleuritis could not be calculated.

In another study, from Spain, follow-up was performed in 53 patients with idiopathic pleuritis after MT/P from a total of 394 patients with pleural effusion (Ferrer et al. 1996). Of these 53 patients, nine (17%) were lost to follow-up, and of the remaining patients, two (5%) appeared

to have malignant pleuritis during follow-up. Similar results were reported by Blanc and co-workers, who observed an erroneous thoracoscopic diagnosis in 10 out of 149 cases, mainly owing to pleural adhesions that limited access to the pleural cavity (Blanc et al. 2002).

The alternative to MT/P in cases of pleural effusions of undetermined origin, after a full diagnostic work-up including thoracentesis and closed needle biopsy of the pleura, is to observe the further course of disease and to use a wait-and-see approach (Rodriguez-Panadero et al. 2006). Maskell states that "the principal aims should be to exclude any treatable causes of the pleural effusion, avoid subjecting frail patients to unnecessary intervention, and at the same time manage patients expectations" (Maskell 2008). Thus, if the clinician expects the results to change patient management, or the patient insists on a clear definition of the underlying disease, MT/P should be the next step.

In a further study, from the United States, patient management was directly affected by thoracoscopy in 85% of patients (Harris et al. 1995). But even after a complete work-up including thoracoscopic biopsies, a clear diagnosis may not be established in quite a significant number of patients. Subsequently, the pleural effusion is defined as "idiopathic," "of indeterminate cause," or as "nonspecific" (Janssen et al. 2004).

The results after open thoracotomy are apparently not much superior, as shown in a study from the Mayo Clinic (Ryan et al. 1981). The cause of pleural effusion remained unclear in 51 cases after thoracotomy. After a period of 12 days to 5 years, malignant pleuritis was eventually found in 13 patients (25%)—including six cases of lymphoma and four cases of mesothelioma. However, in the study from The Netherlands, thoracotomy gave the final diagnosis in 12 of the 31 cases of false-negative MT/P whereas four cases were diagnosed by repeated thoracoscopy, six by repeated thoracentesis, three by autopsy, two by laparoscopy, one by pericardial effusion, and two by other procedures (Janssen et al. 2004).

In conclusion, the most often missed diagnoses in these studies were malignant pleural mesothelioma and malignant lymphoma. Similar results were seen in a retrospective study in a tertiary referal center in the UK with a high incidence of mesothelioma (Davies et al. 2010). In 69% of 142 patients with pleural effusion a definite histological diagnosis was obtained by MT/P, whereas 31% had "nonspecific pleuritis/fibrosis." Five of these 44 patients (12%) were subsequently diagnosed with malignant mesothelioma after a mean interval of 9.8 (±4.6) months. As already mentioned, autofluorescence videothoracoscopy or narrow-band imaging during semirigid pleuroscopy may help in the future to avoid some of the false-negative results (Chrysanthidis and Janssen 2005; Schönfeld et al. 2009). However, a repeated MT/P is also feasible (Breen et al. 2009).

Sometimes, adhesions or thick fibrinous layers prevent the taking of sufficient biopsy specimens during MT/P

(Loddenkemper and Boutin 1993). If this is the case and if pleural thickening on computed tomography strongly suggests mesothelioma, which cannot be diagnosed by multiple closed needle biopsies, a subsequent surgical procedure is warranted in patients with a history of asbestos exposure (Loddenkemper and McKenna 2005).

## Options in the Local Treatment of Pleural Effusions Including Thoracoscopic Talc Pleurodesis

Approximately half of the patients seen by a pulmonologist with undiagnosed pleural effusion are found to have malignancies (Marel et al. 1993; Antony et al. 2000). There are more than 160 000 new cases of pleural effusion annually in the United States. Malignant pleural effusions are most common with lung and breast cancer (Salyer et al. 1975; Chernow and Sahn 1977; Johnston 1985; Hsu 1987; Sears and Hajduh 1987; DiBonito et al. 1992; Martínez-Moragón et al. 1998). The prognosis of lung cancer with malignant pleural effusion is very poor, with a median survival of 2.2–6 months. Certain subtypes of cancer may have better survival; management of these patient presents important challenges in their palliative care (Sanchez-Armengol and Rodriguez-Panadero 1993; Naito et al. 1997; Sugiura et al. 1997).

As has been mentioned, MT/P offers superior sensitivity (>95%) for diagnosis. In addition, one can evaluate the pleural space to assess tumor burden and evidence of trapped lung. However, the more common method of making a diagnosis is by thoracentesis and closed pleural biopsies (Heffner and Klein 2008).

Management goals in malignant pleural effusion are to control symptoms. This palliative goal has to be influenced by patient/family preference and performance status (Antony et al. 2000; Maskell and Butland 2003). There are limited studies comparing treatment options (Tan et al. 2006a; Heffner and Klein 2008), but we will try to present an approach that provides a plan for the palliative care of patients with malignant pleural effusion (as well as for chronic recurrent pleural effusions of other, nonmalignant origin). In the absence of any symptoms, there is usually no need for any therapeutic intervention.

The options available are those of repeated thoracentesis, thoracoscopic pleurodesis, chest tube pleurodesis, or placement of an indwelling pleural catheter (Haas et al. 2007). A thorough understanding and the risk–benefit ratio of each of these procedures should be known prior to performing any of them. Whatever procedure is chosen, it should optimize quality of life. These approaches should be dictated not only by the patient's performance but by the preference and more importantly the availability of expertise to perform the procedures.

Prior to initiating any procedures, the first question should be whether this particular condition is radiotherapy sensitive and/or chemotherapy sensitive (see algorithm **Fig. 3.15**). If this a treatable condition, only a simple thora-

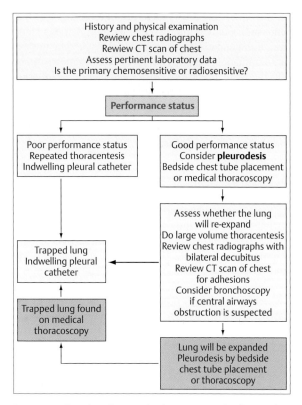

**Fig. 3.15**   Algorithm of options for the treatment of malignant pleural effusions, depending upon the performance score of the patient.

centesis may be needed to alleviate the symptoms. However, if these are nonresponsive conditions then the prognosis and performance status should be ascertained. The median survival is 7.5 months for a patient with malignant pleural effusion due to non–small-cell carcinoma (Sanchez-Armengol and Rodriguez-Panadero 1993; Sugiura et al. 1997). Although certain pleural fluid parameters (Sahn 1985; Rodriguez-Panadero and Lopez-Mejias 1989a,b) have been associated with survival, a multivariate analysis suggests that performance score is the major independent prognosticator of survival. Median survival is 395 days with a Karnofsky performance score of ≥ 70, and is only 34 days with a performance score of ≤ 30 (Burrows et al. 2000). Patients with other malignancies such as lymphoma in general have a better prognosis than lung cancer patients (Elis et al. 1998). Thus, depending on the performance, score procedures can be chosen. If the patient has a poor performance score then the options are serial thoracentesis or an indwelling pleural catheter.

### Serial Thoracentesis

A therapeutic thoracentesis effectively palliates a patient with symptoms (Antony 2000; Maskell and Butland 2003). In a patient with poor performance scores and a short life expectancy, thoracentesis can be repeated. It is safe and can be performed as an outpatient. Depending on the underlying cause, the effusion tends to recur and tends to shorten the interval between interventions. However, if the underlying cause is treatable with chemotherapy or radiation, a limited number of thoracenteses can be effective. A theoretical drawback can be due to adhesion formation, followed by a trapped lung, making future pleurodesis difficult.

### Indwelling Pleural Catheter

The US FDA has approved an indwelling pleural catheter for intermittent drainage: PleurX (Cardinal Health, Dublin, OH, USA). The kit consists of a 15.5 F flexible catheter with multiple fenestrations and a one-way valve. This tunneled catheter can be intermittently drained via attachment to a disposable plastic vacuum bottle. The intention is to leave this in place indefinitely. There are certain advantages: (1) the silicone tube is soft, pliable and small; (2) there is a one-way valve allowing intermittent drainage without the need for a chronic drainage bag; and (3) the catheter has a cuff and is tunneled, potentially reducing the risk of infection and accidental dislodgement. The family or caregivers have to be trained to perform the drainage and maintain the catheter.

In a large retrospective study of 250 sequential patients in a single center, spontaneous pleurodesis occurred in 43% of patients. The catheter stayed in place for a median duration of 56 days. Symptomatic improvement occurred in 89% of patients. No further ipsilateral pleural procedures were needed in 90.1%. The median survival time was 144 days and allowed the patients to be with their family. Complication rates were low: symptomatic loculation (8%), unsuccessful insertion (4%), empyema (3%), pneumothorax, subcutaneous air or bronchopleural fistula (2%), cellulitis (2%), dislodgement (1%), bleeding (0.8%), tumor seeding (0.4%), pain requiring removal (0.4%), and extrapleural catheter placement (0.4%) (Tremblay and Michaud 2006). The drawback of this study and others (Jimenez et al. 2007) was that other options, such as thoracoscopic talc poudrage, were not offered to the patients.

In another study (Warren et al. 2008), in which the goal was to treat all patients as outpatients, 231 Pleur(X) catheters were inserted into 202 patients with a protocol of daily drainage in the initial week, followed by drainage every other day. No sclerosing agents were used. The catheter was removed when drainage was less than 50 mL/day. In all cases the catheter palliated the patient's symptoms and 134 of 231 catheters (58.0%) were removed. Reaccumulation occurred in five of 132 (3.8%), infection in five of 231 (2.2%), and blockage in 11 of 231 (4.8%). In patients who had incomplete reexpansion of the underlying lung, drainage was seen for more than 100 days; thus even trapped lung can be palliated, but the likelihood of needing to remove the catheter is small. Similarly, in a smaller retrospective review, 11 consecutive patients who also had a large pleural drainage up to 1000 mL two or three times weekly did have symptomatic benefit, defined as improved dyspnea and exercise tolerance. In 10 patients, the catheter remained in place until death, for 15–234 days. One patient required revision after catheter occlusion. Thus, in trapped lung syndrome the pleural catheter provided a convenient and effective alternative (Pien et al. 2001).

A randomized, multi-institutional trial comparing standard chest tube thoracostomy and doxycycline pleurodesis with the use of the indwelling catheter found the two methods to have similar recurrence rates, symptom improvement, and survival (Putnam et al. 1999). A retrospective review comparing chest tube thoracostomy and chemical pleurodesis with the use of the indwelling catheter found that 7-day charges were lower for outpatient PleurX catheter placement at $3391 ± 1753 versus $11 188 ± 7830 for inpatient chest tube thoracostomy and chemical pleurodesis (Putnam et al. 2000).

In another study using the same database (Tremblay and Michaud 2006), a retrospective analysis was published. The authors asked the question, whether an indwelling catheter can be the first line therapy. They excluded patients with poor short-term survival and incomplete lung expansion. Thus the study subgroup was defined to include patients whose survival was > 90 days, and in whom 20% residual pleural effusion was noted following 2 weeks of drainage. Spontaneous pleurodesis was perceived to occur when drainage decreased to < 50 mL of fluid on three consecutive drainage attempts. Dyspnea control was determined at a 2-week follow-up. Complete or partial symptom control was achieved in 100% at the 2-week follow-up. No further ipsilateral procedures were required in 87%; pleurodesis was achieved in 64%; empyema occurred in 4.6%. There are certain advantages in terms of both quality of life and cost of treatment. These patients are allowed to remain in their own homes with family and friends without compromising comfort and symptom control.

There is limited information on other forms of indwelling catheters, such as a subcutaneously implanted reservoir (Port-a-Cath) allowing intermittent access (Reed et al. 1999; Verfaillie et al. 2005), and they are not widely accepted. A major drawback is that patients usually require nursing assistance to drain, necessitating either multiple trips to a healthcare facility or sophisticated home health nursing or a hospice.

### Pleuroperitoneal Shunt

Another option in case of failure of pleurodesis due to a trapped, nonexpandable lung is the insertion of a pleuroperitoneal shunt (Cardinal Health, Dublin, OH, USA). With this method, pleural fluid is drained into the peritoneal cavity, where it is absorbed. It has been shown that the method induces effective palliation in a high percentage of patients whose clinical condition is reasonably good (Petrou et al. 1995). However, shunt complications, chiefly occlusion, may occur in more than 10% of the patients; such occlusion is treated by shunt replacement, unless

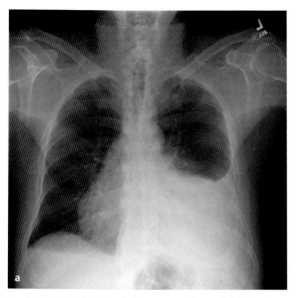
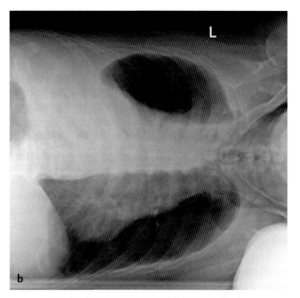
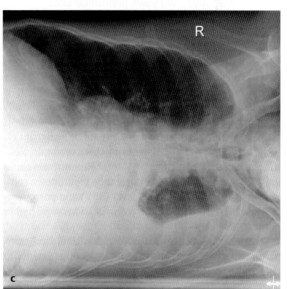

**Fig. 3.16**  Left-sided pleural effusion. AP radiograph (**a**); decubitus film with the patient lying on his right side (**b**); decubitus film with the patient lying on his left side (**c**), demonstrating that the fluid is free-floating toward the apex.

infection has developed (Al-Kattan et al. 1994). The possibility of inducing peritoneal seeding of tumor cells is a potential risk but has not been convincingly documented (Genc et al. 2000).

### Pleurodesis

If the patient has a good performance status, consideration should be given to performing a pleurodesis for local treatment of malignant or other treatment-refractory pleural effusions. This can be achieved by chemical or thoracoscopic talc pleurodesis, by mechanical abrasion or partial resection. The commonly used methods have been chest tube thoracostomy with chemical pleurodesis or thoracoscopic talc insufflation (talc poudrage).

There is controversy about the best sclerosing agent. In a meta-analysis in the Cochrane Review, talc was considered a superior pleurodesis agent compared with bleomycin, tetracycline, mustine, or tube drainage alone, and was not associated with more frequent toxic side-effects than found with the other sclerosing agents (Shaw and Agarwal 2004). Conversely, a more recent meta-analysis confirmed that talc was superior to mustine, but that there was only a trend favoring talc over bleomycin or tetracycline (Tan et al. 2006 a).

Before proceeding to either of the techniques, the physician has to ask whether the lung will reexpand, since this is one of the essential preconditions for the success of pleurodesis. This question can be answered by performing a large-volume thoracentesis of approximately 1–1.5 L to assess not only the capability of the lung to reexpand but

also whether there is any improvement in the symptoms. If there is no improvement in the symptoms after the removal of a large volume of fluid, consideration should be given to alternative reasons for the symptoms (Antony et al. 2000). Also making and reviewing chest radiographs with bilateral decubitus films (**Fig. 3.16 a–c**) can allow one to assess the likelihood that the lung will reexpand. The chest radiograph may also give direct clues (see **Fig. 8.1**, p. 59). A review of the CT scan of the chest should also be performed, to look for adhesions and loculations or visceral pleural thickening. Similar data can be obtained from thoracic ultrasonography.

Bronchoscopy should be considered before pleurodesis is attempted if central airways obstruction is suspected, as in cases with large effusions without contralateral medi-

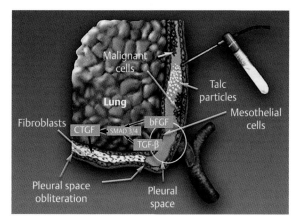

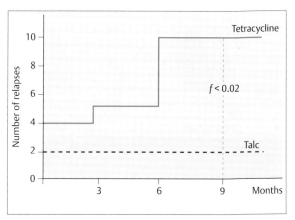

**Fig. 3.19** Schematic drawing of the mechanisms of action of talc pleurodesis. Introduction of particles into the pleural space produces elaboration of TGF-β and bFGF and subsequent production of connective tissue growth factor (CTGF) via the SMAD 3/4 pathway. These growth factors lead to recruitment and proliferation of fibroblasts, which produce pleural fibrosis and obliteration of the pleural space. (From Jantz MA, Antony VB. Pathophysiology of the pleura. Respiration 2008;75(2):121–133, reprinted with permission from S. Karger AG, Basel, Switzerland.)

**Fig. 3.20** Comparison of the long-lasting effect of talc poudrage versus tetracycline pleurodesis ($n = 40$) (number of relapses after 3, 6, and 9 months). There is no significant difference between talc and tetracycline during the first month. As the months pass, however, talc pleurodesis persists whereas relapses occur in patients with tetracycline. (From Boutin C, Viallat JR, Aelony Y. Practical thoracoscopy. Berlin Heidelberg New York: Springer; 1991, reprinted with kind permission from Springer Schiene+Business Media.)

favoring thoracoscopic talc pleurodesis for the end point of recurrence (Yim et al. 1996).

Colt and co-workers compared thoracoscopic talc insufflation (poudrage), talc slurry, and mechanical abrasion in 10 dogs. Although differences were not statistically significant, thoracoscopic talc insufflation consistently produced the most widespread and firm fibrotic adhesions, as evidenced by higher obliteration grades (Colt et al. 1997).

Aelony and co-workers achieved an effective pleurodesis by talc poudrage even when the pleural pH was low (Aelony et al. 1998; Aelony and Yao 2005), which is considered by some authors as a predictor of failure (Rodriguez-Panadero and Lopez-Mejias 1989 a, b). Boutin and co-workers in a prospective randomized study comparing talc poudrage and intrapleural tetracycline achieved a much better long-lasting pleurodetic effect with talc with only 10% relapses as opposed to 50% (Boutin et al. 1985 b) (**Fig. 3.20**). A prospective Dutch study on 100 patients with malignant pleural effusions who were treated with talc slurry according to the guideline showed poor outcome, with fluid recurrence in 36%, underlining the importance of complete apposition of the lung (Burgers et al. 2008).

Talc pleurodesis via either chest tube slurry or thoracoscopic insufflation of dry talc has been reported to induce acute lung injury and acute respiratory distress syndrome (ARDS). The toxic effects of talc are hypothesized to be primarily mediated by smaller talc particles of < 15 μm. A small prospective trial compared a mixed talc preparation with 50% of particles less than 10 μm and a graded talc preparation with < 50% particles smaller than 20 μm and

demonstrated that the mixed talc caused a greater A–a (alveolar–arterial) gradient and systemic inflammatory response (fever and C-reactive protein) than did graded talc (Maskell et al. 2004). However, there is now indisputable evidence that the use of size-calibrated talc is absolutely safe, in short-term (Janssen et al. 2007) as well as long-term follow-up studies (Cardillo et al. 2007; Györik et al. 2007; Hunt et al. 2007; Noppen 2007); that it does not cause cancer, pulmonary fibrosis, or impaired pulmonary function, or impair later thoracic surgery; and that it is by far the cheapest agent!

Janssen and associates, in a prospective multicenter study in 558 patients with malignant pleural effusion, demonstrated that medical thoracoscopic poudrage with large-particle talc (Steritalc) did not cause ARDS (Janssen et al. 2007) (see "Early Complications of Talc Pleurodesis", p. 63). Talc, as well as being the cheapest pleurodesis agent, remains the means preferred by practicing pulmonologists (68%) compared with tetracycline derivatives (26%) and bleomycin (7%) (Lee YC et al. 2003). Similar results were obtained in a survey on pleurodesis practice in South and Central American countries (Marchi et al. 2010). Talc is the preferred agent in Brazil (76%), South America (53%), and Central America (43%), mostly as slurry. Thoracoscopic talc poudrage is used in most cases in Brazil in 31%, and South America and Central America in only 11% and 3% respectively. Existing pleurodesis agents are viewed as less than ideal, and a variety of other agents such as silver nitrate, quinacrine, iodopovidone, and oral forms of doxycycline are under investigation (Dikensoy and Light 2005). As Aelony states in his comment to the *Lancet* article (Aelony 2007) of Janssen and colleagues

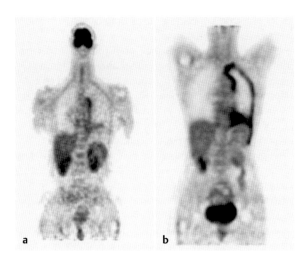

**Fig. 3.21** **a** Before thoracoscopic talcage: high FDG activity at the left lung apex and posterior to the aorta. **b** Three months after thoracoscopic talcage: diffuse and intense tracer activity around the whole left lung. (From De Weerdt S, Noppen M, Everaert H, Vincken W. Positron emission tomography scintigraphy after thoracoscopic talcage. Respiration 2004; 71: 284, reprinted with permission from S. Karger AG, Basel, Switzerland.)

(Janssen et al. 2007), thoracoscopic talc poudrage should be the gold-standard treatment for malignant effusions until controlled observations show a more effective, simpler, and equally safe (local) treatment (Aelony 2007). This opinion has been underlined again by several international experts who participated in the 2007 *Lancet* study (Tschopp et al. 2009).

The uniform distribution of talc after thoracoscopic poudrage was nicely documented by positron emission tomography (PET), which at the same time also demonstrates the distinct inflammatory reaction produced by talc pleurodesis (Fig. 3.21). Thus PET can become false-positive in tumor staging after talc poudrage (De Weerdt et al. 2004).

In addition, talc may have a direct effect on the malignant tumor cells, such as initiation of the events leading to programmed cell death (apoptosis) of the tumor cell (Nasreen et al. 2000). Furthermore, talc has been shown to alter the angiogenic balance in the pleural space from a biologically active and angiogenic environment to an angiostatic milieu. Functional improvements following talc poudrage in patients with malignant pleural effusions may, in part, reflect these alterations in the pleural space (Nasreen et al. 2007).

We advocate the use of MT/P as both diagnostic and therapeutic goals can be achieved in a single session. In addition, MT/P overcomes the limitation of chest tube talc pleurodesis with slurry. This approach is also cost-saving in comparison to needle biopsy, since it avoids the need for separate insertion of a chest drain (after tests have confirmed the need to do this) as well as the need for adequate drainage before administering a sclerosant

to achieve a pleurodesis which is not usually as effective as via MT/P, especially if from lung or breast cancer (Medford 2010). Overall complications from thoracoscopic talc pleurodesis are relatively low, and were not different from those of chest tube talc pleurodesis in the large randomized controlled trial comparing the two methods (Dresler et al. 2005).

Furthermore, it can be decided during the performance of MT/P not to attempt pleurodesis in those cases where the lung is found to have thickened visceral pleura and possibly to be trapped, which would prevent apposition of the parietal and visceral pleural surfaces. Instead, a tunneled indwelling catheter can be placed and the patient can potentially be discharged home immediately afterward.

## The Place of Medical Thoracoscopy/ Pleuroscopy in the Management of Pneumothorax

Pneumothorax is defined as the presence of air in the pleural space. From a clinical standpoint, pneumothorax is classified as spontaneous (no obvious precipitating factor present) or nonspontaneous (**Table 3.8**) (Noppen and Schramel 2002; Baumann and Noppen 2004; Noppen and De Keukeleire 2008).

*Primary* spontaneous pneumothorax is defined as the spontaneously occurring presence of air in the pleural space in patients without clinically apparent underlying lung disease, whereas *secondary* spontaneous pneumothorax is defined as a spontaneous pneumothorax occurring in a patient with known or apparent underlying lung disease. This section describes the management of both types of pneumothorax and the potential role of medical thoracoscopy in treatment and prevention. **Table 3.9** summarizes some of the advantages of MT/P.

**Table 3.8** Classification of pneumothorax

| **Spontaneous** | Primary: no apparent underlying disease |
| --- | --- |
| | Secondary: clinically apparent underlying disease (e.g., COPD, fibrosis, ...) |
| | Catamenial: in conjunction with menstruation |
| | Neonatal |
| **Nonspontaneous** | Iatrogenic: secondary to transthoracic and transbronchial biopsy, central venous catheterization, pleural biopsy, thoracentesis, positive pressure ventilation, etc. |
| | Noniatrogenic: secondary to blunt or penetrating chest injury |

**Table 3.9** Advantages of medical thoracoscopy/pleuroscopy in the management of spontaneous pneumothorax

- Technique similar to chest tube insertion (local anesthesia/neuroleptanalgesia, no intubation)

- Visualization of adhesions, blebs, bullae, air leaks

- Guiding the choice of primary treatment (conservative or surgical approach)

- Additional conservative treatment options: coagulation, talc poudrage, fibrin sealant, mechanical pleural abrasion, etc.

## Primary Spontaneous Pneumothorax

Primary spontaneous pneumothorax (PSP) occurs in 7.4–18 cases (age-adjusted incidence) per 100 000 population per year in males, and in 1.2–6 cases per 100 000 population per year in females (Melton et al. 1979). PSP typically occurs in tall, thin subjects. Other risk factors are male sex and smoking (Bense et al. 1987). A family history may be present. PSP typically occurs at rest. Precipitating factors may include atmospheric pressure changes, and exposure to loud music. In a minority of patients, some pleural fluid is present. Rarely, PSP may be associated with a spontaneous hemothorax.

The exact pathogenesis of PSP is unknown. Most authors believe that spontaneous rupture of a subpleural bleb, or of a bulla, is the cause of PSP (Light 1993), although alternative explanations are available (Sahn and Hefner 2000; Noppen 2003a; Amjadi et al. 2007).

Although the majority of PSP patients have blebs or bullae, usually at the apices of the lungs or at the fissures (Lesur et al. 1990; Bense et al. 1993; Schramel et al. 1997; Amjadi et al. 2007), it is unclear how often these lesions are actually the site of air leakage. Only a minority of blebs are actually ruptured at the time of thoracoscopy or surgery, whereas in the rest of the cases other lesions may be present, often referred to as "pleural porosity" (Masshoff and Höfer 1973; Ohata and Suzuki 1980; Radomsky et al. 1989): areas of disrupted mesothelial cells at the visceral pleura, replaced by an inflammatory elastofibrotic layer with increased porosity, allowing air leakage into the pleural space. The latter phenomenon may explain the high recurrence rates of up to 20% of bullectomy alone as therapy (without associated pleurodesis) (Körner et al. 1996; Hatz et al. 2000; Loubani and Lynch 2000; Horio et al. 2002). Furthermore, blebs and bullae are present in up to 15% of normal subjects (Amjadi et al. 2007). The development of blebs, bullae, and areas of pleural porosity may be linked to a variety of factors, including distal airway inflammation; hereditary predisposition; anatomical abnormalities of the bronchial tree; ectomorphic physiognomy with more negative intrapleural pressures and apical ischemia at the apices; low body mass index and caloric restriction; and abnormal connective tissue. In rare cases, major deformities can be found

at thoracoscopy, including large bullous malformations with systemic arterial supply.

These lesions may therefore predispose to PSP when combined with other abnormalities and precipitating factors. New techniques, such as fluorescein-enhanced autofluorescence thoracoscopy (**Fig. 20.8 a, b** in the *Atlas*) (Noppen et al. 2006) or infrared thoracoscopy (Gotoh et al. 2007), may shed more light on this issue, and may be helpful in the detection of the culprit areas during thoracoscopy or surgery. It should be clear, however, that every therapeutic intervention with the purpose of preventing recurrences of PSP should include a pleurodesis technique, with or without an intervention at the level of the lung parenchyma (Noppen and Baumann 2003). Accordingly, the "old" thoracoscopic classification by Vanderschueren (1981) (type I, no abnormalities; type II, adhesions; type III, small [< 2 cm] blebs; type IV, large [> 2 cm] bullae) has almost no therapeutic significance, although, for example, Japanese authors have observed a high risk of contralateral recurrence of PSP in cases that showed thoracoscopically an aggregation of diffuse and tiny bullae (Tamura et al. 2003).

### Management

A number of therapeutic options are available for treatment of PSP, varying from conservative (observation, oxygen treatment, simple manual aspiration, small-catheter drainage) through intermediately invasive (chest tube drainage, medical thoracoscopic talc poudrage, or pleural abrasion) to invasive measures (video-assisted thoracoscopic surgery with blebectomy or bullectomy, pleural abrasion or partial pleurectomy, or axillary thoracotomy) (Tschopp et al. 2006). An algorithmic approach is usually proposed based on several available guidelines (Baumann et al. 2001; Henry et al. 2003; De Leyn et al. 2005) (**Fig. 3.22**).

A patient presenting with a first episode of a small dehiscence of the lung (i.e., only partial, or complete but less than 15%) should not be treated, but can safely be discharged and followed on an outpatient basis.

In case of complete dehiscence of the lung, and/or in case of pneumothorax symptoms, *air evacuation* treatment is warranted. There is now sufficient evidence that simple manual aspiration should be the first-line treatment approach in these PSP patients (Miller and Harvey 1993; Andrivet et al. 1995; Noppen et al. 2002; Faruqi et al. 2004; Chan and Rainer 2006; Ayed et al. 2006; Camuset et al. 2006; Masood et al. 2007; Wakai et al. 2007; Chan 2008; Zehtabchi and Rios 2008). Success rates vary between 50% and 80% of cases, averaging two-thirds. Complications are absent; pain and discomfort are minimized; recurrence rates are similar to those seen after typical chest tube drainage; outpatient treatment with immediate discharge is possible in over half of cases; and length of stay, when needed, is significantly shortened. Alternatively, because repeat aspiration or insertion of a catheter

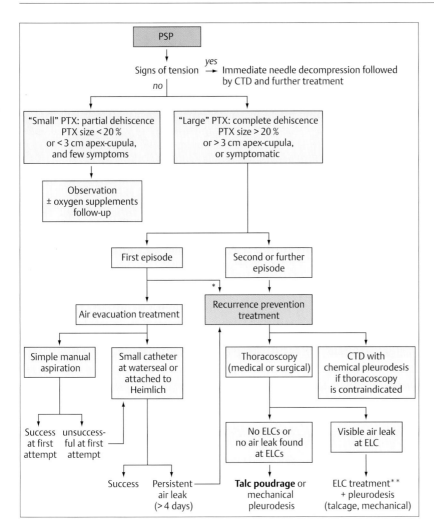

**Fig. 3.22** Algorithm for the approach to the treatment of primary spontaneous pneumothorax. * After informed consent or in certain patient groups (aircraft personnel, divers); ** Staple blebectomy/bullectomy, electrocoagulation, ligation. PSP, primary spontaneous pneumothorax; CTD, chest tube drainage; ELCs, emphysema-like changes; PTX, pneumothorax.

is necessary in one-third of patients, some authors propose immediate placement of a small catheter attached to a Heimlich valve followed by immediate discharge (Marquette et al. 2006; Choi et al. 2007).

There is also good consensus and clinical evidence that PSP *recurrence prevention* should be proposed only after a first recurrence, based on the observation that recurrence occurs in only about one-third of patients but may increase to 62% after a first recurrence, and to 83% after a third. Exceptions may be in patients at occupational risk (aviation personnel, divers), or when it is preferred by anxious patients, or when a prolonged air leak (> 4 days) is present (Baumann et al. 2001; Noppen and Baumann 2003; Baumann and Noppen 2004). The optimal procedure for recurrence prevention remains controversial because of the paucity of prospective, randomized, large, head-to-head comparative studies. Intermediate recurrence prevention success rates can be achieved by administration of a sclerosing agent through a chest tube (e.g., talc slurry, tetracycline, minocycline, doxycycline). This approach is therefore

acceptable only in those patients who are unfit for, or who refuse MT/P or more invasive surgery.

The choice between MT/P, "surgical" thoracoscopy (VATS), or open surgery (usually via anterolateral thoracotomy) as method of access to the pleural cavity depends upon the professional background of the operator (pulmonologist or surgeon) and on local availabilities, preferences, beliefs, and habits. Open surgical approaches are slightly superior to or as effective as "closed" thoracoscopic methods, but they carry a higher morbidity risk. Therefore, unless there are specific clinical indications for more invasive surgery, it would seem reasonable for MT/P to become the recommended approach (Barker et al. 2007; Treasure 2007a,b; Balduyck et al. 2008; Vohra et al. 2008). Also, within the surgical community, there is a trend toward less-invasive VATS approaches, such as uniportal VATS, needle thoracoscopy, or even awake VATS procedures, which narrows the spectrum between surgical and medical thoracoscopy to almost nil (Chang et al. 2007; Pompeo et al. 2007; Salati et al. 2008a).

More important than the technique of access to the pleural space is the procedure that is performed within this space. Treatment of blebs and bullae by means of stapled resection, clipping, ligation, looping, or laser or electrocautery ablation is still the surgical dogma. When performed without associated pleurodesis, recurrence rates are unacceptably high (up to 20%). It is therefore questionable, unless a bleb or bulla is clearly leaking during thoracoscopy, whether a parenchymal procedure is absolutely necessary.

### Thoracoscopic Talc Pleurodesis (Talc Poudrage)

Adequate pleurodesis should be the cornerstone of thoracoscopic recurrence prevention. All pleurodesis techniques are based on the successful induction of some form of pleural inflammation. This can be achieved by mechanical abrasion, partial resection, or thoracoscopic instillation of an abrasive agent, usually talc (Tschopp et al. 2000). There is indisputable evidence that the use of size-calibrated talc is absolutely safe, in short as well as long-term follow-up studies (Alifano et al. 2003; Edenborough et al. 1994; Noppen et al. 1997; Augoulea et al. 2008): it does not cause cancer, pulmonary fibrosis, impaired pulmonary function, or impair later thoracic surgery, and it is by far the cheapest agent. Talc is hydrated magnesium silicate ($Mg_3Si_4O_{10}(OH)_2$), and was first used for pleurodesis in 1935 (Bethune 1935). Since then, talc has increasingly been used by pulmonologists and surgeons because of its effectiveness, availability, and low cost. Talc composition can vary in the amount of calcium, aluminum, and iron according to its origin. Several mineral contaminants may be present, but medicinal talc is asbestos free.

In clinical practice, however, it is the proportion of talc particles < 5 µm in diameter that relates to the severity of local and systemic inflammatory responses, and to safety. In the United States, talc approved by the Food and Drug Administration is provided by the Bryan Corporation (Woburn, MA) in two forms: sterile talc powder (packaged as single dose of 5 g in a 100 mL glass bottle) and as talc aerosol (Sclerosol, a single-dose [4 g] canister) with two delivery tubes and using dichlorofluoromethane (CFC-12, 26 g per canister) as a propellant. In Europe, commercial talc for pleurodesis is manufactured by Novatech (La Ciotat, France), and is available in four forms: Steritalc F2 (2 g of sterile talc powder in a glass vial), Steritalc F4 (4 g of sterile talc powder in a glass vial), Steritalc Spray (3 g in a spray canister with propellant gas), and Steritalc PF4 spray (4 g in a hand/air-driven pump). The particle size distribution is not stated by Bryan for the FDA-approved talc; the French Novatech talc (not approved for use in the United States) is size-calibrated, with a median particle diameter of 31.3 µm.

Talc insufflation (synonym: thoracoscopic talc poudrage) is performed during an MT/P procedure (see **Figs. 11.33** and **11.34**). The latter can be performed under local anesthesia, under conscious sedation and spontaneous ventilation, under total intravenous anesthesia with spontaneous breathing, or under total intravenous anesthesia and mechanical ventilation (using a single-lumen or double-lumen endotracheal tube). Talc insufflation in spontaneous pneumothorax is painful since the parietal pleura is normal; intravenous injection of a bolus of an opiate and/or intrapleural administration of 250 mg of 1% lidocaine via spray are necessary when performed under local anesthesia. For pneumothorax pleurodesis, 2–3 g of talc is sufficient.

After talc insufflation, a chest tube (16–24 F) is left in place, and negative pressure is applied (5–20 cm $H_2O$). The chest tube can be removed when there is complete lung expansion and absence of an air leak.

Thoracoscopic recurrence prevention techniques, whether "medical" or "surgical," usually show recurrence rates between zero and 10%.

## Secondary Spontaneous Pneumothorax

A multitude of respiratory disorders have been described as causes of spontaneous pneumothorax. The most frequent underlying disorders are chronic obstructive pulmonary disease (COPD) with emphysema, cystic fibrosis, tuberculosis, lung cancer, HIV-associated *Pneumocystis jirovecii* (*carinii*) pneumonia, followed by rare but "typical" disorders such as lymphangioleiomyomatosis and pulmonary Langerhans cell histiocytosis (Table 3.**10**). Because lung function in these patients is already compromised, secondary spontaneous pneumothorax (SSP) may present as a potentially life-threatening disease, requiring immediate action, in contrast with PSP which is more a nuisance than a dangerous condition. The general incidence is similar to that of PSP. Depending upon the underlying disease, the peak incidence of SSP can occur later in life, e.g., 60–65 years of age in the emphysema population.

Dyspnea is the most prominent clinical feature in SSP; chest pain, cyanosis, hypoxemia, hypercapnia, sometimes resulting in acute respiratory failure, can also be present. Diagnosis is confirmed on a PA chest radiograph; in bullous emphysema, the differential diagnosis from a giant bulla can be difficult, necessitating CT confirmation. At times, it may be difficult to distinguish radiologically between pneumothorax and a large bulla. Here, MT/P may be helpful in the differentiation (Brezler and Abeles 1975).

### Management

Secondary spontaneous pneumothorax requires immediate air evacuation, followed by recurrence prevention at the first episode, since recurrence rates are usually higher than those for PSP, ranging up to 80% of cases as is observed in cystic fibrosis (Noppen et al. 1994). All patients with SSP should be hospitalized. Awaiting recurrence prevention treatment, air evacuation can be achieved by simple manual aspiration in younger patients (< 50 years old)

**Table 3.10** Frequent and/or typical causes of secondary spontaneous pneumothorax

| Airway disease | Emphysema |
|---|---|
| | Cystic fibrosis |
| | Severe asthma |
| Infectious lung disease | Pneumocystis jirovecii pneumonia |
| | Tuberculosis |
| | Necrotizing pneumonia |
| Interstitial lung disease | Idiopathic pulmonary fibrosis |
| | Sarcoidosis |
| | Langerhans cell histocytosis |
| | Lymphangioleiomyomatosis |
| Connective tissue disease | Rheumatoid arthritis, scleroderma, ankylosing spondylitis |
| | Marfan syndrome |
| | Ehlers–Danlos syndrome |
| Malignant disease | Lung cancer |
| | Sarcoma |

with small pneumothoraces, but most authors and guidelines recommend immediate insertion of a chest tube (Baumann et al. 2001; Henry et al. 2003; De Leyn et al. 2005). Small-bore chest tubes and even pigtail catheters are usually sufficient; large-bore chest tubes are recommended when large air leaks are suspected or when mechanical positive pressure ventilation is required.

Recurrence prevention using a thoracoscopic approach (medical or surgical) is recommended; in case a visible air leak is present, for example, a ruptured emphysematous bulla, air leak closure using electrocautery or stapling is indicated. In any case, a pleurodesis procedure such as talc poudrage (as described above), pleural abrasion, or partial pleurectomy should be performed (Johnson 1996; Noppen and Schramel 2002; Noppen and Baumann 2003; Baumann and Noppen 2004; Lee et al. 2004). In patients in whom lung transplantation is a possible future option (e.g., cystic fibrosis, some cases of COPD), the transplant team should be consulted on the opportunity to perform pleurodesis or not. For most transplant teams, former pleurodesis does not represent a contraindication for later transplantation (Judson and Sahn 1996; Noppen and De Keukeleire 2008).

## Catamenial Pneumothorax

Catamenial pneumothorax occurs typically within 24–72 hours after onset of menstruation. It is often recurrent, and may be more common than previously thought. In most cases, catamenial pneumothorax is related to pelvic or thoracic endometriosis (Alifano et al. 2003; Augoulea et al. 2008). Recurrence prevention treatment is indicated after even a first episode of catamenial pneumothorax, because recurrences are frequent (Alifano et al. 2007). Hormonal suppression treatment is often added. Even tetracycline pleurodesis may be successful (Kropp and Loddenkemper 1985).

### Traumatic Noniatrogenic Pneumothorax

Pneumothorax ranks second to rib fracture as the most common sign of chest trauma, occurring in up to 50% of chest trauma victims (Bridges et al. 1993). In half of these cases, pneumothorax may be occult; in chest trauma patients requiring mechanical ventilation, CT of the chest should therefore always be performed. Most surgeons and emergency physicians will place a chest tube in occult and nonoccult traumatic pneumothoraces. However, studies suggest that carefully selected patients may be treated conservatively, ultimately requiring chest tube placement only in approximately 10% of cases (Johnson 1996). If positive pressure ventilation is anticipated, placement of a chest tube is mandatory. In these cases, and in case of an associated hemothorax (20% of patients), placement of a large-bore chest tube (28–36 F) is advocated (and can be combined with MT/P).

### Traumatic Iatrogenic Pneumothorax

Iatrogenic pneumothorax occurs most often following transthoracic needle biopsy (24%), subclavian vein catheterization (22%), thoracentesis (20%), transbronchial lung biopsy (10%), pleural biopsy (8%), and positive pressure ventilation (7%). Diagnosis of iatrogenic pneumothorax is often delayed, which should prompt physicians to vigilance. Small and asymptomatic iatrogenic pneumothoraces often need no treatment, and resolve spontaneously. In larger or symptomatic pneumothoraces, simple manual aspiration or placement of a small catheter or chest tube attached to a Heimlich valve are usually successful (Brown et al. 1997). Larger tubes may be necessary in emphysematous patients, or when mechanical ventilation is indicated.

In cases with diffuse lung disease and iatrogenic pneumothorax, usually following transbronchial lung biopsy, this situation can be used for MT/P with taking of lung biopsies before the insertion of the tube, if drainage is indicated.

# The Place of Medical Thoracoscopy/ Pleuroscopy in the Diagnosis of Diffuse Lung Diseases

Diffuse lung diseases are of great clinical interest because of the increasing prophylactic and, in particular, therapeutic potential. There are more than 100 possible causes, and many of them can be diagnosed by the specific history of the patient, by laboratory tests, by typical changes in high-resolution computed tomography (HRCT), and by bronchoalveolar lavage and/or transbronchial lung biopsies through flexible bronchoscopy. However, in a certain proportion of patients larger biopsy specimens of the lungs are required for a definite histological diagnosis and will provide better prognostic and therapeutic information (American Thoracic Society/European Respiratory Society 2002). Surgical lung biopsy, either by open thoracotomy or by video-assisted thoracic surgery (VATS), is regarded as the gold standard for obtaining a definite histological diagnosis (Hunninghake et al. 2001; Fishbein 2005).

Forceps lung biopsies taken during MT/P have also been shown to be quite efficient, and the technique has been used for many years by pulmonologists as an integral part of the method now termed medical thoracoscopy (Brandt 1981; Boutin et al. 1991; Loddenkemper and Boutin 1993; Mathur et al. 1995; Mathur and Loddenkemper 1995; Tassi et al. 2006). In a study at Lungenklinik Heckeshorn, thoracoscopic lung biopsies have provided useful histological information in 87% of 252 cases of diffuse lung disease. In the remaining 13% of cases, open lung biopsy was performed, but in only 50% of these were pathological findings obtained that differed from those at thoracoscopy (Liebig and Freise 1977).

An overview of the total lung surface assisted by the magnification of the thoracoscope allows harvesting of abnormal areas of parenchyma, as is well illustrated in the *Atlas* section. But the use of the technique for this indication has considerably decreased with the advent of VATS (Loddenkemper 1998; Tassi et al. 2006).

Heine in Germany was the first, in 1957, to report excellent biopsy results in diffuse lung diseases (Heine 1957). Subsequently, he and others obtained an almost 100% success rate in the diagnosis of stage II sarcoidosis (Brandt 1964b; Heine 1965; Diwok et al. 1974; Kapsenberg 1981; Voellmy 1981). Today pulmonary sarcoidosis can also be so successfully diagnosed by transbronchial lung biopsy that more invasive biopsy procedures are rarely necessary. However, with the exception of a very few other pathological entities such as lymphangitis carcinomatosa, transbronchial lung biopsy has a failure rate in excess of 50% (Wall et al. 1981).

A review of the literature comprising 1030 cases up to 1999 in diffuse lung diseases of varying etiologies demonstrated an overall sensitivity of thoracoscopic biopsies of 85% with a range between 75% and 100%, with a low com-

**Table 3.11**  Literature review of the diagnostic yield of pulmonary biopsies taken during medical thoracoscopy (*n* = 1030)

|  | Diagnostic yield (%) | No. of Patients |
|---|---|---|
| Brandt (1981) | 87 | 467 |
| Dijkman (1989) | 98 | 65 |
| Faurschou (1985 a) | 100 | 7 |
| Guy et al. (1983) | 100 | 14 |
| Janik et al (1982) | 100 | 17 |
| Kapsenberg (1981) | 95 | 115 |
| Rodgers (1981) | 94 | 81 |
| Voellmy (1981) | 75 | 32 |
| Wetzer et al. (1980) | 89 | 63 |
| Boutin (unpublished) | 96 | 170 |
| Total | 93 | 1031 |

Modified from Boutin et al. (1991).

plication rate (**Table 3.11**) (Boutin et al. 1991). In the largest published series of 585 cases (**Fig. 3.23**) a varying sensitivity, depending on the etiology, between 96% (sarcoidosis) and 42% (Langerhans cell histiocytosis) was found (Schaberg et al. 1989). Tumor-conditioned diffuse lung diseases were clarified in 88% of the cases; proof of an interstitial pulmonary fibrosis or interstitial pneumonia was established in 85%; the results in Langerhans cell histiocytosis (*n* = 12) were poor, possibly because the pathognomonic lesions are not always manifested in the periphery of the lung (although other authors have achieved better results [Bayle et al. 1988]). In the 15% of cases not diagnosed by thoracoscopic biopsy, open lung biopsy was performed, but in only half of these cases were pathological findings obtained that differed from those at MT/P.

In another large series (*n* = 170), positive diagnostic results were achieved in 96% (Boutin et al. 1991). Dijkman and co-workers reported a sensitivity of 93% in 81 patients with diffuse interstitial pulmonary disease (Dijkman et al. 1982). In 1989, Dijkman presented the results of thoracoscopy in 65 immunosuppressed patients suffering from pulmonary complications in immunosuppression and in whom he needed an urgent diagnosis while surgeons were not available (Dijkman 1989). Here, the sensitivity was as high as 98%. The most frequent complication was a slowly resolving pneumothorax (10 out of 65). In this very high-risk group, two leukopenic patients developed a staphylococcal sepsis and two patients died (one from perforation of the large leukemic spleen and one from bleeding after multiple deep parenchymal biopsies). Fifteen patients needed post-thoracoscopic ventilation treatment because of their already pre-thoracoscopi-

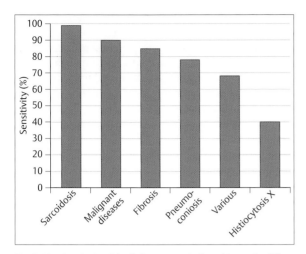

**Fig. 3.23** Sensitivity (%) of thoracoscopic lung biopsy in diffuse lung diseases of various origins (mean 86%, *n* = 585) (From Schaberg et al. 1989).

cally reduced respiratory function (see also Chapter 9, "Complications and Their Prevention").

With regard to both the invasiveness of the method and its sensitivity, medical thoracoscopic biopsy occupies an intermediate position between bronchoscopic transbronchial biopsy and open lung biopsy/VATS, including the modifications according to Maassen (Maassen 1972, 1981). In comparison with transbronchial lung biopsy, the results are much better owing to larger biopsies and visual selection of the best biopsy site, while it is usually possible to survey the whole pleural surface. Furthermore, hemorrhage can be controlled by means of electrocautery, although in practice this is rarely necessary since only minimal hemorrhage occurs from the small peripheral vessels, especially if the biopsies are taken from the edge of the lung lobes.

However, transthoracoscopic lung biopsy invariably produces small bronchopleural fistulae necessitating post-thoracoscopically prolonged drainage. Schaberg et al., using the single-entry technique without a coagulation forceps, on average took three biopsies from different areas per patient and observed a mean drainage time of 4.5 days (Schaberg et al. 1989). Boutin et al. (1991), using the two-entry technique with a coagulation forceps, had an average length of chest tube drainage of 4 days, and Dijkman (1989) (single entry) an average of 4.6 days. Reports from Japan describe the successful application of cyanoacrylate tissue cement to seal fistulas post biopsy (Hatakenaka 1976; Hitomi et al. 1984). Boutin and co-workers successfully used laser coagulation after removing samples of pulmonary parenchyma (Boutin et al. 1991). They observed shrinkage of the lung around the biopsy hole, ensuring both hemostasis and aerostasis.

Today, if larger lung biopsies are needed in diffuse pulmonary diseases, usually a VATS procedure is requested.

However, for those familiar with the technique, MT/P is a valuable alternative (Loddenkemper and Boutin 1993).

A necessary prerequisite for MT/P in diffuse lung disease is a pneumothorax, which has to be induced before the introduction of the thoracoscope. This can be achieved by different methods, such as the use of a pneumothorax apparatus, as outlined in the section "Access to the Pleural Space," Chapter 11, p. 78ff. If the pleural space is obliterated and a pneumothorax cannot be induced, MT/P is not possible. However, this occurs only rarely in diffuse pulmonary disease. As has been mentioned already, an excellent indication for MT/P is in patients in whom a pneumothorax is present or has developed as a complication of transbronchial peripheral biopsy, and in whom the introduction of a pleural drainage is necessary anyway. Before inserting the chest tube through a cannula, the thoracoscope can be introduced through this cannula and forceps biopsies can be taken from the lung.

Bradley Rodgers, a pediatric thoracic surgeon, has performed "medical" thoracoscopy in children starting at age 2 years using local anesthesia and additional blockade of the stellate ganglion to suppress the cough reflex during examination of the mediastinum (Rodgers and Talbert 1976). He suggested thoracoscopic biopsies for diagnosis of *Pneumocystis carinii* pneumonia and other pulmonary infections in immunosuppressed children (Rodgers et al. 1979a). In his hands, the diagnosis has been obtained in 98% of immunosuppressed children and, as a result of early and reliable diagnosis, the cure rate has been increased considerably. In other diffuse lung diseases of his series the diagnostic success rate was 93% (see also Chapter 4, "Medical Thoracoscopy/Pleuroscopy in Children").

Boutin and co-workers studied thoracoscopic lung biopsy first in animals and then in humans, demonstrating a high diagnostic yield with low morbidity (Boutin et al. 1982). They also found thoracoscopic pulmonary (and pleural) biopsies, examined by electron microscopy, to be very useful for mineralogical studies in the search for asbestos fibers (Boutin et al. 1981b).

In an excellent study, Vansteenkiste and co-workers harvested 118 samples from 24 consecutive patients in whom medical thoracoscopic lung biopsies in interstitial lung disease had been taken, using a diathermy coagulation cup forceps. Chest tube drainage averaged 5.3 ± 4.7 days and was related to the total lung capacity, which mirrors the severity and stiffness, respectively, of interstitial lung disease (**Fig. 3.24**). A good quality biopsy was obtained in 23 of the 24 patients, and in 78% of the 118 samples. They concluded that lung biopsy sampling can be performed safely by interventional pulmonary endoscopists and has a good diagnostic yield in interstitial lung disease of unknown origin (Vansteenkiste et al. 1999).

Colt and co-workers compared the gross and histological findings of wedge lung biopsy with those of forceps video-thoracoscopic lung biopsy in five adult swine, using a 5 mm endoscopic cupped forceps. One hundred and thirteen forceps biopsy specimens and 24 sections from eight

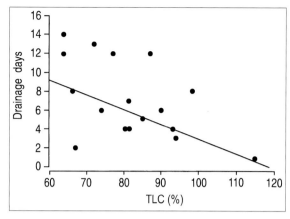

**Fig. 3.24** Relationship between preexisting total lung capacity (TLC) (% normal) and duration of drainage in the 17 patients in whom drainage lasted at least 1 day. A significant correlation was found ($p = 0.008$). (From Vansteenkiste et al. 1999, reprinted with permission from ERS Journals Ltd.)

wedge biopsy specimens were examined. They detected no major differences in overall microscopic specimen quality (Colt et al. 1995).

Marchandise and co-workers performed medical thoracoscopic lung biopsies in interstitial lung diseases in 33 nonimmunocompromised patients. A diagnosis was obtained in all patients and no severe complication was observed. The average time of drainage was 4 days. They concluded that this technique has advantages over open lung biopsy (Marchandise et al. 1992).

In conclusion, medical thoracoscopic lung biopsies are a suitable alternative for those who are familiar with the technique, which is easy and safe. The advantage of medical thoracoscopic biopsy is that it is less invasive, using local anesthesia and no intubation. The disadvantage is a longer drainage time. Taking biopsy samples of honeycomb lung from end-stage pulmonary fibrosis should be avoided as it contributes to high incidence of bronchopleural fistula. Contraindications for pulmonary biopsy are suspicion of arteriovenous pulmonary aneurysm, vascular tumors, and hydatid cysts.

In comparison with bronchoscopy, MT/P is more invasive but presents several advantages. It provides significantly larger samples and allows the physician to choose the biopsy site—at least three biopsy samples should be taken. In addition, it is possible to take numerous biopsies from various lobes, particularly in cases that are difficult to characterize macroscopically. However, it is likely that the limits of visualization and evaluation using the thoracoscope have not yet been achieved and it may be that, eventually, a form of microscopic in-vivo examination via the endoscope could become possible, as it is applied already with confocal laser endomicroscopy in gastrointestinal endoscopy (Hoffmann et al. 2006), or by fiber confocal fluorescence microscopy as applied during bronchoscopy (Thiberville et al. 2009).

Furthermore, unlike in transbronchial biopsy, hemorrhage can be controlled by means of electrocautery (or laser), although in practice this is rarely necessary since only minimal hemorrhage occurs from the small peripheral vessels when using forceps with or without coagulation (see "Biopsy Techniques," Chapter 11, p. 89 ff.).

With regard to sensitivity and invasiveness, MT/P ranks between open lung biopsy and transbronchial biopsy. In contrast to open lung biopsy, which provided a diagnosis in 92 % of cases (Gaensler and Carrington 1980), and to VATS, which provides similar results (Bensard et al. 1993; Carnochan et al. 1994; Molin et al. 1994), the advantage of medical thoracoscopic biopsy is that it can be performed under local anesthesia, while rarely producing significant pleural reactions or scars on the skin (Mathur and Loddenkemper 1995). Thus, it is important that interventional pulmonologists remain familiar with a technique that still can be relevant (Tassi et al. 2006).

## Medical Thoracoscopy/Pleuroscopy in Other Indications

MT/P will most often be used in the diagnosis and treatment of pleural exudates, recurrent pleural transudates, and spontaneous pneumothorax. With increasing expertise, other indications may follow: lung biopsies (e.g., for diffuse interstitial lung disease), empyema, diffuse pleural thickening, or pleural tumors, as described in the respective chapters. In some instances, trained medical thoracoscopists will also tackle other clinical problems. These include interventions at the sympathetic chain (sympathectomy, e.g., for the treatment of essential hyperhidrosis; splanchnicectomy, e.g., for the treatment of chronic pancreatic pain) (Tassi et al. 2006), and pericardial fenestration for the treatment of pericardial tamponade (Vogel and Mall 1990).

### Medical Thoracoscopic Sympathectomy

Thoracoscopic sympathectomy is defined as the anatomical interruption of the thoracic sympathetic chain by means of thoracoscopic techniques. The level of interruption depends upon the indication and the desired therapeutic effects (Noppen 2004b). Thoracoscopic sympathectomy techniques are currently standard approaches for sympathectomy since open surgical approaches have become obsolete. Percutaneous ablation techniques are not widely used because of lower efficacy and higher complication rates (Wilkinson 1984).

Most thoracoscopic sympathectomy techniques are performed and described by surgeons; classically, unilateral three-entry-port VATS interventions using single-lung, double-lumen ventilation, pleural and sympathetic chain dissection and resection, and postoperative chest drainage is proposed (Hashmonai et al. 2001). Recently, however, there is a trend toward less cumbersome, less extensive, simplified one-time bilateral surgical approaches using clipping or diathermy cauterization, single-lumen intubation, and smaller-diameter trocars (Goh et al. 2000; Lin 2001; Atkinson and Fealy 2003). It is noteworthy that thoracoscopic sympathicolysis using simple medical thoracoscopic instrumentation and techniques can safely be performed by trained interventional pulmonologists (Noppen et al. 1996; Noppen 2004b).

## Indications

The most frequent indications for thoracoscopic sympathectomy include refractory essential hyperhidrosis (palmar, axillar, facial). Other indications include facial flushing, vascular disorders of the upper limbs (Raynaud's phenomenon, acrocyanosis, arterial insufficiency, Buerger disease), causalgia, thoracic outlet syndrome, and some cardiac arrhythmias (e.g., long QT syndrome) (Noppen 2004b).

## Equipment and Technique

No standard guidelines on equipment and technique are available, and very few comparative studies on this subject have been done: most authors therefore have developed and gained experience with original technical approaches. In general, bilateral thoracoscopic sympathetic interventions today (whether performed by surgeons or by interventional pulmonologists) should be performed in a one-day setting, under total intravenous anesthesia. A one-time bilateral procedure using one to three small-diameter trocars should be standard of care. The sympathetic chain can be dissected and resected, cauterized, interrupted, or clipped. The level and extent of anatomical interruption depends upon the clinical indication, and should also be kept to a minimum. For example, for essential hyper-

hidrosis, sympathetic interruption can be limited to the T3 level (Lin and Teleranta 2001).

At the University Hospital UZ Brussels (M.N.), this is a 1-day procedure, under total intravenous anesthesia, single-lumen tube intubation, and high frequency jet ventilation delivered through the endotracheal tube. Patients are positioned in dorsal decubitus, arms abducted and supported at 90° (**Fig. 3.25**). The thorax is elevated at 30°. Both armpits are disinfected. The procedure is commenced at the right hemithorax. A pneumothorax is induced using a blunt 2-mm pneumothorax needle. A 1 cm skin incision is made at the third intercostal space, just below the pectoral muscle. The 7-mm trocar is introduced gently. A second incision is made 2 cm cranially, and a 5-mm trocar is inserted (**Fig. 3.26**). A 0° rigid telescope is introduced through the first trocar, and the sympathetic chain is identified. A 5-mm cautery forceps is introduced through the second trocar, and the sympathetic ganglion of choice (T2 for facial flushing, T3 for palmar hyperhidrosis, and T4 for axillar hyperhidrosis) is cauterized above the rib head using a few bursts of 60-watt monopolar current. Thereafter, the forceps and 5-mm trocar are withdrawn, and the skin is closed. A flexible 5-mm catheter is then inserted through the first trocar, all air is aspirated, and the trocar and catheter are withdrawn, followed by skin closure. No chest tube is left in place. Thereafter, a similar procedure is performed on the left side. The total procedure takes approximately 12–15 minutes. After a control chest radiograph, the patient is discharged the same day. No major complications have been encountered in more than 1000 procedures up to the present.

## Results and Complications

Although very few comparative studies are available, short- and long-term results are excellent in hyperhidrosis patients: relief of palmar, axillar, and/or facial sweating is obtained in 90–100% of cases (Noppen 2004b). Recurrence rates vary between 5% and 10%, but repeat interventions

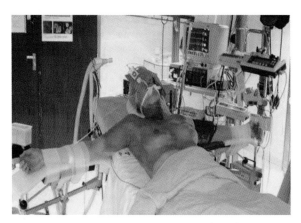

**Fig. 3.25** Positioning of the patient for medical thoracoscopic sympathicolysis.

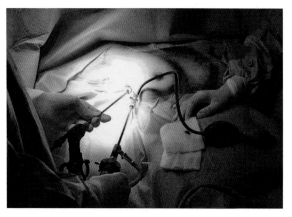

**Fig. 3.26** Two-port axillary approach for thoracoscopic sympathicolysis.

are often successful. Sporadic (< 1%) complications include Horner syndrome, complicated pneumothorax, and hemorrhage necessitating conversion to thoracotomy. No procedure-related mortality has been reported. Compensatory sweating occurs in the majority of patients after sympathetic interruption, and may be related to the level (for example, T2 interruption increases its likelihood) and extent (for example, extensive-level interruption increases its likelihood) of interruption. Patients should be informed in detail about the probable occurrence of compensatory sweating, though, in general, this is considered no more than a nuisance, not affecting overall patient satisfaction. A small percentage (1–2%) of patients, however, regret the intervention afterward (Milanez de Campos et al. 2003; Young et al. 2003; Doolabh et al. 2004; Licht and Pilegaard 2004; Ojimba and Cameron 2004).

## Conclusion

Thoracoscopic sympathectomy, sympathicotomy, or sympathicolysis today is a minimally invasive, accepted intervention for patients with a variety of autonomous nervous system disturbances. Essential hyperhidrosis patients, and well-selected patients with other disorders, can be helped with this procedure, which can be performed by surgeons or interventional pulmonologists (Tassi et al. 2006). Short- and long-term results are excellent, severe complications are extremely rare, and side-effects are usually limited to a certain (but acceptable) degree of compensatory hyperhidrosis.

## Splanchnicectomy

Intractable pain is the most incapacitating symptom in patients suffering from chronic pancreatitis. Anatomical interruption of the major afferent pain nerves is indicated in severe refractory cases. Among the various techniques and sites of interruption, thoracoscopic splanchnicectomy has emerged as an efficient alternative for the more aggressive open surgical splanchnicectomy, and for the (only temporarily effective) transcutaneous neural blocks. Thoracoscopic splanchnicectomy is usually performed by a surgical procedure, using video-assisted thoracoscopic surgery techniques, double-lumen intubation, and so on. We have, as pulmonologists, and in analogy with thoracoscopic upper dorsal sympathicolysis for essential hyperhidrosis as described above, developed a simplified thoracoscopic splanchnicolysis technique (Noppen et al. 1998 b). All procedures are performed in the operating theater, under total intravenous anesthesia and single-lumen endotracheal intubation. A left-sided procedure is always performed; in case of incomplete or unsatisfactory results, a right-sided procedure can be performed subsequently. The patient is positioned in lateral decubitus, left arm elevated at a 90° angle. After skin preparation, a pneumothorax is induced using a 2-mm blunt needle, and air insufflation if necessary. A 7-mm trocar is introduced in the sixth or seventh intercostal space, midaxillary. A 0° rigid telescope is introduced, and the pleural cavity is inspected. Two additional 5-mm trocars are inserted at the fifth through seventh intercostal spaces, anteriorly and posteriorly to the original trocar. A lung retractor is inserted through one port, a cautery forceps coupled to a 60-watt monopolar electrocautery apparatus through the second. While retracting the lung, the splanchnic fibers can be visualized running through the posterior costovertebral region; they are cauterized on the rib surfaces, from the fifth to the tenth or eleventh rib. Thereafter, both 5-mm trocars are removed and the skin is closed. A flexible suction catheter is introduced through the 7-mm trocar, the air is aspirated, and the trocar is removed and the skin closed. No chest tube is left in place. Pain control (allowing for discontinuation of opiate use) can be achieved in the majority of patients with chronic pancreatitis with a short intervention (20 ± 8 minutes), short hospitalization (2 days), and a simple procedure (single-lumen intubation, no chest drains). There have been no complications.

## Pericardial Fenestration

Pericardioscopy was proposed by Jacobaeus in his first publication (Jacobaeus 1910). One report (Vogel and Mall 1990) describes successful pericardial fenestration by the use of a laser (see **Fig. 22.1a, b** in the *Atlas* section).

Creation of pericardial fenestration can be indicated in cases of recurrent pericardial effusions and tamponade, both for diagnosis (microscopic examination of pericardial tissue) and treatment (prevention of tamponade). At the University Hospital UZ Brussels, this procedure is performed by the medical thoracoscopist (M.N.), but usually in a team with the cardiothoracic surgeon. The procedure is performed under total intravenous anesthesia and single-lumen endotracheal intubation with high-frequency jet ventilation, in left lateral decubitus with the arm elevated and abducted at 90°. After induction of a pneumothorax, the 7-mm trocar for the telescope is introduced at the fifth intercostal space, midaxillary. Two 5-mm trocars are inserted in a "triangular" position at the fifth to seventh intercostal space. One port serves for the insertion of a retractor, pulling the pericardium gently away from the heart. Care must be taken to grasp a pericardial region away from the coronary arteries and phrenic nerve. The pericardium is then incised with 5-mm scissors, and a 2 cm × 2 cm window is created. A 24-gauge chest tube is left in the pleural space.

## Solitary Lung Lesions

Obtaining a diagnosis in solitary lung disease by means of medical thoracoscopy is not nearly as likely as in diffuse pulmonary disease. However, thoracoscopy might occasionally be worthwhile if abnormal areas are close to the pleura, if other methods (bronchoscopy, needle aspiration) are unsuccessful, and if, for various reasons, surgery including VATS cannot be undertaken or can only be undertaken with great risk and especially if a pneumothorax has developed after nondiagnostic biopsy procedures.

At Lungenklinik Heckeshorn in Berlin, in a retrospective analysis of 240 patients with a solitary lung lesion adjacent to the visceral pleura, the overall diagnostic sensitivity was 0.47, varying with different etiologies: in 129 cases with a malignant tumor, the sensitivity was 0.37; in 23 cases with benign tumor it was 0.68; and in 88 cases with various other diseases it was 0.55. If only those patients are considered in whom MT/P was performed merely for diagnostic reasons, the sensitivity was as high as 0.63. In contrast, the sensitivity was low (0.46) in those patients ($n = 93$) in whom a pneumothorax as sequela of a previous biopsy procedure was used for the thoracoscopic attempt (Raffenberg et al. 1990, 1992).

This indication has become very rare (**Fig. 3.27** shows the trend up to 1994) and VATS has become the preferred method (if a thoracotomy is not indicated), since the lesions can thus be removed by a wedge resection with a much higher diagnostic yield.

## Diseases in the Region of the Chest Wall, Diaphragm, and Thoracic Spine

Pathological changes in the chest cage previously provided a good indication for MT/P if the pleural space was not obliterated. Hyaline pleural plaques, pleural fibroma, lipoma, neurinoma, rib metastases, rib erosions, etc. can almost always be macroscopically characterized and, if necessary, biopsied. In the retrospective study of the Lungenklinik Heckeshorn in Berlin, 133 cases with chest-wall

lesions of different origin were analyzed (Raffenberg et al. 1990). The overall diagnostic yield was as high as 80%. However, today, these indications have almost completely disappeared, due to improved imaging techniques, which often allow the diagnosis without biopsy, and due to the introduction of VATS, which allows the simultaneous removal of the lesion if necessary.

## Mediastinal Tumors

In the past, mediastinal tumors provided quite a good indication for diagnostic thoracoscopy (Brandt 1964a; Mai et al. 1989). Lipomas, bronchial cysts, pleuropericardial cysts, neurinoma, and endothoracic goiters, for example, are readily recognized.

However, the new imaging techniques often already provide the diagnosis, and VATS allows the simultaneous removal of the tumor/cyst, making MT/P obsolete in these indications.

## Postoperative Cavities

MT/P has been employed only rarely for evaluation of postoperative cavities. It has been performed for rapid diagnosis of tumor recurrence (Brandt and Kund 1964; Brandt and Mai 1971). In cases of chronic pneumothorax or pneumolysis cavities containing increasing exudates, medical thoracoscopy helped to exclude reactivation of tuberculosis. In one case, a small rubber drain, overlooked at surgery, was removed (Brandt and Kund 1964). In **Figure 3.28a, b** the radiographs are shown of a patient in whom the broken tip of an intrapleural small-bore catheter was removed thoracoscopically.

An extremely rare indication was a case of cardiac herniation that occurred following radical left-sided pneumonectomy with resection of the pericardium. This was rapidly recognized at thoracoscopy and immediately corrected surgically (Rodgers et al. 1979b).

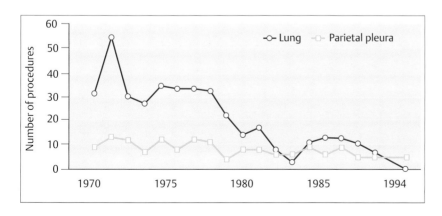

**Fig. 3.27** Decline in the number of medical thoracoscopies in localized lung and pleural lesions at the Lungenklinik Heckeshorn in the period 1971–1994.

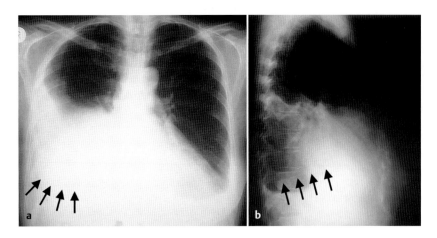

**Fig. 3.28a, b**  Chest radiographs (PA and lateral) showing the broken tip of an intrapleural suction catheter (arrows), which was removed during medical thoracoscopy.

# 4 Medical Thoracoscopy/Pleuroscopy in Children

Indications for medical thoracoscopy/pleuroscopy (MT/P) in children are rare, and there are only a few publications. Rodgers and Talbert, pediatric surgeons, were the first who reported on their experience with thoracoscopy in nine children, ranging in age between 17 months and 16 years, which they used for diagnosis of various intrathoracic lesions (Rodgers and Talbert 1976). In 1979 they published their results on 65 (medical) thoracoscopies in 57 children (Rodgers et al. 1979c); 34 procedures were performed in immunosuppressed patients to diagnose or rule out *Pneumocystis carinii* pneumonia with an accuracy of 100%. In 12 patients, the indications were persisting pulmonary infiltrates of undetermined origin, again with an accuracy of 100%; and in 15 cases the procedure was performed for the diagnosis of intrathoracic tumors. In four cases, a therapeutic thoracoscopy was performed, three times for pulmonary cysts and once for talc insufflation for malignant pleural effusion.

In additional publications, Rodgers and co-workers reported exclusively on their excellent results in 24 children with interstitial pneumonitis accompanying immunosuppression (Rodgers et al. 1979a), and in 23 children with suspected intrathoracic neoplasms (Ryckman and Rodgers 1982). Also in 1982 another group published their positive experience with thoracoscopy in children, with a variety of localized or diffuse intrathoracic lesions (Janik et al. 1982).

Rodgers was invited to the Thoracoscopy Symposium in Marseille where he gave an impressive lecture on his thoracoscopic technique in children (Rodgers 1981). He also showed there a very exciting video on thoracoscopy in a horse! To the *Atlas of Diagnostic Thoracoscopy* he contributed an endoscopic photograph of a pneumocystis pneumonia in a 15-year-old patient (case 54 in Brandt et al. 1985).

The indications for the single-entry technique are similar to those in adults. However, there are differences in instruments and in anesthesia: the instruments have to be smaller, as manufactured by Storz Company, with trocars of 4.0 or 5.5 mm diameter. In addition, optics and instruments similar to those for infant rigid bronchoscopy can be used. Although Rodgers performed his first thoracoscopies under local anesthesia and with additional blockade of the stellate ganglion (to suppress the cough reflex during examination of the mediastinum), later he (and Janik) more often used general anesthesia with endotracheal intubation. The final decision on whether local or general anesthesia was used depended on the age, the ability to cooperate, and the pulmonary function of the children.

Successful thoracoscopic treatment has also been reported in children for pulmonary cysts and for talc poudrage in malignant pleural effusion (Rodgers et al. 1979c) and in spontaneous pneumothorax due to cystic fibrosis (Tribble et al. 1986) as well as for empyema (Kern and Rodgers 1993; Stovroff et al. 1995) and sympathicolysis for essential hyperhidrosis (Noppen et al. 1996, 1998).

Today the technique has become adopted widely by pediatric surgeons and is currently considered to be the optimum technique for management of many intrathoracic disorders in children. The most common indications include pleural debridement for empyema, mediastinal lymph node biopsy, and pulmonary parenchymal biopsy for inflammatory infiltrates or nodules (Rodgers 2003).

# 5   Medical Thoracoscopy/Pleuroscopy in Animals

Thoracoscopy in animals relates to three different topics: use for diagnosis and treatment in animals, use for research in animals, and use for teaching of the technique.

## Use for Diagnosis and Treatment in Animals

In veterinary medicine, thoracoscopy has been mainly applied in the horse, first for diagnostic purposes (Mackey and Wheat 1985; McCarthy 1990), but also for treatment, e.g., for drain placement in pleural effusions and abscesses, transection of pleural adhesions, and decortication as well as for window pericardectomy (Vachon and Fischer 1998). In an experimental study in six healthy, conscious horses, the pleuropulmonary and cardiovascular consequences of thoracoscopy were investigated and no detrimental effects or significant complications were found (Peroni et al. 2000). The advances in instrumentation enabled the use of video-assisted thoracic surgery in horses (Klohnen and Peroni 2000).

Thoracoscopy for evaluating the etiology of pleural effusions is used successfully in dogs and cats as well, and is seen as a less-invasive alternative to thoracotomy (Kovak et al. 2002).

## Use for Research in Animals

Boutin and co-workers tested the technique of thoracoscopic lung biopsy (TLB) in 14 dogs using two entries, one for the telescope, and one for a coagulating forceps. TLB yielded a high rate of adequate samples (up to 5 mm × 5 mm × 5 mm) without major complications (Boutin et al. 1982). In the same article, they report on the subsequent application of TLB in 75 patients, with a high diagnostic yield and few minor complications.

Viallat and co-workers, using TLB with instruments adapted to the size of animals, investigated the bacteriological diagnostic yield in 84 immunosuppressed and/or infected NZ rabbits (Viallat et al. 1985). They compared the results with those of surgical biopsies made in the same animals, and found similar sensitivities of both methods (approx. 90% versus 100%).

Seitz and co-workers, again from Christian Boutin's group in Marseille, performed an experimental study in dogs to test whether the instillation of a fibrin sealant (Tissucol) was effective in the treatment of pneumothorax. The result was negative since no pleurodesis was noted (Seitz et al. 1989).

Colt and co-workers compared the gross and histological findings of wedge lung biopsy to forceps video-thoracoscopic lung biopsy in five adult swine, using a 5-mm endoscopic cupped forceps. One hundred and thirteen forceps biopsy specimens and 24 sections from eight wedge biopsy specimens were examined. They detected no major differences in overall microscopic specimen quality (Colt et al. 1995).

In another animal study, Colt and co-workers compared thoracoscopic talc insufflation (poudrage), talc slurry, and mechanical abrasion in 10 dogs. Although differences were not statistically significant, thoracoscopic talc insufflation consistently produced the most widespread, firm fibrotic adhesions as evidenced by higher obliteration grades (Colt et al. 1997).

Another talc pleurodesis study was done in six young swine in which the effects on respiratory mechanics were measured (McGahren et al. 1990). The authors found that talc pleurodesis causes a temporary impairment in dynamic transpulmonary and transrespiratory compliance that resolves with time and growth. Several other studies on thoracoscopic talc pleurodesis were performed in dogs (Mathlouthi et al. 1992) and pigs (Cohen et al. 1996; Whitlow et al. 1996).

## Use for Teaching of the Technique

A variety of animal models have been used in training courses along with didactic lectures including videos. The most common animal model is the goat or the pig. The animal is intubated with single-lumen tube ventilation and is then placed in the lateral decubitus position and allowed to breathe spontaneously, or occasionally has to be placed on a ventilator with low tidal volume. The pleural space is opened in standard manner as for medical thoracoscopy. The instruments are then placed in the chest for observation. The biopsies of the pleura are again done in a standard manner but are somewhat difficult because the pleura is normal and the forceps tend to slip. The biopsies have to be taken over the rib. The normal pleura allows visualization the rib and the neurovascular bundle during the procedure, which is not the case in the human as the diseased pleura are thick and painless. Occasionally the procedure has to be stopped for ventilation of the animal as needed. The whole procedure should be done with a veterinarian responsible for the well-being of the animal, and the procedure should have been approved by the institutional board. Proper animal care is essential and euthanasia should be performed in a standard manner as suggested by the veterinary services.

# 6 Medical Thoracoscopy/Pleuroscopy in Research

Medical thoracoscopy/pleuroscopy (MT/P) is a valuable tool for research in pleural diseases. It allows macroscopic inspection of the whole pleural cavity, including the surface of the lungs, and selective sampling of biopsies from the pleura or lung under visual control; it thus can diagnose or exclude several pathologies with high sensitivity and specificity. MT/P is the pulmonologist's gold standard for diagnosis of pleural effusions.

Research domains for MT/P in normal subjects include performance of pleural lavage in otherwise normal subjects undergoing MT/P for other reasons than pleuropulmonary disease (e.g., treatment of essential hyperhidrosis), which enables the examination of the normal pleura and its contents (Noppen et al. 2000; Noppen 2004a) and the examination of pleural changes in pleuropulmonary disease not associated with pleural effusions, such as spontaneous pneumothorax (De Smedt et al. 2004).

There are numerous examples of the research value of MT/P in the diagnosis of pleural effusions. Prospective studies have been performed in malignant pleural effusion (Loddenkemper et al. 1983a; Canto et al. 1985; Boutin and Rey 1993), which showed the high diagnostic yield compared with pleural cytology and closed needle biopsy. Prospective studies in tuberculous pleurisy have also shown the superiority of MT/P in comparison with pleural fluid examinations and closed pleural biopsies (Loddenkemper et al. 1978; Loddenkemper 1983b; Walzl et al. 1996; Diacon et al. 2003).

MT/P is also superior in the diagnosis of diffuse malignant mesothelioma (Boutin and Rey 1993). The technique of autofluorescence thoracoscopy has been evaluated for the improved detection of otherwise invisible pleural lesions (Chrysanthidis and Janssen 2005). MT/P allows better staging and has prognostic implications in malignant mesothelioma (Boutin et al. 1993c). Narrow band imaging has also been applied to MT/P in order to facilitate the detection of otherwise invisible malignant lesions (Schönfeld et al. 2009; Ishida et al. 2009). MT/P allows the grading of pleural involvement, which is correlated with survival (Sanchez-Armengol and Rodriguez-Panadero 1993) and also with the success of talc pleurodesis (Rodriguez-Panadero and Antony 1997; Dresler et al. 2005; Antony et al. 2004). It also allows study of the mechanisms of talc pleurodesis in malignant pleural effusion (Nasreen et al. 2000, 2007; Antony et al. 2004). After several experimental animal studies, the safety of talc poudrage was demonstrated in a large prospective multicenter study (Janssen et al. 2007).

Research has been done on the role of MT/P in the management of pneumothorax (van de Brekel et al. 1993; Boutin et al. 1995a; Schramel et al. 1997; Tschopp et al. 2002, 2006), including the role of talc poudrage in comparison with other pleurodesis techniques (Boutin et al. 1995a; Schramel et al. 1997; Tschopp et al. 2002). New techniques under research include (fluorescein-enhanced) autofluorescence thoracoscopy in the study of spontaneous pneumothorax (Noppen et al. 2006) and exudative pleural effusion (Chrysanthidis and Janssen 2005).

Vansteenkiste and co-workers in a prospective study analyzed the quality and diagnostic value of lung biopsies for the diagnosis of interstitial lung disease (Vansteenkiste et al. 1999). Thoracoscopic autopsy has been compared with conventional autopsy and yielded excellent results (sensitivity of 87%) (Avrahami et al. 1995).

Research using thoracoscopy in animal experiments has been described in Chapter 5.

## Future Areas of Research

- Prospective studies on the diagnostic accuracy of MT/P should be performed to determine its value in so-called idiopathic pleural effusions.
- New methods in the early diagnosis of malignant pleural effusions should be evaluated using autofluorescence or narrow-band imaging.
- Prospective studies to compare the role of MT/P in tuberculous pleurisy are needed to evaluate the potential benefits of MT/P regarding early diagnosis, complete drainage, and early drug treatment compared with drug treatment alone.
- Prospective studies of different pleurodesis techniques in malignant pleural effusions as well as in pneumothorax are needed.
- There are no prospective studies on the role of MT/P in the management of empyema. It is an open question whether pleuroscopy in addition to pleural drainage is helpful, in particular in patients with multiple loculations in whom fibrinopurulent membranes can be removed by MT/P.
- MT/P may also be used in the future for intrapleural gene therapy (Sterman 2005).

# 7 Clinical Prerequisites for Medical Thoracoscopy/Pleuroscopy

Medical thoracoscopy/pleuroscopy (MT/P) should be considered an invasive procedure that the chest physician should use only when other, simpler methods fail to yield a diagnosis or when less-invasive therapeutic measures are not available or are less promising. For each individual, the risk/benefit ratio must be considered. Therefore, a careful evaluation of the patient a well as of the indications and contraindications to the procedure is mandatory. MT/P is safe if the patient is evaluated carefully, the thoracoscopist is adequately trained, the contraindications are observed, and complications are prevented.

The history of the patient reveals information about the acute or chronic evolution of the disease, effort intolerance, and possible underlying previous or concomitant pulmonary or extrapulmonary disease such as tumor, asthma, COPD, deep venous thrombosis, coagulation disorders, congestive heart failure, myocardial infarction, renal insufficiency, liver cirrhosis, pancreatitis, diabetes mellitus, HIV, or rheumatoid arthritis. It is well known that the lung and pleura may be involved in many of these diseases. The patient's history may also provide important information on possible risk factors. For example, in case of idiosyncratic or allergic sensitivities to local anesthetics, general anesthesia should be planned.

There should be knowledge of the preceding drug therapy, in particular of anticoagulant treatment, which may be an absolute or relative contraindication to the investigation. Systemic immunosuppressive treatment, especially with corticosteroids, may cause a delayed closure of biopsy sites of the lung. It is important to notify the pathologist about previous therapy with cytostatic agents or radiotherapy as well as about occupational exposures, e.g., to asbestos. The microbiologist needs information on previous antibiotic therapy.

Besides a detailed history a thorough physical examination is a vital component of any preoperative evaluation. Routine posteroanterior and lateral chest radiography has frequently to be supplemented with a CT scan, bilateral decubitus films, or ultrasonography, which also provide the basis for determining the optimum point of insertion of the thoracoscope. They often also prove or exclude the presence of pleural thickening, which points to a possible symphysis by adhesions. This could be a contraindication for MT/P, since the presence of an adequate pleural space is an absolute prerequisite. However, neither CT scan (Mason et al. 1999) nor ultrasonography (Sasaki et al. 2005) provides 100% accuracy in excluding adhesions.

The respiratory status is evaluated, at a minimum, with blood gas analysis and, if necessary, with pulmonary function tests. An electrocardiogram should be obtained to exclude a recent myocardial infarction or significant arrhythmia. The clinical laboratory will provide the coagulation parameters, serum electrolytes, serum creatinine, glucose, liver function studies, and a complete blood count as well as a blood group typing.

If convinced, by applying strict criteria, that MT/P is indicated, the physician should have little difficulty explaining the need for the procedure to the patient and obtaining informed consent. To be certain that the patient fully understands what is to be done and why the procedure is necessary, a hand-out with detailed explanations of the procedure should be provided, followed by verbal explanation and discussion. This includes an explanation of the planned technique, the management of postoperative pain and other possible, so-called typical complications, as well as the expected diagnostic or therapeutic results. It is only then that the patient can truly provide informed consent.

# 8 Contraindications

Medical thoracoscopy/pleuroscopy (MT/P) is a safe procedure with only a few absolute and relative contraindications (Table 8.1), and these follow logically, for the most part, from the preceding chapter describing the clinical prerequisites for the procedure.

An absolute contraindication is lack of pleural space resulting from extensive adhesions of the pleural layers (e.g., in pleural fibrosis, after infections, or previous pleurodesis) since it is impossible to carry out the procedure if the pleural space has been obliterated (often this can be suspected from the patient's history or from ultrasound or radiography (**Fig. 8.1**). A partial pneumothorax of at least 100–200 mL, or of approximately 2–4 cm in depth, must be present or induced. Otherwise, the thoracoscope/pleuroscope cannot be inserted safely without danger of injuring the lung or other organs. Sometimes this technical difficulty may be overcome by enlarging the skin incision and digitally dissecting the lung away from the chest wall, a technique originally described as so-called "extended thoracoscopy" (Janssen and Boutin 1992). For details see "Access to the Pleural Space," Chapter 11, p. 78 ff.

Coagulopathies usually provide only relative contraindications. More severe coagulopathies are a contraindication at least to biopsy procedures that do not allow immediate local control. The platelet count should be in excess of 60 000, and the International Normalized Ratio (INR)

less than 1.2 (Rodriguez-Panadero et al. 2006), otherwise a correction of the coagulopathy must be undertaken prior to the procedure. There are no MT/P studies on the risk of bleeding in patients with aspirin or clopidogrel medication. A report on the risk after transbronchial biopsies did not reveal increased bleeding with aspirin (Herth et al. 2002). The risk of bleeding is also higher in patients with renal insufficiency and elevated nitrogen urea (> 30 mg/dL) or creatinine (> 3 mg/dL).

Great care should be taken in the face of hypoxemia, and particularly in the presence of hypercarbia. Depending on the severity of the respiratory insufficiency, this may provide an absolute contraindication. The only exception would be patients with massive pleural effusion or tension pneumothorax, in whom it can be anticipated that the procedure will provide therapeutic benefit with improvement of gas exchange due to the reexpansion of the compressed or collapsed lung. Under these conditions, (pre)medication should be administered judiciously to minimize respiratory center depression. Although these are relative contraindications, inability to adequately collapse the lung away from the chest wall due to intolerable hypoxemia not only limits exploration but also increases the risk of lung injury and bleeding from instrumentation. In such instances, MT/P is not recommended unless good control of airways, respiration, and oxygenation can be achieved. The same may apply if the patient does not tolerate the lateral decubitus position. However, even in very ill patients on a ventilator, MT/P can be performed without significant complications.

Several other factors may make it necessary to postpone the procedure but are rarely prohibitive; for example, persistent cough, fever, or an unstable cardiovascular status.

MT/P should not be performed following a recent myocardial infarction or in the face of serious arrhythmia, unless the latter is due to marked hypoxemia as in patients with tension pneumothorax. The patient should be free of infection unless a parapneumonic effusion or empyema is present, which provides the therapeutic indication to carry out MT/P.

Contraindications for pulmonary biopsy are suspicion of arteriovenous pulmonary aneurysm, vascular tumors, and hydatid cysts. Taking biopsy samples of honeycomb lung from end-stage pulmonary fibrosis should also be avoided as it contributes to a high incidence of bronchopleural fistula.

**Table 8.1** Absolute and relative contraindications to medical thoracoscopy/pleuroscopy

| Absolute | Relative |
| --- | --- |
| Lack of pleural space due to:<br>• Advanced empyema<br>• Pleural thickening of unknown etiology<br>• Suspected mesothelioma where the visceral and partial surfaces are fused | Inability to tolerate lateral decubitus position<br><br>Unstable cardiovascular or hemodynamic status<br><br>Presence of severe, uncorrectable hypoxemia despite oxygen therapy<br><br>Bleeding diathesis<br><br>Pulmonary arterial hypertension<br><br>Refractory cough<br><br>Drug hypersensitivity<br><br>Reduced general health status with short suspected survival |

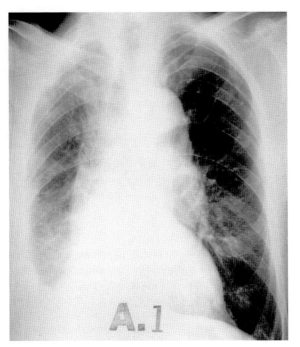

**Fig. 8.1** Chest radiograph of a patient with right-sided pleural thickening suggesting obliteration of the pleural space.

A markedly reduced general health status with an expected short survival should exclude the performance of the examination unless it is likely to improve the patient's situation—for example, in case of pneumothorax or empyema.

MT/P is very similar to the technique of chest tube insertion with the trocar. The only difference is that before insertion of the chest tube, a thoracoscope is introduced through the trocar shaft for inspection of the pleural cavity, for taking biopsies, etc. (**Fig. 8.2**). Nevertheless, the need for adequate and satisfactory training cannot be overemphasized.

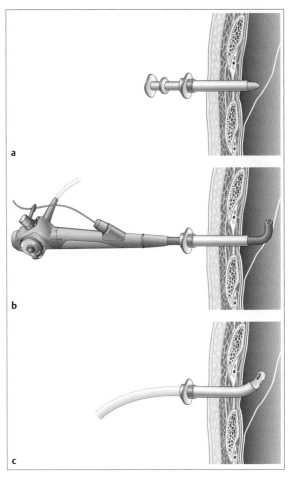

**Fig. 8.2a–c** Drawings illustrating that the technique of medical thoracoscopy is similar to the trocar technique of insertion of a pleural drain.

# 9 Complications and Their Prevention

Medical thoracoscopy/pleuroscopy (MT/P) is a safe and effective modality in the diagnosis and treatment of several pleuropulmonary diseases if certain standard criteria are fulfilled. Complications of thoracoscopy were well known to earlier phthisiologists. The advantages of the technique should be weighed against the discomfort to the patient and the slight potential for morbidity and mortality. Although the risks are low, it is important that adequate precautions are taken, including the recommended technical procedure as well as monitoring of cardiac and hemodynamic parameters and oxygen saturation during the procedure.

As for all conscious sedation protocols, patients undergoing MT/P should refrain from eating and drinking 6–8 hours before the procedure to reduce the risk of aspiration.

Complications that may be associated with MT/P can be separated into those that may occur before, during, or after the procedure (**Table 9.1**). These potential complications, although rare, will be described in detail because their knowledge and their prevention will enable the thoracoscopist/pleuroscopist to avoid them in great part.

## Prethoracoscopic/Prepleuroscopic Complications

### Air Embolism

The most serious complication of *pneumothorax induction* is air or gas embolism that can occur during pneumothorax induction. Fortunately it happens very rarely (< 0.1%) and can be prevented if appropriate precautionary measures are taken (see "Access to the Pleural Space," Chapter 11, p. 78 ff.). However, in older reports the frequency of air embolism in therapeutic pneumothorax, often performed under less-optimal conditions, varied between 0.1% and 0.5% (Schmidt 1938). In more than 3000 diagnostic thoracoscopies, one of the authors (R. L.) observed only one case of transient neurological abnormality, presumably due to cerebral gas embolism ($CO_2$ was used for pneumothorax induction) (Brandt et al. 1985). Otherwise, incorrect needle position during filling with a pneumothorax apparatus can produce *subcutaneous emphysema*.

**Table 9.1** Potential complications of medical thoracoscopy/pleuroscopy before, during, and after the procedure

| Prethoracoscopic/prepleuroscopic complications | Complications during thoracoscopy/pleuroscopy | Postthoracoscopic/postpleuroscopic complications |
|---|---|---|
| • Air embolism, subcutaneous emphysema and pain during pneumothorax induction<br>• Shortness of breath after pneumothorax induction<br>• Hypersensitivity reaction to local anesthetic | • Pain<br>• Hypoxemia<br>• Hypoventilation<br>• Cardiac arrhythmias<br>• Hypotension<br>• Hemorrhage<br>• Injury to lung or other organs | • Reexpansion pulmonary edema<br>• Pain<br>• Postoperative fever<br>• Wound infection<br>• Hypotension<br>• Empyema<br>• Subcutaneous emphysema<br>• Persisting pneumothorax<br>• Prolonged air leakage<br>• Continuing pleural fluid production<br>• Early and late complications after talc pleurodesis<br>• Seeding of chest wall by tumor cells<br>• Mortality |

The patient may experience a short *pain* during penetration of the parietal pleura by the pneumothorax needle. Additional pain may occur in patients with dense adhesions, but this is always associated with an increase in the intrapleural pressure, since the lung cannot collapse sufficiently.

## Hypersensitivity Reaction to Local Anesthetic

The patient should be asked whether there are known idiosyncratic or allergic sensitivities to local anesthetics. In this case general anesthesia should be planned.

## Complications during Medical Thoracoscopy/Pleuroscopy

### Pain

In the presence of effective local anesthesia (see "Technique of Local Anesthesia," Chapter 11, p. 84 ff.) and well-titrated sedation, little discomfort is felt, even when instruments with a larger diameter (11 mm) are used. When biopsies of the parietal pleura are taken, patients must be warned of the associated brief discomfort, and should be advised that they may cough when the lung is biopsied.

**Prior to talc insufflation**, which may be painful, additional analgesics (alternatively intrapleural lidocaine spray) should be given to the patient (see "Technique of Thoracoscopic Talc Pleurodesis," Chapter 11, p. 92 ff.). Although an average total dose of 600 mg of lidocaine appeared safe in bronchoscopy (Langmack et al. 2000), the total dose should be limited to approximately 300 mg, which should be sufficient for local anesthesia. *Methemoglobinemia* is an uncommon complication of topical anesthetics, particularly of lidocaine (Weiss et al. 1987).

### Hypoxemia

The procedure may cause hypoxia for several reasons: depression due to the anesthesia, healthy lung in the lateral decubitus position, and collapse of the investigated lung due to the induced pneumothorax. Oxygen saturation usually decreases only insignificantly during the procedure (Oldenburg and Newhouse 1979; Faurschou et al. 1983; Cho et al. 2000). Nasal oxygen may be provided prophylactically.

### Hypoventilation

Some advocate the simultaneous cutaneous measurement of carbon dioxide tension ($P_cCO_2$), since significant hypoventilation might occur due to the sedation (Chhajed et al. 2005).

### Cardiac Arrhythmias

Except for a slight sinus tachycardia, cardiac arrhythmias are rare (Faurschou et al. 1983, Cho et al. 2000).

### Hypotension

With the removal of large pleural effusions, one should be alert to the development of hypotension because of the associated considerable volume loss. Some authors recommend atropine (0.25–0.8 mg) to suppress vaso-vagal reflexes (Boutin et al. 1991; Rodriguez-Panadero 2008), but it is not clear whether atropine is necessary as routine premedication (Cho et al. 2000; Loddenkemper 2000).

During the procedure, cardiorespiratory functions should be monitored by electrocardiography (ECG), measurement of blood pressure, and continuous oximetry. Many complications such as benign cardiac arrhythmias, low-grade hypotension, or hypoxemia can be prevented by administration of oxygen and intravenous fluids.

### Hemorrhage

A major concern often expressed regarding MT/P is the risk of bleeding and the need for surgical back-up. In this regard, the reported incidence of significant bleeding—i.e., requiring transfusion or surgical intervention—is exceedingly low. Superficial bleeding at the site of introduction ceases as a result of compression following the introduction of the trocar. If hemorrhage occurs after the taking of biopsies, this is in general only very slight and ceases spontaneously if the suggested precautions are observed. If bleeding does not stop or if an intercostal vessel has been biopsied inadvertently, the bleeding area should be compressed and/or cauterized with electrocoagulation (see "Biopsy Techniques," Chapter 11, p. 89 ff.). Contraindications for pulmonary biopsy are suspicion of arteriovenous pulmonary aneurysm and highly vascularized pulmonary lesions.

### Injury to Lung or Other Organs

Injury to the lung and other organs is almost always avoided by proceeding carefully, in particular when adhesions between the chest wall and the lung are present. It has to be kept in mind that the diaphragm is elevated in the recumbent position, and it is important to observe the suggested sites of introduction of the cannula to avoid dangerous areas (see "Selecting the Point of Entry," Chapter 11, p. 78). One fatal complication caused by injury to an enlarged leukemic spleen has been reported (Dijkman 1989). One of the authors (R. L.) performed an unintended "pericardioscopy" in a case where the pericardium was fixed to the left anterior chest wall by a small postinflammatory adhesion (without further complication).

# Postthoracoscopic/Postpleuroscopic Complications

## Reexpansion Pulmonary Edema

This rare possibility may arise in particular when a large amount of pleural fluid has caused an atelectatic lung, when a stiff or trapped lung is present, in the case of a complete endobronchial obstruction, or in the case of a long-lasting pneumothorax. In these situations, negative pressure through the drainage tube should be applied very cautiously, and the patient should be observed closely (see also "Knowledge of the Pathophysiology of the Pleura," Chapter 10, p. 67 ff. and "Chest Tube Care," Chapter 11, p. 95 ff.).

## Pain

Analgesics should be given as needed. The correct position of the chest tube should be monitored.

## Postoperative Fever

Low-grade fever (37.5–38.5 °C), which often occurs in the following days, does not signify an infection but rather an inflammatory tissue reaction (Viskum 1989). Higher fever and stronger systemic reactions are noted after talc poudrage (Froudarakis et al. 2006).

## Wound Infection

Wound infection as a complication is not mentioned in any study. It does of course occur, but must have been considered too insignificant to be mentioned (Viskum and Enk 1981). The chest tube site should be regularly inspected and, if necessary, dressings should be changed.

## Empyema

Postthoracoscopic empyema is a rare complication, but may occur after a long drainage duration or due to a bronchopleural fistula. It has been reported in 12 cases in three studies comprising 652 patients (2%) (Viskum and Enk 1981).

## Subcutaneous Emphysema

Subcutaneous emphysema is usually only slight and resolves spontaneously if the suction drainage functions appropriately.

## Persisting Pneumothorax

Here, first it must be checked whether the chest tube drainage functions properly. Otherwise, this complication is most likely to occur when lung biopsies are taken from a fibrotic lung (see "The Place of Medical Thoracoscopy/Pleuroscopy in the Diagnosis of Diffuse Lung Diseases," Chapter 3, p. 46 ff. and "Biopsy Techniques," Chapter 11, p. 89 ff.), which may necessitate additional chest tubes. In cases of trapped lung or of pneumothorax with persisting pleuropulmonary fistulas, the appropriate measures have to be taken, as described in the sections on "Options in the Local Treatment of Pleural Effusions Including Thoracoscopic Talc Pleurodesis," Chapter 3, p. 35 ff. and "The Place of Medical Thoracoscopy/Pleuroscopy in the Management of Pneumothorax," Chapter 3, p. 41 ff., respectively.

## Prolonged Air Leakage

Prolonged air leakage is a potential complication after lung biopsies have been taken, particularly with a stiff or trapped lung. Therefore, taking biopsy samples of honeycomb lung from end-stage pulmonary fibrosis should be avoided as it contributes to a high incidence of bronchopleural fistulae with prolonged suction. Biopsies should also be avoided in cases of bullous lung disease. However, air leakage can also occur in patients with necrotic tumor nodules, especially those with prior chemotherapy, even if no biopsies of this area have been taken (Antony et al. 2000). In these cases very gentle suction should be applied through the chest tube (see "Chest Tube Care," Chapter 11, p. 94 ff.). Empyema with a bronchopleural fistula needs appropriate surgical intervention (see the section on "Parapneumonic Effusions and Pleural Empyema," Chapter 3, p. 31 ff.).

## Continuing Pleural Fluid Production/Pleurodesis Failure

In cases where pleural fluid is still produced in a considerable amount after the procedure without performance of talc poudrage, the usual pleurodesis procedures are indicated (see "Chest Tube Thoracostomy with Chemical Pleurodesis," Chapter 3, p. 38). Initial failure of thoracoscopic talc pleurodesis (poudrage) can occur as a result of suboptimal techniques or inappropriate patient selection (e.g., a patient with trapped lung or mainstem bronchial occlusion). When initial pleurodesis fails, several alternatives may be considered. Repeat pleurodesis may be performed either with instillation of sclerosants through the chest tube or by repeat MT/P and talc poudrage (Antony et al. 2000). Other alternatives are described in "Options in the Local Treatment of Pleural Effusions Including Thoracoscopic Talc Pleurodesis," Chapter 3, p. 35 ff. Recurrence after pleurodesis is unusual with talc but does occur occasionally. In these cases, one of the other options that have been mentioned should be tried. If the patient is receiving corticosteroid therapy, the drug should be stopped or the dose reduced if possible because of concerns of decreased efficacy of pleurodesis (Kennedy et al. 1994).

## Early Complications after Talc Pleurodesis

Talc pleurodesis via either chest tube slurry or thoracoscopic insufflation of dry talc, has been reported to induce acute lung injury and the acute respiratory distress syndrome (ARDS) (Kennedy and Sahn 1994; Campos et al. 1997; Rehse et al. 1999; Light 2000; Sahn 2000). The toxic effects of talc are hypothesized to be mediated primarily by smaller talc particles < 15 μm. A small prospective trial compared a mixed talc preparation with 50% of particles less than 10 μm and a graded talc preparation with < 50% particles smaller than 20 μm and demonstrated that the mixed talc caused a greater A–a (alveolar–arterial) gradient and systemic inflammatory response (fever and C-reactive protein) than did graded talc (Maskell et al. 2004). Meanwhile, a large prospective multicenter study in more than 500 patients with malignant pleural effusion has shown that the use of size-calibrated talc (Steritalc with a mean particle size of 24.5 μm and only 11% having size < 5 μm) prevents the development of ARDS, probably due to a substantially reduced systemic distribution (Janssen et al. 2007). Talc poudrage causes more fever and systemic inflammatory reactions than does thoracoscopy alone (Froudarakis et al. 2006).

## Late Complications after Talc Pleurodesis

Potential long-term sequelae such as reduced pulmonary function and cancer have been excluded by long-term follow-up studies that confirmed the safety of talc (Lange et al. 1988; Cardillo et al. 2007; Györik et al. 2007; Hunt et al. 2007; Noppen 2007).

## Seeding of Chest Wall by Tumor Cells / Implantation of Tumor Cells

To prevent the potential late complication of contamination of the entry site(s) by tumor cells, particularly in mesothelioma cases, prophylactic radiotherapy 10–12 days after MT/P has been recommended (Boutin et al. 1995 b), although this is controversial (Low et al. 1995; Bydder et al. 2004; O'Rourke et al. 2007; Davies et al. 2008).

## Mortality

Mortality is reported to be an extremely rare event of MT/P with only one death in 8000 cases, for a mortality rate of 0.01 (Viskum and Enk 1981); in another series reviewing 4300 cases, the mortality rate was 0.09% (Boutin et al. 1981b). The mortality rate of 0.24% for MT/P is comparable to that reported for transbronchial biopsies (0.22–0.66%) (Boutin et al. 1985 a).

However, in the prospective multicenter study on medical thoracoscopic talc poudrage in malignant pleural effusions, published in *The Lancet* in 2007, 11 out of 558 patients died within 30 days after the procedure. Thus the 30-day mortality (2%) was higher than in the above articles. This is explained by the limited life expectancy and serious co-morbidity of these patients, in a small proportion of whom postthoracoscopic complications and mortality can be expected (Janssen et al. 2007). All causes of death, listed in detail, were due to severe co-morbidities. Serious adverse events were observed in seven cases (1.24%): two patients developed a reexpansion edema, one had a transient cardiogenic pulmonary edema, one had an acute respiratory insufficiency due to unexplained contralateral pneumothorax on the day of thoracoscopy, one had a pulmonary embolism on day 8, one developed pneumonia with high fever, and one developed nonpulmonary sepsis. No acute respiratory distress syndrome (ARDS) was observed.

Dijkman, who, between 1976 and 1987, performed MT/P in 65 patients suffering from pulmonary complications in immunosuppression of various non-HIV origins reported two fatal complications (3%), one following injury of an considerably enlarged leukemic spleen and one following uncontrollable bleeding after several deep parenchymal lung biopsies at the same site. Fifteen of these severely ill patients, who already had compromised respiratory function, needed postthoracoscopic mechanical ventilation (Dijkman 1989).

Menzies and Charbonneau in their study of 102 patients registered a major complication rate of 1.9% including ventricular tachycardia responding to resuscitation, subcutaneous emphysema, and persistent air leakage, while the minor complication rate was 5.5% including transient air leakage, fever, and minor bleeding at the biopsy site (Menzies and Charbonneau 1991).

In a review of four studies (including the study of Menzies and Charbonneau 1991), comprising 819 MT/Ps, using conscious sedation and local anesthesia, no fatal case was reported. The most severe complications were subcutaneous emphysema in 39 patients (5%); transient cardiovascular complications in 10 patients (1%); empyema in two patients; excessive bleeding and air embolism in one patient each (Rodriguez-Panadero et al. 2006).

Another large series including 360 patients reported morbidities of fever in 9.8%, empyema in 2.5%, pulmonary infection in 0.8%, and malignant invasion of the scar in 0.3% (Viallat et al. 1996).

In a prospective study, Colt demonstrated safety of MT/P when performed by an experienced pulmonologist (Colt 1995a). In 52 procedures he observed no mortality, one major adverse event (recurrent pleural effusion requiring chest tube drainage in a patient with scleroderma and trapped lung), and minor adverse events in 10 instances (19.2%) including seven with talc-related fever and one each with fever, with wound infection at the chest tube insertion site in a patient who underwent thoracoscopy for empyema, and with a small clinically insignificant pneumothorax after chest tube removal.

Major uncontrollable bleeding requiring thoracotomy was not reported in any of these large series and appears to be extremely rare. However, the safety of the procedure depends on the physician's technique and skill, and on careful observation of the patient.

It has to be decided individually whether heparin prophylaxis for prevention of venous thrombosis (and pulmonary embolism) should be started postthoracoscopically, which some authors recommend because a strong activation of the coagulation system has been observed after the procedure with and without talc pleurodesis (Rodriguez-Panadero 1995).

## Summary

Complications can best be prevented by observing a few simple rules:

- Postpone for several days if the patient is coughing.
- Measure blood gases; monitor cardiac status.
- Oxygenate the patient during the procedure.
- Coagulate and ensure hemostasis if hemorrhage exceeds 20 mL.
- Insert a chest tube until no air leakage is detected, to prevent subcutaneous emphysema.
- Start a lung expansion protocol on the day of MT/P to prevent atelectasis.
- Start gentle suction to avoid reexpansion pulmonary edema
- To prevent invasion of the insertion tract of the thoracoscope in malignant mesothelioma, consider radiation therapy of 7 grays/day for 3 days to the incision area; if thoracentesis or closed needle biopsies were taken, their tracts may also receive radiation.

# 10 Knowledge and Skills Required

To learn medical thoracoscopy/pleuroscopy (MT/P), a pulmonologist needs to know the exact topographical anatomy of the thorax, the pathophysiology and pathology of respiratory diseases, their diagnostic approach and their management options, in particular of pleural diseases, as well as the clinical prerequisites, the contraindications, and the complications that have been described in detail in the preceding chapters. He or she must also know the details of the technique of medical thoracoscopy/pleuroscopy including all instruments used, the different options of access to the pleural space, the technique of coagulation, and so on, as outlined in the following chapters. In addition, he or she should already have adopted certain skills in the diagnosis and treatment of respiratory diseases, particularly pleural diseases (Lamb et al. 2010).

## Knowledge of Respiratory Diseases

- The diagnostic approach, the differential diagnosis, and the management options of the respective diseases are described in detail in Chapter 3, pp. 22–52.
- Typical pathological changes are demonstrated in the *Atlas* part of this book.

## Knowledge of Thoracic Anatomy

- The interior anatomical topography of the left and right hemithoraces is shown in **Figures 10.1** and **10.2**.
- How to find the exact orientation during the endoscopic exploration of the pleural cavity is described in Chapter 11, p. 86 ff. and p. 91 ff.

Several important anatomical landmarks of the chest cage must be kept firmly in mind:
- The anteromedial end of the second intercostal space is located by palpating the angle formed by the manubrium and the body of the sternum.
- The ribs can then be counted from top to bottom.
- In the axillary hollow, the second intercostal space is the highest space that can be felt in a nonobese patient.

- The ribs can also be numerated in the back, using the dorsal spinous processes. The reference point here is the prominent C7 spine, from which the vertebrae and ribs may easily be counted.
- The ribs of a patient in the lateral position can be counted along the mid-axillary line: the lowest rib that can be felt is the tenth; the eleventh and twelfth, floating ribs, are behind. The ribs can then be counted from the bottom upward.
- The male nipple is generally situated near the level of the fourth rib.
- If an anterior point of entry is selected, remember that the internal mammary artery and vein pass just posterior to the ribs some 16–18 mm lateral to the sternal margin.
- When erect, the liver is very high within the thorax: reaching as far as the fourth intercostal space during forced exhalation. However, in the left lateral decubitus position, gravity pulls the liver away from the chest wall and there is little possibility of injuring it. Avoiding the liver should be a simple matter once the insertion levels of the diaphragm and the dimensions of the costophrenic angle are appreciated radiographically. Lateral decubitus films or, preferably, fluoroscopy/ultrasonography "on the table," provide an extra margin of safety when a low entry site is planned.
- Radiographic review is mandatory in each patient. One should keep the typical diaphragmatic anatomy in mind: the diaphragm is more or less symmetrical on both sides; it starts anteriorly just below the sixth costal cartilage at about the same height as the xiphoid process, slopes downward toward the side, and reaches its lowest point level with the end of the eleventh rib and the second lumbar vertebra, approximately in the mid-axillary line. Then it rises again toward the back, crossing the twelfth rib 8–9 cm from the spine and joins the upper edge of the first lumbar vertebra.
- Remember that the major fissure crosses the mid-axillary line at the fourth intercostal space on the right.
- The minor fissure begins at this point and at the fifth intercostal space on the left.

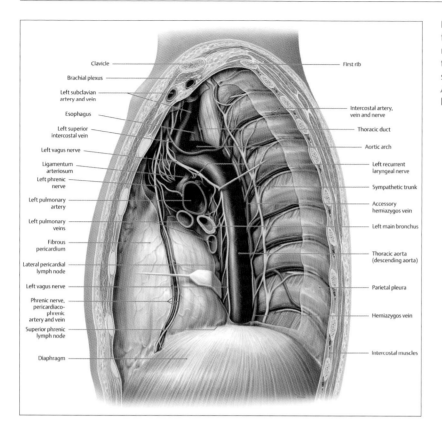

Clavicle
Brachial plexus
Left subclavian artery and vein
Esophagus
Left superior intercostal vein
Left vagus nerve
Ligamentum arteriosum
Left phrenic nerve
Left pulmonary artery
Left pulmonary veins
Fibrous pericardium
Lateral pericardial lymph node
Left vagus nerve
Phrenic nerve, pericardiaco-phrenic artery and vein
Superior phrenic lymph node
Diaphragm

First rib
Intercostal artery, vein and nerve
Thoracic duct
Aortic arch
Left recurrent laryngeal nerve
Sympathetic trunk
Accessory hemiazygos vein
Left main bronchus
Thoracic aorta (descending aorta)
Parietal pleura
Hemiazygos vein
Intercostal muscles

**Fig. 10.1** Mediastinum seen from the left side. The lung has been removed, and after stripping away the parietal pleura, retropleural structures are visible. (From *Atlas of Anatomy*, © Thieme 2008. Illustration by Marcus Voll.)

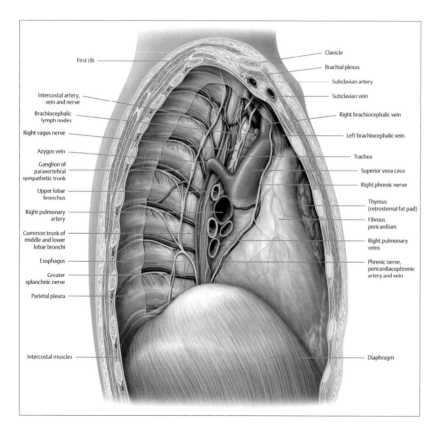

First rib
Intercostal artery, vein and nerve
Brachiocephalic lymph nodes
Right vagus nerve
Azygos vein
Ganglion of paravertebral sympathetic trunk
Upper lobar bronchus
Right pulmonary artery
Common trunk of middle and lower lobar bronchi
Esophagus
Greater splanchnic nerve
Parietal pleura
Intercostal muscles

Clavicle
Brachial plexus
Subclavian artery
Subclavian vein
Right brachiocephalic vein
Left brachiocephalic vein
Trachea
Superior vena cava
Right phrenic nerve
Thymus (retrosternal fat pad)
Fibrous pericardium
Right pulmonary veins
Phrenic nerve, pericardiacophrenic artery and vein
Diaphragm

**Fig. 10.2** Mediastinum seen from the right side. The lung has been removed, and after stripping away the parietal pleura, retropleural structures are visible. (From *Atlas of Anatomy*, © Thieme 2008. Illustration by Marcus Voll.)

# Knowledge of the Pathophysiology of the Pleura

The pleural space lies between the visceral pleura, which covers the external surface of the lung, and the parietal pleura, which covers the internal surface of the chest wall, the diaphragm, and lateral parts of the mediastinum. It is the coupling system between the lungs and the chest wall and diaphragm and thus a crucial feature of the respiratory apparatus. Normally, only a very small amount of fluid is present in the pleural space, which serves as lubricant between the two pleural layers. A unique characteristic of the pleural space is that it is a potential space within a closed environment (Jantz and Antony 2008).

The lung has a tendency to collapse due to its elastic recoil, but is kept in close apposition to the chest wall with its opposed recoil. A negative pleural pressure results that increases during inspiration and decreases during expiration. Collapse of the lung occurs when air enters the pleural space (pneumothorax) and the pleural pressure becomes positive (atmospheric).

Pleural fluid formation depends on the difference in pressures (hydrostatic and oncotic) between the pleural space and the visceral and parietal capillaries. Extrapolating from animal models, it is assumed that pleural fluid is normally produced at a rate of approximately 0.01 mL/kg/h and is primarily formed from capillaries on the parietal pleura. Pleural fluid is removed via stomata, also on the parietal pleura, that drain into lymphatics, which have the ability to absorb fluid at a rate of approximately 0.28 mL/kg/h (Feller-Kopman et al. 2009).

For fluid to accumulate in the pleural space, one of the following three things must happen: the disease process must overwhelm the ability of the lymphatics to reabsorb fluid by substantially increasing pleural fluid production (this requires a change of at least a factor of 28, based on the figures above); the process must reduce the ability of the lymphatics to clear the fluid; or the process must both increase production and decrease lymphatic clearance (Feller-Kopman et al. 2009). In addition, pleural capillaries are not the only source of pleural fluid; in disease states, other sources include the interstitial spaces of the lung and the peritoneal cavity.

Thus, pleural effusion may result from several pathophysiological mechanisms, all of which disturb the physiological balance between the formation and removal of pleural fluid (Zocchi 2002). Most effusions develop from both an increase in the entry rate of liquid into the pleural space and a decrease in the maximal exit rate of liquid from the pleural space. Transudative effusions are caused either by increased hydrostatic pressure (e.g., in cardiac failure) or by reduced plasma-oncotic pressure because of protein deficiency (e.g., liver cirrhosis, nephrotic syndrome). The pleura itself remains intact. Rarely, transudates may arise from the entry of liquids with low protein concentrations (e.g., urine [ipsilateral obstructive uropathy], cerebrospinal fluid [duropleural fistula], or iatrogenic intrapleural infusion of fluids). In contrast, pathological changes in the pleura result in exudation and are caused by diffuse increase of capillary permeability, or are related to localized ruptures (e.g., of blood vessels, lymphatic vessels, a lung abscess, the esophagus) or to disturbed absorption (e.g., lymphatic blockage). Thus, a wide spectrum of diseases may be associated with pleural effusion.

When performing a therapeutic thoracentesis, careful attention should be paid to the symptoms of the patient—in particular cough, since this may signal too negative a pleural pressure. This can be induced by the removal of a large amount of pleural fluid or if the lung is not able to reexpand due to trapped lung or lung entrapment. (Lung entrapment is defined as inability of the lung to fully reexpand during thoracentesis as a result of either pleural or nonpleural disease; trapped lung, on the other hand, represents the sequelae of prior pleural inflammation resulting in visceral pleural scarring or thickening [Feller-Kopman et al. 2009].)

If the pleural pressure becomes too negative during the removal of large volumes of pleural fluid, the risk of reexpansion pulmonary edema is present. During thoracoscopy, large volumes of pleural fluid—up to several liters—can be removed without the immediate danger of reexpansion pulmonary edema since air will enter through the trocar, thus creating a pressure equilibrium.

However, after the procedure, there is the risk of reexpansion pulmonary edema when the chest tube has been placed and negative pressure is applied by suction via the drainage system. The possibility that the lung does not reexpand appropriately applies, in particular, when a large amount of pleural fluid has compressed the lung, in case of lung entrapment or trapped lung, in case of endobronchial obstruction, or in case of a complete pneumothorax that has existed already for some time. In all these situations, negative pressure should be applied in a very gentle manner, and the patient should be observed closely (see "Chest Tube Care", Chapter 11, p. 95 ff.).

# Skills

The learner should already have acquired skills in the following (see also Chapter 13, "Teaching Methods"):
- Application of the above knowledge.
- Diagnostic and therapeutic thoracentesis.
- Performance of local anesthesia.
- Closed needle biopsy of the pleura.
- Familiarity with chest tubes and pleural drainage.
- Closed chest tube insertion.
- Pleurodesis techniques.
- Flexible bronchoscopy.
- Rigid bronchoscopy (optional).

- Use of either the semirigid pleuroscope or the rigid thoracoscope (or both).
- Use of biopsy forceps and other instruments.
- Use of coagulation systems.
- Use of the talc atomizer/talc spray.
- Use of video-endoscopic equipment.
- Ultrasonography and/or fluoroscopy (optional).

As with all technical procedures, there is certainly a learning curve before full competence in MT/P is achieved (Boutin et al. 1981a; Rodriguez-Panadero 1995).

# 11 Techniques of Medical Thoracoscopy/Pleuroscopy

The principles and technique of medical thoracoscopy using rigid instrumentation were developed in continental Europe during the second half of the last century. They have proven their value ever since (Brandt 1964; Boutin et al. 1980, 1991; Enk and Viskum 1981; Loddenkemper 1981; Brandt et al. 1985), and have been introduced into the pulmonological community of North America by pioneers such as Aelony, Colt, Mathur, and others (Aelony et al. 1991; Colt 1992; Mathur 1994). These principles remain valid for the use of the newer generation of semirigid (semiflexible) pleuroscopes (Lee and Colt 2005; Munavvar et al. 2007).

In many centers, and for most indications, medical thoracoscopy/pleuroscopy (MT/P) will be performed under local anesthesia and with conscious sedation. For the most part, the method is similar to that of tube thoracostomy with the addition of thorough inspection of the pleural space and the adjacent organs. For most indications, MT/P will start as a single-port, single-instrument rigid procedure, as first described by Jacobaeus for diagnostic purposes.

An alternative approach, as used by Jacobaeus for lysis of adhesions, is the two-entry-site technique, one entry for the examination telescope and the other for the introduction of accessory instruments, including the biopsy forceps. For this technique, neuroleptic deep sedation or general anesthesia is preferred (the technique for "Medical Thoracoscopic Sympathectomy," see Chapter 3, p. 48 ff.).

With the introduction of the semirigid pleuroscope (LTF 160, Olympus, Japan), similar in design, accessory equipment, and handling to the flexible bronchoscope, MT/P can now be performed in a fashion analogous to flexible bronchoscopy. Thus, this technique is now increasingly used by pulmonologists who are experienced with video-controlled flexible bronchoscopy.

## Endoscopy Room

MT/P can be performed either in an operating room or in a (clean) endoscopy suite (Harris et al. 1995). Cleanliness requirements are greater than for endoscopy via natural orifices, for example bronchoscopy, but less than in cardiac catheterization. Thus, the procedure is best performed in rooms used for laparoscopy or in operating rooms or in a clean bronchoscopy unit. Electrical systems should be properly isolated and protected against overload, and ideally should be attached to a voltage regulator and auxiliary electrical supply independent of the mains. Additionally, a premedication area, a washroom, and an area for cleaning and sterilizing instruments should be provided.

A properly equipped endoscopy room and arrangement of the personnel has already been shown in **Figure 1.13**. See also **Figure 11.1**. The room must contain the following:

- Thoracoscopy table: This may be a simple operating table, preferably radiolucent, or, ideally, may have a height adjustment and a back that can be raised for operating in the semisitting position. Some tables can be adjusted laterally along a longitudinal axis, which allows the patient to be repositioned easily. Although these sophisticated tables are very useful, they are certainly not essential.
- On a separate sterile table, the thoracoscope, trocar, forceps, talc atomizer, and all other accessories are placed (**Fig. 11.2**).
- A pneumothorax apparatus (optional).
- Adjustable aspiration equipment for the pleural fluid, with 2-L or larger collecting bottles connected to negative pressure (suction pump, electric pump, or central vacuum system with negative pressure regulator).
- Simple anesthetic equipment, with air-feed (nasal prongs) and oxygen.
- An overhead light with adjustable brightness.
- A (Mayo) stand placed sideways across the surgical table to hold the instruments.
- Electrocautery.

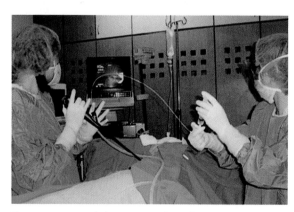

**Fig. 11.1** Semirigid pleuroscopy in the endoscopy room.

**Table 11.1**   Equipment for the resuscitation trolley

| Cardiac management | Airway management | Drugs | Antagonists |
| --- | --- | --- | --- |
| Electrocardiogram and leads | Laryngoscope, different size blades, batteries | Epinephrine (adrenaline) | Naloxone (narcotic) |
| Defribrillator, paddles, and gel pads | Ambu bag, and masks (small, medium, large) | Atropine | Flumazenil (benzodiazepine) |
| Blood pressure monitor | Endotracheal tubes (6–9) and stylets | Lidocaine (lignocaine) | |
| | Oral and nasopharyngeal airways | Bretylium tosylate | |
| | Suction catheters | Calcium chloride | |
| | Oxygen (wall outlet with adaptor or cylinder) | Sodium bicarbonate | |
| | | Narcotics | |
| | | Benzodiazepines | |
| | | Propofol | |
| | | Succinylcholine | |
| | | Neuromuscular blockers: suxamethonium, vecuronium, atracurium | |

- Laser equipment (optional).
- Separate mobile carts for endoscopic light sources, video equipment, and equipment for color photography.
- A viewing box or electronic medical records to display the patient's radiographs during the procedure.
- A fluoroscope with an image intensifier and C-mount (optional).
- An alternative is ultrasonography (optional).

In addition, a trolley equipped with resuscitative drugs, endotracheal and chest tubes, and equipment for cardioversion and airway intubation should be easily accessible (**Table 11.1**).

## Sterile Conditions

MT/P must be performed under strictly sterile conditions: All materials have to be sterilized, after careful cleansing, including all instruments, light conducting cables, and video cameras.

The method of disinfecting, cleaning, and sterilizing instruments and cannulas should be based on the local state and federal regulations. However, since many errors are made in handling the optics, we stress several important points:

- Predisinfecting cleaning is best accomplished before secretions have dried on the instruments by submersion in protein-dissolving, hypochlorite-containing, disinfecting and cleansing solutions. Operating channels in the instruments should be filled with this solution by means of a syringe. Cleaning should continue for at least 15 minutes.
- For the mechanical cleaning of predisinfected instruments, clean, demineralized water should be used. Preferably, instruments are rinsed with water and cleaned with soft brushes.
- The final stage of disinfection is best performed with an aldehyde-containing solution, e.g., Cidex, to which a commercially available activator is added. Large containers are needed and manipulation of the instruments with gloved hands is easier than the use of forceps. This disinfection stage should take about 15 minutes.
- Instruments should then be rinsed in a bath of fresh demineralized water. The washed and dried instruments are then sterilized by placing them, for 24 hours, into gas-tight cabinets containing formalin tablets. Following this, the optics are sterile and ready for use.

Some companies suggest autoclaving the optics in an autoclave or by means of ethylene oxide. These methods, which require high and low pressures, may damage older instruments with hairline cracks. Sterilization by means of ionizing radiation may turn the glass of normal optics brown. All video equipment is sterilized by soaking in Cidex. The semirigid (semiflexible) pleuroscope can be autoclaved (Munavvar et al. 2007) (**Table 11.2**).

Talc is sterilized by dry autoclaving at 160 °C, or by gamma-irradiation or by ethylene oxide gas. All have proved to be effective sterilization methods (Kennedy et al. 1995; Mattison et al. 1996).

**Table 11.2**   Parameters for the steam sterilization (autoclaving) of semiflexible pleuroscopes

| Process | Parameters | | |
|---|---|---|---|
| Prevacuum<br>Vacuum drying phase | Prevacuum pressure: − 0.085 MPa<br>Prevacuum pulses: 3 times<br>Temperature: 132–134 °C (270–274 °F)<br>Exposure time: 5 min | | |
| Steam pulses<br>Vacuum drying | **Parameters** | **Steam pulses 1** | **Steam pulses 2** |
| | Vacuum pressure | − 0.06 MPa | − 0.065 MPa |
| | Steam pulse pressure | + 0.17 MPa | + 0.13 MPa |
| | Prevacuum pulses (no.) | 3 | 2 |
| | Temperature | 132–134 °C (270–274 °F) | |
| | Exposure time | 5 min | |

The physician and the assistant clean their hands with the standard surgical scrub technique and then put on sterile gown/cap/mask and gloves.

The patient's skin is prepared by shaving and disinfecting a large area, so that different points of entry are possible, reaching from the sternum up to the clavicle, across the axilla, past the scapula to the spinous processes, and down as far as the base of the thorax. Then the patient is covered with sterile sheets.

### Patient Monitoring during the Procedure

The pulse, blood pressure, and respiration are carefully monitored. Depending on the equipment available, local custom, and the clinical condition, ECG and continuous pulse oximetry monitoring are used. Oxygen is administered as required (Cho et al. 2000; Loddenkemper 2000).

### Personnel

Personnel required for this procedure are the physician performing the MT/P and an endoscopy assistant (or an endoscopy nurse) to assist with the instrumentation, and additionally a circulator nurse outside the sterile field to bring necessary equipment (see **Fig. 1.13**). Finally, depending on local custom, a nurse responsible for monitoring the patient's oxygenation, cardiac, and ventilatory parameters as well as for titration of sedation according to patient comfort is desirable when the procedure is performed in the bronchoscopy room, or in the operating room with the support of the full anesthesia team. In an emergency, the procedure can be performed with only a physician and a nurse, but this is less efficient and may prolong the procedure.

All members of the team should be familiar with MT/P procedures and have the knowledge, competence, and resources necessary to respond to an emergent situation.

Nurses who take care of patients following MT/P should have sufficient knowledge of the procedure to provide optimal patient outcomes (Davidson and Colt 1997).

### Equipment

Since the first detailed description by Jacobaeus in 1910; rigid endoscopic instruments such as stainless-steel trocars and telescopes have been pivotal in the performance of thoracoscopy (**Fig. 11.2**) and VATS. With the introduction of the semirigid (semiflexible) pleuroscope, similar in design and handling to the flexible bronchoscope, pleuroscopy is now frequently performed with this technique, analogous to flexible bronchoscopy. An additional advantage of the pleuroscope is that parts of the bronchoscopy equipment (e.g., the light source) can be used, reducing the acquisition cost.

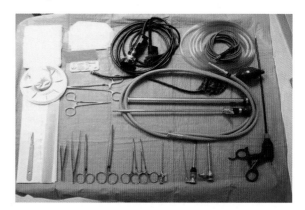

**Fig. 11.2**   Instruments for rigid thoracoscopy (Storz company).

The equipment requirements include trocar, thoracoscope/pleuroscope, biopsy forceps, unipolar coagulation forceps, light sources, video system, aspiration system, talc, chest tubes, and pleurovacs. The usual diameter of the rigid thoracoscope is 7–9 mm, that of the semirigid pleuroscope 7 mm.

Corresponding to the historical development, we will describe first the rigid technique, followed by the flex-rigid technique.

## Rigid Thoracoscopes

One type of rigid thoracoscope is manufactured by the German company Storz (in the United States available from Karl Storz Endoscopy America Inc, Culver City, CA). The diameter of the trocar most commonly used is 10 mm and of that the thoracoscope 9 mm (7–12 mm thoracoscopes are also available) with a working channel of 3 or 5 mm. The trocar consists of an obturator and cannula with a blunt conical tip, adjacent to which there is a small hole connected to the trocar lumen, open to the exterior, so that penetration into the pleural cavity is signaled. Unlike the instruments for laparoscopy, this trocar does not have to be airtight. Air should be allowed to enter and leave the thoracic cavity freely. Examination will be limited by pain if the trocar is larger than 10 mm. Trocars are also available with diameters of 5 and 3.75 mm for performing thoracoscopy in children. In infants, optics and instruments similar to those used in infant rigid bronchoscopy are used.

**Figure 11.3** shows a selection of thoracoscopy instruments. Besides the biopsy forceps, needle biopsy, and suction catheter, the working channel also accommodates

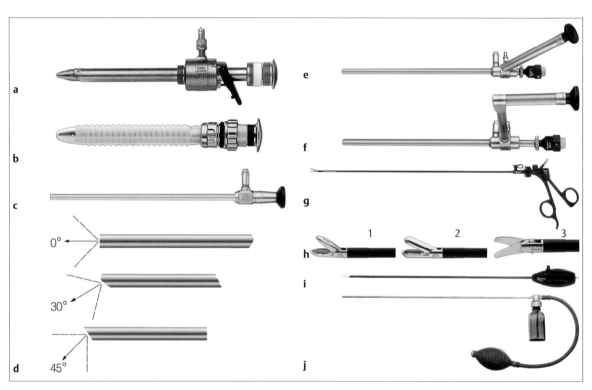

**Fig. 11.3**   Selection of instruments for rigid medical thoracoscopy. (Reprinted with kind permission from Karl Storz GmbH & Co. KG, Tuttlingen, Germany.)

**a** Trocar with multifunctional valve with insufflation stopcock, 11 mm, autoclavable.

**b** Trocar with silicone leaflet valve, 11 mm, autoclavable.

**c** Telescope, particularly suited for single-incision thoracoscopy, here with light shaft for photography, diameter 10 mm, length 31 cm, trocar size 11 mm.

**d** Various fields of view. (**1**) Straight-forward telescope 0°, diameter 10 mm, length 31 cm, autoclavable. (**2**) Forward-oblique telescope 30°, diameter 10 mm, length 31 cm, autoclavable. (**3**) Telescope 45°, diameter 10 mm, length 31 cm, autoclavable.

**e** Straight-forward telescope 0° with angled eyepiece, diameter 10 mm, working length 27 cm, with instrument channel 6 mm, trocar size 11 mm, single puncture.

**f** Straight-forward telescope 0°, with parallel eyepiece (bayonet optic), diameter 10 mm, working length 27 cm, with instrument channel 6 mm, trocar size 11 mm, single puncture.

**g** Dissecting and biopsy forceps, rotational, that can be dismantled, with connector pin for unipolar coagulation, 5 mm.

**h** Single-action jaws: (**1**) dissecting and biopsy forceps; (**2**) biopsy forceps; (**3**) scissors.

**i** Dissecting electrodes, with connector pin for unipolar coagulation, L-shaped, size 5 mm, working length 43 cm.

**j** Powder blower, with rubber bulb, size 5 mm, working length 42 cm.

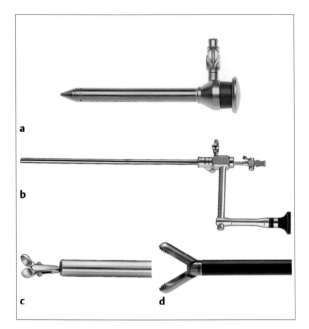

**Fig. 11.4** Selection of instruments for rigid medical thoracoscopy. (Reprinted with kind permission from Richard Wolf GmbH, Knittlingen, Germany.) **a** Trocar sleeve with lateral tap, metal, straight distal tip. **b** Straight-forward telescope with parallel eyepiece (bayonet optic). **c** Biopsy forceps with double-spoon jaws. **d** Grasping biopsy forceps.

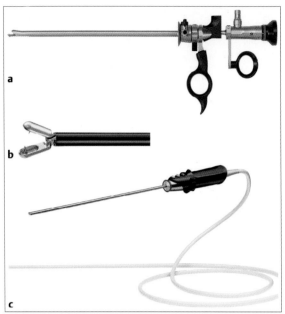

**Fig. 11.5** Selection of instruments for rigid medical thoracoscopy. (Reprinted with kind permission from Olympus Medical Systems Europa GmbH, Hamburg, Germany.) **a** Rigid optical biopsy forceps with 4-mm diameter OES Pro Telescope. **b** Biopsy forceps. **c** 5-mm scope with distal video chip (endo eye).

electrocautery. Thoracoscopes are available with various angles of vision including 0°, 45° or 90°. Direct viewing is more natural when moving the thoracoscope in a circular manner: most of the thoracic cavity can be viewed. With an oblique thoracoscope, one can also obtain a panoramic view of the whole chest cavity as well as of areas difficult to view. The 3- or 5-mm insulated coagulation forceps can be introduced through the working channel for biopsies. A bayonet optical system with an instrumentation channel and the appropriate instruments may facilitate directed fluid suction, electrocautery or directed insufflation of talc.

A xenon light source satisfies the requirements for high-quality visual exploration and video documentation.

The instruments of the German company Richard Wolf GmbH are very similar (**Fig. 11.4**). They are most commonly used with the two-entry-site technique. Since instruments used for laparoscopy are practically identical, laparoscopic equipment as produced, for example, by Olympus Corporation, can also be used for one-entry rigid medical thoracoscopy (**Fig. 11.5**).

Rigid minithoracoscopes (Tassi and Marchetti 2003) (or arthrocopes as used by Ash and Manfredi 1974) are much less suited for thoracoscopy since they have the disadvantage that a second point of entry is necessary for biopsy purposes and insertion of a large drainage catheter through the same channel post thoracoscopy is impossible (Janssen et al. 2003; Rodriguez-Panadero et al. 2006).

## The Semirigid (Semiflexible) Pleuroscope

A semirigid (semiflexible, flex-rigid) pleuroscope must satisfy two requirements:
1. To provide high-quality visual exploration and video documentation.
2. To allow multiple, large pleural biopsies of sufficient size to ensure a definitive histopathological diagnosis, while accommodating electrocautery when necessary.

The equipment used has been developed by the Japanese company Olympus in conjunction with pulmonologists for a single-puncture technique (Ernst et al. 2002; Lee and Colt 2005; Wang et al. 2008). These instruments comprise several parts, as discussed below.

### Pleuroscope

The semirigid pleuroscope (Pleuravideoscope model LTF-160 or -240 (Olympus, Japan) consists of a handle that is similar to the standard flexible bronchoscope, and a shaft that measures 7 mm in outer diameter and 27 cm in length (**Fig. 11.6**). The shaft is made up of two sections: a 22-cm proximal rigid portion and a 5-cm flexible distal end. The flexible tip is movable by a lever on the handle, which allows two-way angulation capability of 160° up and 130° down. It also has a 2.8-mm working channel that accommodates biopsy forceps, needles, and other

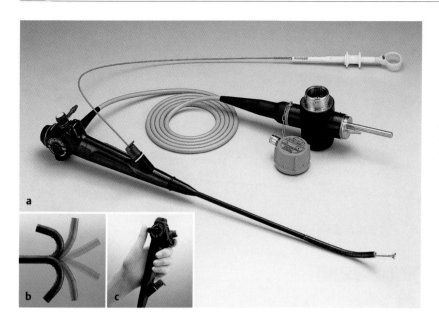

**Fig. 11.6    a** The semirigid (semi-flexible) pleuroscope (Olympus Corporation). Control section allows handling as with the flexible bronchoscope. **b** Angulation capability 160° upward/130° downward. **c** Diameter of the pleuroscope 7-mm, with a 2.8-mm diameter of the working channel. (Reprinted with kind permission from Olympus Corporation.)

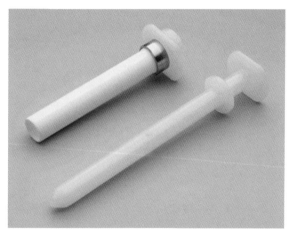

**Fig. 11.7**    Rigid trocar and cannula with valve for the semiflexible pleuroscope (Olympus). Outer diameter 10 mm, inner diameter 8 mm.

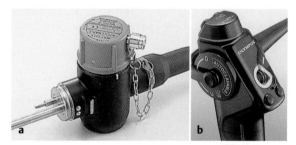

**Fig. 11.8    a** A dedicated, green waterproof cap protects the electrical connections of the LTF 160 pleuroscope during autoclaving. **b** Waterproof control section. (Reprinted with kind permission from Olympus Corporation.)

accessories, and is compatible with various electrosurgical and laser procedures. The instrument is used with a single-port technique. A single 1-cm skin incision that accommodates a disposable 8-mm inner diameter flexible trocar suffices (**Fig. 11.7**).

Moreover, the LTF 160 model allows autoclaving, thereby obviating important questions and issues related to asepsis (**Fig. 11.8a, b**). The other notable advantage of the semirigid pleuroscope over rigid instruments is that it interfaces easily with existing processors (CV-160, CLV-U40,) and light sources (CV-240, EVIS-100 or 140, EVIS EXERA-145 or 160) made by the manufacturer for flexible bronchoscopy or gastrointestinal (GI) endoscopy, which are available in most endoscopy units without additional cost (**Fig. 11.9**).

The optical quality allows excellent visual exploration as well as good video recording or photographic documentation. The flexible tip will allow various angles of vision, including straight-ahead and oblique angles of view. The lateral or oblique angles of view are essential to endoscopic examination. As with a bronchoscope, one very quickly becomes accustomed to movement of the tip simply by rotating the pleuroscope and manipulating the tip so that a superb panoramic view of the entire pleural cavity can be achieved.

### Forceps

The 3-mm forceps for biopsy under direct vision, using a single point of entry, is ideal for sampling the parietal pleura. The coagulation forceps is especially well suited for biopsy of the diaphragmatic pleura and thick, hard, or fibrous pleural lesions, including asbestosis pleural plaques (**Fig. 11.10a, b**). Other accessories for electrosurgical and laser procedures are shown in **Figure 11.11a–c**.

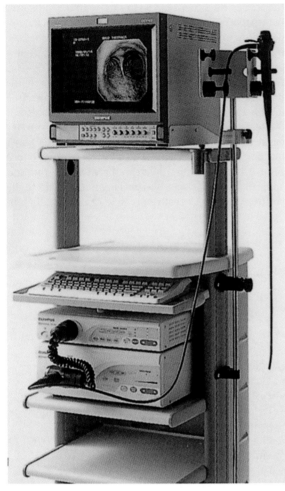

**Fig. 11.9** Light source, processor, and monitor used with the bronchovideoscope. (Reprinted with kind permission from Olympus Corporation.)

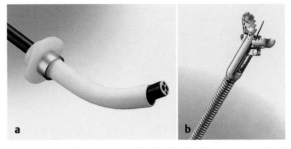

**Fig. 11.10 a** Pleuroscope with the flexible forceps, introduced through the trocar shaft. **b** Swing jaw needle forceps (alligator jaw type). (Reprinted with kind permission from Olympus Corporation.)

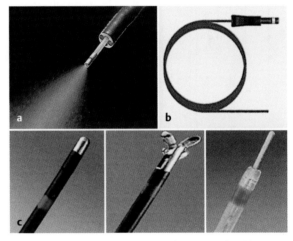

**Fig. 11.11** Additional accessories for electrosurgical and laser procedures that can be introduced through the semirigid (semiflexible) pleuroscope. **a** Spray catheter. **b** Argon plasma coagulation catheter (Erbe). **c** (Left to right) coagulation electrode, hot biopsy forceps, electrosurgical knife. (**a** and **c** reprinted with kind permission from Olympus Corporation.)

## Auxiliary Instruments and Accessories for Medical Thoracoscopy/Pleuroscopy

- Sterile sheets (e.g., Laparotomy Pack IV, Johnson & Johnson Medical Inc. Arlington TX, USA).
- Sterile gowns and gloves for the physician and assistant.
- Needles, syringes, local anesthetics, scalpels, 4 × 4, suture.
- Various forceps, needle holders, clamps, hemostats (usually all available in a chest tube insertion tray).
- Electrocautery/laser.
- Talc can or talc atomizer.
- Chest tubes between 24 F and 32 F (self-contained chest tube set with inner stylet).
- Underwater drainage systems.
- Anti-fog solution.

- Light sources, light cables.
- Video camera, video tapes, photo camera (optional).
- Manometer to measure pleural pressure (optional).
- Laser equipment (optional).
- Equipment for autofluorescence thoracoscopy or narrow-band imaging (optional).
- Pneumothorax apparatus and pneumothorax needles (optional).

Pneumothorax instruments that operate according to the principle of communicating tubes and utilize a water manometer are the simplest and least prone to malfunction. Electronic instruments, such as for filling the peritoneum, are unsuitable since they do not allow immediate switching from filling to suction. (See **Fig. 11.12** for a diagram of the historical pneumothorax apparatus.)

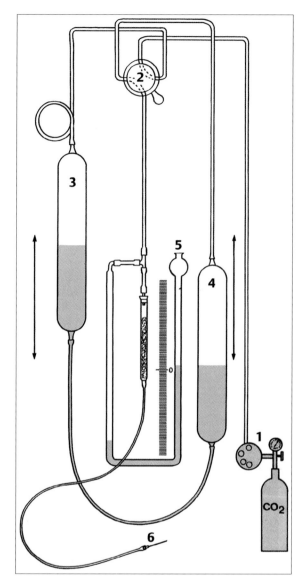

**Fig. 11.12** Schematic diagram of the pneumothorax apparatus according to the principle of communicating tubes in the position "fill." (**1**) $CO_2$ lung automat; (**2**) stopcock in position "fill"; (**3**) upper reservoir bottle from which water is draining; (**4**) lower reservoir bottle into which the water drains and thus pushes the fill gas through the pneumothorax needle into the fill gas tube; (**5**) water manometer which in the position "fill" indicates the back pressure before the pneumothorax needle into the fill gas tube; (**6**) cannula with pneumothorax needle. (From Brandt et al. 1985.)

The fluid reservoirs are graduated and filled with sterile water. By raising and lowering the bottles and appropriately setting the multidirectional stopcock, the filling gas can be directed from a gas reservoir or so-called Lung Automat (Dräger) directly from the compressed gas cylinder (if carbon dioxide is used as filling gas, this may minimize the effects of possible air embolism due to its more rapid absorption). By repeatedly changing the position of the bottles, the system can be flushed with the filling gas. In the stopcock position "fill," the water runs from the upper bottle into the lower one and as a result, pushes the filling gas into the nozzle and via the connecting tubing to the pneumothorax needle. While the gas is flowing, the attached water manometer shows the pressure in the tubing and needle. In the stopcock position "measure," the intrathoracic (intrapleural) pressure can be recorded. If the scales are graduated in centimeters, then positive or negative pressure can be read directly from the water manometer (the centimeter scale must be multiplied by 2 since it is the pressure *difference* between the two columns that is important). By switching the stopcock to the position "suction," negative pressure can be rapidly produced to provide suction.

# Phases of Medical Thoracoscopy/Pleuroscopy

- Preparation of the patient (information, fasting status, shaving of the skin).
- Premedication (optional).
- Radiographic review is mandatory in each patient.
- Positioning of the patient.
- IV line, nasal oxygen, ECG electrodes, blood pressure meter, oximeter.
- Choice of entry site on the basis of radiography/CT or ultrasound/fluoroscopy "on the table."
- Careful aspiration of fluids in case of pleural effusion.
- Insufflation (or spontaneous entrance) of air if necessary.
- Induction of pneumothorax if indicated.
- Careful local anesthesia plus sedation as needed.
- Introduction of the trocar.
- Inspection of the thoracic cavity using thoracoscope/pleuroscope.
- Documentation by photography or video.
- Insufflation of additional air/$CO_2$ into the pleural cavity if necessary.
- Section of adhesions preventing inspection if necessary.
- Obtaining multiple biopsy samples.
- Control of bleeding.
- Talc pleurodesis if necessary after additional analgesics.
- Systematic suction drainage.
- Surveillance during recovery.

## Patient Positioning

The patient lies usually on the healthy side in a lateral decubitus position with the involved side up; the head is resting on a pillow (**Fig. 11.13**). The patient's movement is minimized with cushioned support; the arm is raised over the head with the help of a sling. A rolled-up sheet or a pillow is placed on the table under the patient's flank, causing the spine to flex laterally, thus widening the intercostal spaces at the procedural site. This axillary roll also protects the brachial plexus provided it is not placed too high in the axilla.

The final position of the patient, e.g., in the case of localized lesions, will be determined by the chosen point of entry depending on the location of the lesion as shown by chest radiography/CT or ultrasound (see "Selecting the Point of Entry" below). **Figure 11.14** shows, by means of a CT image, how the force of gravity can be used to encourage the lung to fall out of the field of view. The most often used lateral position (**Fig. 11.14a**) provides the best view in cases of pleural effusion and diffuse lung disease. The prone position (**Fig. 11.14b**) is best for inspecting the posterior abnormalities. The supine position (**Fig. 11.14c**) is optimal for visualizing abnormalities of the lung, chest wall, and mediastinum located anteriorly.

A special situation is given for bilateral sympathectomy where the patient is placed in the supine position (see "Medical Thoracoscopic Sympathectomy," Chapter 3, p. 48 ff.).

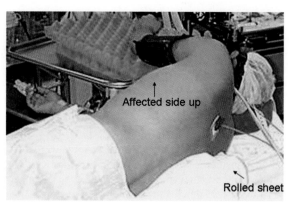

**Fig. 11.13** Patient lying in the lateral decubitus position with the healthy side up; the head rests on a pillow; the arm is raised over the head with the help of a sling; a rolled-up sheet is placed on the table under the patient's flank; the axillary roll protects the brachial plexus.

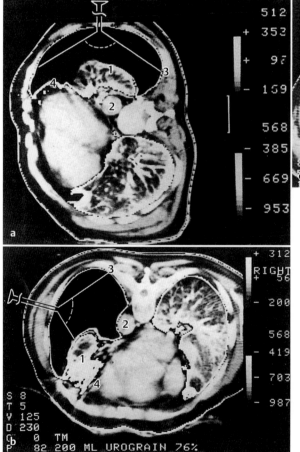

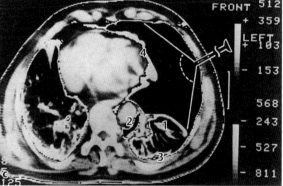

**Fig. 11.14** Computed tomography images with two-window technique at the level of the ninth thoracic vertebra in a patient with a complete, left-sided pneumothorax for the purpose of demonstrating the influence of position on the thoracoscopic visualization of various structures (CT: H. Witt, Berlin). (From Brandt et al. 1985.)

**a** *Lateral position:* If entered laterally, visualization of the lung surface (**1**) is optimum, of the anterior mediastinum (**4**) is partial, of the posterior mediastinum (**2**) is not possible, and of the paravertebral space (**3**) is fairly good.

**b** *Prone position:* The lung (**1**) has retracted and fallen forward. The dorsum of the posterior lung and mediastinum with aorta (**2**) and paravertebral space (**3**) are easily accessible via the lateral approach.

**c** *Supine position:* The lung falls toward the back. Complete visualization of the anterior mediastinum (**4**) and of the anterior portions of the lung (**1**) with lateral approach. The posterior mediastinum (**2**), and the paravertebral space (**3**) cannot be visualized.

## Selecting the Point of Entry

An axillary point of entry is selected as standard in most cases. The axillary triangle has no large muscle obstructing passage of the instruments: it is bordered anteriorly by the lower edge of the pectoralis major muscle, posteriorly by the anterior edge of the latissimus dorsi muscle, and inferiorly at the level of the diaphragmatic insertions. Its apex reaches the second intercostal space.

Thoracic and specifically intercostal anatomy is depicted on many of the figures included in the *Atlas* part. The skin overlies subcutaneous adipose tissue, which is superficial to the fascial lining of the intercostal muscles. Three layers of intercostal muscles lie over and between the ribs. Lining the inside of the thoracic cavity is the parietal pleura. The intercostal neurovascular bundle traverses the chest wall from the vertebral body around the circumference of the chest and again to the midline anteriorly in a depression on the inferior aspect of each rib, the intercostal groove. Obviously, in certain areas other muscle groups may be present between the skin and thoracic cage, such as the pectoralis group anteriorly and the latissimus dorsi posteriorly; thus the axillary triangle has no large muscles obstructing the passage of the instruments.

The point of entry is generally near the mid-axillary line, within this triangle. The final location of this insertion port will be determined by the indication: for pleural effusions most commonly in the fifth, sixth, or seventh intercostal space. The last two spaces are especially preferred when metastatic tumor and diffuse malignant mesothelioma are suspected to reach the most common sites of these malignancies. This provides an excellent view of both the diaphragm and the costovertebral gutter where malignant lesions (if present) will usually be reachable.

In case of spontaneous pneumothorax, the entry port will be located at the third or fourth intercostal space, to allow a thorough inspection of the lung apex and because a leak, if present, is usually in the upper lobe (see "The Place of Medical Thoracoscopy/Pleuroscopy in the Management of Pneumothorax," Chapter 3, p. 41 ff.).

### Point of Entry for Specific Localized Lesions

An axillary point of entry is selected in most cases. In the few exceptions, the site of entry depends on the anticipated location of the pathological lesion. To provide a good view of the lesion, the patient has to be placed in such a position that the lung falls out of the field of view (**Fig. 11.14a–c**).

The entry in the mid-axillary line at the level of the fourth or fifth intercostal space, in the lateral position, allows best the complete thoracic cavity inspection. Metastatic tumors or diffuse malignant mesothelioma are commonly found in the inferior costovertebral angles and on the diaphragmatic surfaces. Therefore, entry in the fifth or sixth or seventh intercostal space allows direct visualization of these lesions.

In unusual cases, other points of entry are used depending on the clinical setting and/or the chest radiography/CT or ultrasound results. For instance, the second or third anterior intercostal spaces are chosen in cases of pneumothorax when anterior and superior blebs are suspected; one must bear in mind that a pleural lesion that is too close to the point of entry cannot be viewed.

The lesion is approached most easily from the opposite side. Therefore, one should choose:

- For posterior lesions: the anterior axillary line.
- For anterior lesions: the posterior axillary line.
- For lateral lesions: the mid-clavicular line.

Every effort must be made to identify the precise level of the lesion on the radiograph/CT image so that the appropriate intercostal space can be used for the point of entry.

# Techniques for Introduction of the Endoscope in Pleural Effusion, Pneumothorax, and Other Conditions

The single-puncture technique is the easiest method to learn and is commonly used by pulmonologists. A double-puncture method will increase the diagnostic and therapeutic benefit of the procedure in selected cases. With the double-puncture method, the second site of entry is selected closer to the area of interest. This will permit the viewing of areas difficult to reach, such as the mediastinal pleural surfaces and the apex of the lung. This may also be facilitated by the use of the semirigid pleuroscope with its flexible tip.

However, one (or two) additional points of entry can be made under direct thoracoscopic guidance as needed. This may be the case when extensive adhesions are present (**Fig. 11.15**), when the single entry site does not allow for complete inspection or does not allow one to reach a suspect lesion for biopsy, when more elaborate procedures are indicated (e.g., extensive adhesiolysis, visceral pleural/lung biopsies, sympathicolysis, …), or when it is necessary to control hemorrhage after biopsy. When medical thoracoscopy is performed under general anesthesia, the two-port technique is most often used. The accessory instrumentation usually is passed through a 5- or 7-mm insulated trocar. The principles of biopsy of the parietal pleura are the same as described above. Usually, a 5-mm double-spoon insulated coagulation forceps is used (see "Biopsy Techniques", p. 89 ff.).

### Access to the Pleural Space

Since it is impossible to perform the procedure if the pleural space is completely obliterated, the lack of a sufficiently large pleural space is an absolute contraindication. Thus,

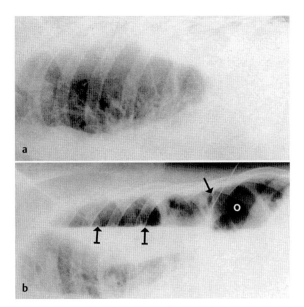

**Fig. 11.15** Radiological monitoring before and after induction of pneumothorax in pleural effusion with adhesions. **a** Fluoroscopy in the lateral decubitus position before induction. **b** After induction of pneumothorax, puncture needle (→) within the adhesions, air–fluid level (↦). Point of insertion (o) of the trocar away from the adhesions. (From Brandt et al. 1985.)

the most important prerequisite for medical thoracoscopy/pleuroscopy is a freely accessible pleural space that allows introduction of the trocar and thoracoscope/pleuroscope without injury to the lung or other organs (it should be recalled that the diaphragm lies in a much higher position in the supine patient than in the upright patient).

We list here some important points to be considered before the insertion of the thoracoscope/pleuroscope as well as several possibilities for providing a safe entry to the pleural space:

- A pleural symphysis can be suspected from the patient's history (previous pleurisy or thoracic surgery) or/and from imaging (radiography, CT, MRI, ultrasound, and/or fluoroscopy).
- A partial pneumothorax of at least 100–200 mL should be present or induced to permit the introduction of instruments without risk.
- The simplest access is available in case of a preexisting *complete pneumothorax.*
- If the preexisting *pneumothorax is only partial,* due to adhesions, these should be localized by the imaging techniques to avoid the introduction of the trocar in the area of the adhesions.
- In the presence of a *large pleural effusion,* the trocar can also be introduced directly without producing a pneumothorax (if fluid is readily aspirated as the pleural space is entered), although this may carry a somewhat greater risk of injury in case of unsuspected adhesions.
- In the presence of a *smaller pleural effusion,* a needle puncture should be performed at the level of greatest

opacification/dullness or, ideally, under sonographic (Macha et al. 1993; Hersh et al. 2003; Noppen 2003 b) or fluoroscopic guidance (Brandt et al. 1985; Loddenkemper 1998). When pleural fluid is aspirated, the syringe is removed from the needle and air will enter into the pleural space either spontaneously or when asking the patient to take a few deep breaths. The entry of air causes the lung to collapse away from the chest wall, and creates a pleural space for safe trocar insertion.

- Alternatively, if one is certain that the needle is well positioned in the pleural fluid (and not, for example, in the lung), air can be introduced into the pleural space by means of a syringe. Most often a few milliliters of air are sufficient to provide good ablation of the lung from the chest wall pleura.
- Some authors recommend aspirating 200–300 mL of fluid from the pleural cavity using a needle, angiocatheter, arrow thoracentesis catheter, or reusable Boutin pleural puncture needle (2 mm × 80 mm reusable trocar with side tap) and injecting an equivalent amount of ambient air (Lee and Colt 2005).
- Some experienced teams regularly perform MT/P in pleural effusions without any form of image-guided induction of a pneumothorax. In one series of more than 700 MT/P procedures conducted without preprocedural imaging of the entry site, induction of a pneumothorax was impossible in only 10 patients, due to extensive adhesions. No major complications such as bleeding were observed (Noppen 2003 b). Furthermore, in these cases biopsies could be performed using the extended thoracoscopy technique (Janssen and Boutin 1992) (see below).
- Greater safety is provided under ultrasound guidance, which allows the operator to localize the pleural effusion and to avoid transecting significant adhesions, with possible complications such as bleeding and injury to the lung, diaphragm, and other thoracic structures (Macha et al. 1993; Hersh et al. 2003; Noppen 2003 b).
- An alternative approach is fluoroscopy "on the table" after introducing air into the pleural cavity, which will show the air–fluid level as well as adhesions if present (**Fig. 11.15**). This is done with the patient in the lateral decubitus position and the hemithorax to be studied facing upward (**Fig. 11.16**) (Brandt et al. 1985; Mathur et al. 1994; Loddenkemper 1998).
- If it is difficult to aspirate pleural fluid, the pneumothorax can be induced with special pneumothorax needles (of different types, all with a blunt tip and a side hole as in the Deneke and Veress needles [**Fig. 11.17**], or the Saugmann or Boutin needles), under pressure control, ideally with a manometer or a pneumothorax apparatus (see **Fig. 11.12**).
- In case of difficulties in creating a pneumothorax because of *adhesions,* the blunt dissection technique is recommended, as first described by Janssen and Boutin

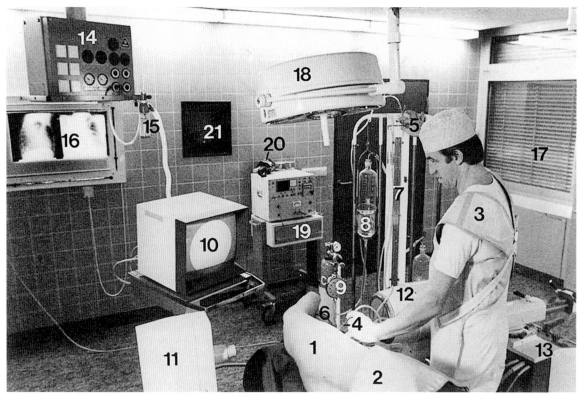

**Fig. 11.16** Set-up for induction of pneumothorax. (**1**) Patient in the lateral decubitus position with lead apron (**2**) on his abdomen. (**3**) Physician (the author) with lead apron. The left hand guides the pneumothorax needle (**4**), the right hand the stopcock (**5**) of the pneumothorax apparatus. In the field of view of the physician are: the patient's face (**6**), water manometer (**7**), meniscus of the graduated filling flask (**8**), lungautomat with $CO_2$ cylinder (**9**), monitor (**10**) of the radiographic image intensifier. (**11**) X-ray tube and (**12**) picture tube on the C arm which runs under the table. The radiography equipment (**13**) is controlled with a footswitch. (**14**) Central service unit with oxygen, compressed air and oxygen humidifier (**15**). (**16**) Radiograph view box with PA and lateral chest radiographs. (**17**) Window blind (**17**); (**18**) surgical light; (**19**) resuscitation unit with ECG monitor and defibrillator; (**20**) bag ventilator; (**21**) lead glass window for observation. (From Brandt et al. 1985.)

in 1992 as "extended thoracoscopy: a biopsy method to be used in case of pleural adhesions" (Janssen and Boutin 1992). This usually involves gentle dissection of the pleural adhesions with a finger to verify the existence of a free pleural space before advancing the instruments into the pleural space (Mares and Mathur 1997): The skin, subcutaneous tissues, intercostal muscles, periosteum of the ribs, and pleura are anesthetized as for the other techniques. The skin is incised superficial to the ribs below the desired interspace. A (Kelly) forceps is used for blunt dissection through the subcutaneous tissues, intercostal muscles, and pleura. Once the pleura is penetrated by the forceps, a finger is placed through the site and the nearby thoracic structures are palpated (**Fig. 11.18**). Palpation is performed to ensure that there are no pleural adhesions that would misdirect the trocar tube toward the lung and possibly cause the tube to penetrate the visceral pleura and enter the lung parenchyma. If fibrinous adhesions are found, they may be gently broken down with the probing finger. This ability to manually palpate the pleura and break down adhesions constitutes

one of the advantages of this particular technique. Disadvantages include the greater trauma to skin and intercostal muscles, with greater risk of bleeding. However, local control of bleeding can be more easily accomplished.

- If unbreakable, dense adhesions are felt, another point of entry should be selected (or the whole procedure should be stopped and a closed needle biopsy or a surgical approach substituted).

- In patients with *previous symptomatic pleural effusions* who have derived relief from chest tube drainage, MT/P can still be performed despite complete removal of fluid and reexpansion of the underlying lung. This is possible by first disconnecting the chest tube and opening it to the atmosphere while the patient takes in several deep breaths. The pneumothorax that ensues causes the lung to collapse away from the chest wall, thereby allowing safe insertion of the trocar (**Fig. 11.19**).

- The guide-wire technique, introduced for placement of a thoracostomy tube, has also been used and with this technique, also, commercially prepared kits are available in multiple sizes. Based on the Seldinger technique

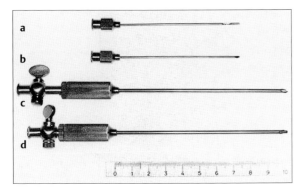

**Fig. 11.17** Pneumothorax needles. Denecke: **a** Side hole visible, **b** turned without side hole visible, Luer-Lock pneumothorax cannula; Veress: **c** Luer-Lock and tap with retracted inner cannula and **d** with the blunt inner cannula containing a side hole protruding. (From Brandt et al. 1985.)

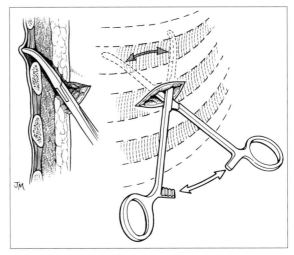

**Fig. 11.18** Schematic drawing of the access to the pleural cavity using a "Kelly" forceps for blunt dissection through the subcutaneous tissues, intercostal muscles, and pleura. Once the pleura is penetrated by the forceps, a finger is placed through the side and the nearby thoracic structures are palpated. (From P. Mathur in Beamis JF Jr, Mathur PN, eds. Interventional pulmonology. New York: McGraw-Hill; 1999. Reprinted with kind permission from McGraw-Hill.)

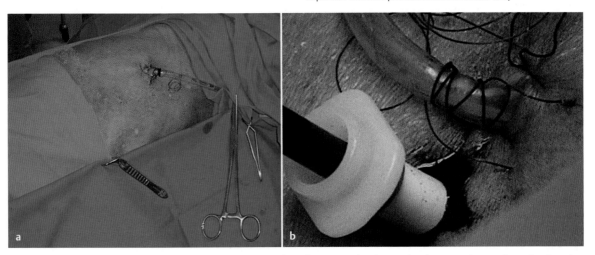

**Fig. 11.19** Pleuroscopy after chest tube drainage. **a** The chest tube is disconnected and opened to the atmosphere as the patient breathes spontaneously. A sterile field for the procedure is created. **b** After confirming the presence of pneumothorax, the trocar is inserted in the sixth intercostal space, a space below the chest tube.

for vascular catheter placement, a needle is first used to enter the pleural space in a similar fashion to the needle-over-catheter technique. The needle is oriented in the desired direction and the guide wire is advanced through the needle to a depth of several centimeters deeper than the needle tip. The needle is removed by retracting it along the length of the wire. Each dilator is serially placed over the guide wire to a depth to ensure dilation of the full thickness of the chest wall. Several dilators may be necessary to progressively enlarge the thoracostomy site to allow passage of a trocar of the desired size. Overall, this technique provides a rapid and minimally traumatic way to place thoracostomy tubes. However, there are some potential concerns. This technique is a relatively blind access to the pleural space, so the chance to manually palpate the pleura and break down adhesions or verify their absence is lost. Another possible concern is that the guide wire is relatively long and the free end of the wire might easily contact an object outside of the sterile field and potentially compromise the sterility of the procedure.

- If *neither effusion nor pneumothorax* is present (e.g., in diffuse lung disease), an artificial pneumothorax must be created either by the blunt dissection technique using the finger or by the technique of pneumothorax induction as introduced by Forlanini as early as 1888.

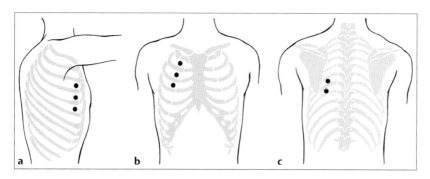

**Fig. 11.20** Typical sites for induction of a pneumothorax in order of preference. **a** In lateral decubitus position in the anterior axillary line from the third to the fifth ICS. **b** In supine position in the mid-clavicular line from the first to the third ICS. **c** In prone position in the midscapular line immediately adjacent to the abducted scapula from the sixth to the seventh ICS. (From Brandt et al. 1985.)

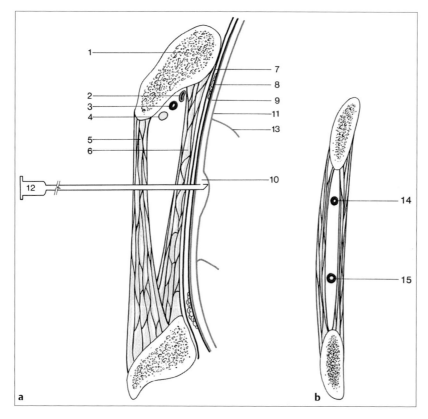

**Fig. 11.21** Correct position of the pneumothorax needle and anatomy of the intercostal nerve. **a** Section through the chest wall in the anterior axillary line showing correct position of the pneumothorax needle (Denecke) in the pleural space. Injury to the intercostal artery is very unlikely because it lies protected in the intercostal sulcus. The intercostal nerve is located caudally at the rib margin and is accessible for local anesthesia. **b** Section through the intercostal space in the mid-clavicular line. The artery has divided into a cranial and caudal branch so that needle puncture at right angles to the chest wall is virtually free of risk.

**1** Rib; **2** intercostal vein; **3** intercostal artery; **4** intercostal nerve; **5** external intercostal muscle; **6** internal intercostal muscle; **7** intercostal fascia; **8** internal endothoracic fascia with pleural fat tissue; **9** parietal pleura; **10** pleural space; **11** visceral pleura; **12** pneumothorax needle with side hole in the pleural space; **13** interlobular pleura (endopleura); **14** ramus cranial intercostal artery; **15** ramus caudal intercostal artery. (From Brandt et al. 1985.)

Although this technique of pneumothorax induction (in the past mainly applied for pneumothorax treatment of tuberculosis) is nowadays rarely used, it will be described here in detail, since it is difficult to find a description in the newer literature (see the description of the pneumothorax apparatus under "Auxiliary Instruments and Accessories for Medical Thoracoscopy/Pleuroscopy" above).

**Figure 11.20a–c** shows the best sites for inducing the pneumothorax depending upon the position of the patient. The lateral thoracic region in the third, fourth, and fifth intercostal spaces (see **Fig. 11.20a**) are best because the intercostal vessels are well protected by the rib margins (**Fig. 11.21a**). More anteriorly, arterial branches lie both above and below the edge of the ribs and are therefore more readily injured (**Fig. 11.21b**). The paramediastinal area should also be avoided because of the internal mammary artery, the axillary region because of the lateral

thoracic artery, and the infraclavicular fossa, which contains the subclavian artery. In supine position, the mid-clavicular line from the first to the third ICS should be selected (see **Fig. 11.20b**). The region of the diaphragm is unsuitable, not only because adhesions are frequent but also because the liver or spleen may be accidentally injured. A pneumothorax may be induced in the mid-scapular line (see **Fig. 11.20c**) if, in the prone position, the scapula falls obliquely forward. However, the thickness of the skin of the back usually requires that an incision be made after infiltration with local anesthetic before the needle can be introduced. Special pneumothorax needles with a side hole are used (see **Fig. 11.17**).

If a pneumothorax apparatus is used (**Fig. 11.12**, **Fig. 11.16**) immediately prior to establishing the pneumothorax, the pneumothorax needle is flushed with a filling gas since obstruction or even a small amount of humidity in the needle could prevent optimal monitoring of the needle position. With the stopcock in the "fill" position, the needle lumen is held near the eye, allowing a stream of air to be easily felt. When the stopcock is turned to the "measure" position, the system pressure should immediately fall to zero.

After sterile preparation, the skin of the intercostal space is fixated with two fingers and the needle is inserted through the cutis at right angles with a short jab. Then, with the stopcock in the "measure" position, the needle is slowly advanced up to the internal thoracic fascia. There, a slight negative pressure is measured. Upon gently perforating the internal thoracic fascia and the pleura, the sensation of resistance to the needle is suddenly overcome, and at the same time the patient experiences a short, sharp pain. **Figure 11.21a, b** shows schematically the anatomical situation and the correct intrapleural position of the pneumothorax needle.

In the presence of a patent pleural space, the breathing-related negative pleural pressure should lie between $-15$ and $-5$ cm $H_2O$ (1 cm $H_2O \approx 1$ mbar). Briefly turning the stopcock to "fill" will introduce a few milliliters of filling gas. The resulting positive system pressure should, after switching to "measure," again immediately indicate negative pressure swings. The pneumothorax can now be filled under fluoroscopic monitoring optionally, interrupted only briefly from time to time to assess the slowly decreasing negative pressure. If the patient complains of feeling unwell, associated with a rise in intrathoracic positive pressure, the discomfort can be rapidly relieved by switching the stopcock to position "suction." A 4–5 cm pneumothorax is sufficient. If no positive pressure results, 1–2 L of filling gas may be introduced without difficulty. Possible adhesions noted at fluoroscopy are marked on the chest wall (**Fig. 11.15**).

The pressure swings in the water manometer at various stages during the procedure are shown in **Figure 11.22**. The slightly negative pressure noted before penetrating the internal thoracic fascia would, during an attempt to induce filling in that position, immediately change to a persistent positive pressure.

As previously noted, a clearly negative pressure with free movement of the water manometer during respiration is always seen when the needle is in the pleural space. If the needle enters the lung, as may occur whether the pleural space has been obliterated or not, a weakly negative pressure is again seen, although usually without free movement of the water manometer column during respiration. Furthermore, the negative pressure does not stabilize since the filling gas is continually lost via the airways (the most serious complication of pneumothorax induction is air or gas embolism; see Chapter 9, p. 60). Should the peritoneal cavity be entered in error, paradoxical respiratory pressure variations occur because during inhalation positive pressure is seen and during exhalation negative pressure develops.

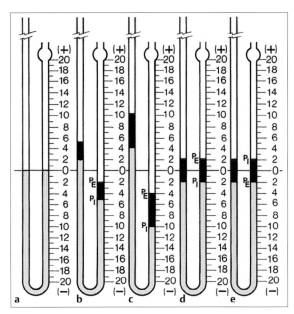

**Fig. 11.22** Schematic diagram of the water manometer of the pneumothorax apparatus. Testing the position of the needle tip during induction of pneumothorax in the "measure" position. The tip of the arrow indicates the end inspiratory pressure ($P_I$) and the end expiratory pressure ($P_E$). Water levels are for the water manometer during quiet spontaneous respiration. The pressures indicated in centimeters should be doubled, since the pressures indicate the *difference* in cm $H_2O$ between the water levels. Typical manometer deflections according to the location of the needle opening. **a** Needle subcutaneous, no deflections. **b** Needle before the endothoracic fascia; minimal negative deflections; administration of filling gas produces immediate positive pressure. **c** Needle opening intrapleural; free movement of the water level between pressures of $-8$ to $-20$ cm $H_2O$; on administration of filling gas, the pressure changes only slowly. **d** Needle lies in the lung parenchyma; minimal deviations about zero; on administration of filling gas, no change in pressure difference. **e** Needle lies intraperitoneally; minor deviations around zero; paradoxical pressure changes in relation to breathing; on inspiration, the pressure becomes positive and on expiration it becomes negative. (From Brandt et al. 1985.)

- If a pneumothorax apparatus and carbon dioxide are used, the pneumothorax should be induced immediately before undertaking medical thoracoscopy/pleuroscopy, because the gas will be absorbed rapidly. Fluoroscopy allows evaluation of adhesions between the lung and chest wall that might complicate introduction of the thoracoscope (**Fig. 11.15**).
- Some authors may alternatively induce the pneumothorax the same day or the day before the procedure (Boutin et al. 1991). This would allocate ample time to pressure measurements, and the presence of pleural obliteration is more likely to be anticipated. It also would reduce the actual time spent in a busy operating/endoscopy room or even clarify whether the thoracoscopy is not possible at all due to extensive pleural symphysis. It may also be desirable to induce the pneumothorax on the previous day when general anesthesia

is planned, so that a general anesthetic is not given unnecessarily to a patient with an obliterated pleural space.

## Anesthesia for Medical Thoracoscopy/Pleuroscopy

The anesthesia technique varies: MT/P is commonly performed under local anesthesia with moderate sedation, which is quite well tolerated by patients. The term "conscious sedation" is widely used in the literature, and refers to patients who remain awake or arousable during the procedure while given mild anxiolytics and pain medications (Rodriguez-Panadero et al. 2006). With conscious sedation, an anesthetist is not needed, which saves costs.

MT/P, in contrast to VATS, does not normally require tracheal intubation with either a single- or double-lumen tube. However, general anesthesia may be preferable in some special indications, such as in case of idiosyncratic or allergic sensitivities to local anesthetics, in very anxious or uncooperative patients including children, or for advanced procedures such as sympathectomy and others.

An excellent alternative today is intravenously administered propofol (with or without premedication), which provides sedation similarly to midazolam but with a faster onset of action and a more rapid recovery (Clarkson et al. 1993; Clark et al. 2009).

MT/P may be a painful and unpleasant procedure:
- Unpleasant because of the position of the patient, instrument manipulations, and vagus-mediated reflexes (which can occasionally produce hypoventilation, hypotension, and syncope).
- Painful during certain well-defined periods:
  - at the beginning of local anesthesia
  - during examination, i.e., by the pressure of the endoscope acting as a lever on the ribs
  - during removal of adhesions by coagulation
  - at biopsies of the parietal pleura
  - in particular, in the minutes following the insufflation of talc
  - at insertion of the chest tube and its suturing to the skin.

Thus, moderate sedation in addition to local anesthesia is useful for the following reasons:
- To improve patient comfort.
- To suppress pain.
- To induce amnesia of the procedure.
- To improve conditions for the physician by preventing motor reactions and diminishing cough reflexes.

The recommended steps are as follows:
- **Preanesthesia examination:** In addition to pulmonary examination, a clinical cardiovascular examination and ECG and routine blood work, including for hemostasis, is performed. Blood gases are useful to identify hypoxemia and hypercapnia. Physicians should use their judgment for other associated tests similarly to other endoscopies they perform. The patient is asked to refrain from eating and drinking 6–8 hours before the procedure to reduce the risk of aspiration.
- **Preparation of the patient:** The best "premedication" is an explanation of the procedure, starting with the pneumothorax induction to the postoperative phase. All details that worry the patient should be explained, including chest pain and the chest drain.
- **Premedication** (both optional) with atropine to minimize the chance of vasovagal reaction and/or with hydrocodone to suppress coughing (which, combined with midazolam, markedly reduces cough during flexible bronchoscopy without causing significant desaturation (Stolz et al. 2004).
- **Patient in the suite:** Once the patient is in decubitus position, an ECG monitor, intravenous fluids of normal saline on the arm opposite the procedure, automated blood pressure cuff, and pulse oximetry are placed ($SaO_2$ is noted in decubitus position before sedation as well as before and after placement of a nasal oxygen prong).
- **Placement of the patient:** Then the patient is placed in the lateral decubitus position, the upper arm is cleared of the hemithorax being examined and attached in a vertical position on a flexible and mobile support, which can be moved if it interferes with the operator. Meticulous placement of the patient is indispensable since discomfort is a frequent cause of patient agitation.
- **Induction of medication** is performed during cleaning and preparation of the operating field. It consists of a combination of an analgesic (e.g., morphine, demerol or fentanyl) and/or a sedative (e.g., propofol, midazolam). The medication should be titrated to patient comfort without compromising respiration (Migliore et al. 2002).
- According to the patient's reactions (movement, respiratory rate) during skin injection for the local anesthesia and insertion of the trocar, reinjections of morphine and/or midazolam/propofol can be given (usually older patients experience less pain than younger ones).
- Other thoracoscopists may prefer IV propofol and assisted ventilation either with laryngeal mask airway or single-lumen endotracheal tube.
- Table 11.**3** lists in detail all drugs used during and after medical thoracoscopy/pleuroscopy as well as their actions, route/dose, onset, duration, and adverse effects, and in addition the antagonistic drugs.

## Technique of Local Anesthesia

The recommended steps for the performance of local anesthesia are as follows:

**Table 11.3**   Drugs for use during and after medical thoracoscopy/pleuroscopy

| Drug | Actions | Route/dose | Onset | Duration | Adverse effects |
|---|---|---|---|---|---|
| **Sedatives** | | | | | |
| Benzodiazepines | Sedation<br>Anterograde<br>Amnesia<br>Antiepileptic | | | | Respiratory depression<br>Hypotension |
| Midazolam | | IV, IM<br><br>5–10 mg<br>(0.075 mg/kg) | IV: 5 min<br><br>IM: 15 min | IV, IM: 2 h<br><br>2 h | IV, IM: Paradoxical aggression |
| Diazepam | | IV: 5–10 mg<br>IM: not advised<br>PO: 5–10 mg | IV: < 3 min<br>IM: 15 min to hours | IV: min to hours | Coma at high doses<br>Thrombophlebitis |
| Narcotics | Analgesia<br>Sedation<br>Anxiolysis<br>Antitussive | | | | Respiratory depression<br>Drowsiness<br>Seizures<br>Bronchospasm<br>Bradycardia<br>Hypotension<br>Nausea, vomiting<br>Constipation<br>Biliary spasm |
| Morphine | | IV, IM, SC<br>1–10 mg | IV: 5 min<br>IM: 15 min<br>SC: 30 min | 1–4 h | |
| Fentanyl | | IV, IM<br><br>50–100 µg | IV: 2 min<br><br>IM: 10–15 min | 30–45 min | Adverse effects less common than with morphine |
| Alfentanil | | IV, IM<br>250–1000 µg | < Fentanyl | < Fentanyl | Similar to fentanyl |
| Sufentanil | | IV, IM<br>5–70 µg | < Fentanyl | < Fentanyl | Similar to fentanyl |
| Propofol | Sedation | IV<br>50 µg/kg/min | < 1 min | 10 min | Respiratory depression<br>Hypotension<br>Bradycardia |
| **Antagonists** | | | | | |
| Naloxone<br>(Narcotic antagonist) | | IV 1–4 µg/kg | < 1 min | 30 min | Tachycardia<br>Hypertension |
| Flumazenil<br>(Benzodiazepine) | Reversal<br>of sedation | IV | 5 min | 1–4 h | |

- The previously marked site of entry in the intercostal space is palpated with the index and middle finger of one hand.
- Between the two fingers a syringe with 20 mL of 2% lidocaine attached to a small-bore needle (25 or 27 gauge, ½ inch) for intradermal injection produces a small wheal (approx. 0.2 mL).
- The local anesthetic is infiltrated subcutaneously and in the intercostal muscle down to the parietal pleura, using a larger needle (0.8 or 0.9 mm). The path of the needle should be kept perpendicular to the chest wall to ensure that the entire path of the instruments will be pain free. This deeper anesthetic should only be injected after the plunger has been withdrawn partially to ensure that the needle has not penetrated a vascular structure.
- As the needle penetrates the parietal pleura, the patient usually experiences transient pain. Entry into the pleural cavity is confirmed by drawing back on the syringe, which will fill with air or pleural fluid (when aspirating pleural fluid, it is advisable to change the needle and syringe because of the risk of implanting tumor cells in the chest wall).
- The depth, established as a result of withdrawing the needle until the gas bubbles are no longer obtained, later serves as an indication for placement of the trocar.
- At this location of the parietal pleura, about 8–10 mL of lidocaine is infiltrated. Subsequently, the caudal rim of the upper rib is infiltrated to anesthetize the intercostal nerve as well as the periosteum of the rib itself, while taking care, again by repeated aspiration, that the tip of the needle is not located in the adjacent intercostal artery.
- A further lidocaine depot of about 8–10 mL is then injected around the cranial rim of the lower rib.

### Additional Technical Suggestions

- Local anesthesia is administered with care for each site of entry with 1% or 2% lidocaine (optionally with epinephrine when there are no cardiovascular contraindications).
- Maneuvers that are known to cause the most pain (in particular insufflation of talc) require a preventive injection of morphine.
- Monitoring results of cardiac rate, blood pressure, and respiratory rate are noted at least every 5 minutes. $SaO_2$ is continuously monitored and nasal oxygen is provided as needed.
- The procedure may cause hypoxia for several reasons: depression due to the anesthesia, healthy lung in the lateral decubitus position, and collapse of the investigated lung due to the induced pneumothorax.
- Most frequently, agitation and coughing may interfere with the procedure; additional morphine will help with this problem.

- Apnea is very rarely encountered.
- When the patient snores in a deep sleep due to relaxation of the pharyngeal muscles, it is sufficient to pull the lower jaw toward the front to clear the airways, or if necessary, insert a pharyngeal cannula.
- Arrhythmia: a few extra systolic beats may be noted when the pericardium is touched.
- Mediastinal shift: when air is injected (under pressure) into the hemithorax, the amplitude of ECG tracing will vary with respiratory movements. The operator should decompress the hemithorax.
- At the end of the procedure the lung should be very slowly expanded back to the chest wall by gentle negative pressure suction.
- For recovery (see "Antagonists" in **Table 11.1**), the patient can be immediately woken with flumazenil, a benzodiazepine antidote. However, since flumazenil has a shorter action than that of midazolam, there is a risk of the patient going back to sleep with the need for reinjection of flumazenil in the recovery room. Morphine is reversed by naloxone.
- Observation in the recovery room is obligatory as for any anesthetized patient. Continuous oxygenation can be titrated down according to need. The intravenous line is maintained for the next few hours until the patient is fully awake.
- It is mandatory to prescribe a postoperative analgesia.

## Performance of Rigid Thoracoscopy

The physician and assistant clean their hands with the standard surgical scrub technique and then put on a sterile gown and gloves. Every patient is monitored with automated blood pressure monitoring and cardiac and cutaneous oxygen saturation monitors. The patient's skin is prepared by shaving and disinfecting a large area to include from the sternum to the clavicle and across the axilla past the scapula to the spinous processes and down to the base of the thorax. Then the patient is covered with sterile sheets. Usually, the thoracoscopist faces the patient during the procedure (but may change the position if needed), while the assistant is across the table. Then the following steps are taken:

- With a scalpel, a vertical incision is made through the skin and subcutaneous tissue, appropriate to the size of the trocar tube used, usually of approximately 10 mm, parallel with and in the middle of the selected intercostal space (**Fig. 11.23**).
- The incision is relatively small so that the trocar fits tightly and bleeding from the incision is automatically stopped due to the resulting compression.
- The handle of the trocar should be held firmly in the palm of the hand, while the extended index finger, for safety's sake, limits the depth of insertion previously established with the local anesthetic needle.

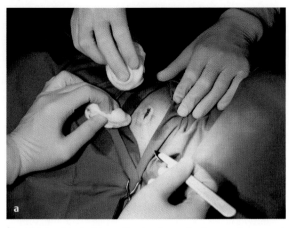

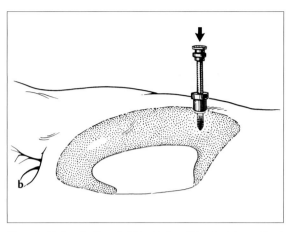

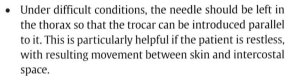

**Fig. 11.23** Skin incision after local anesthesia, usually approximately 10 mm, parallel with and in the middle of the selected intercostal space (**a**). The trocar being placed in the pleural cavity (**b**).

(From P. Mathur in Beamis JF Jr, Mathur PN, eds. Interventional pulmonology. New York: McGraw-Hill; 1999. Reprinted with kind permission from McGraw-Hill.)

- Under difficult conditions, the needle should be left in the thorax so that the trocar can be introduced parallel to it. This is particularly helpful if the patient is restless, with resulting movement between skin and intercostal space.
- While fixating the intercostal space with two fingers, the trocar is advanced in a corkscrew motion until the sudden release of resistance is felt.
- Optional: Blunt dissection is performed with a hemostat through the intercostal muscles and parietal pleura.
- The process is identical to inserting a chest tube, with the exception that a tunnel is not created as this would limit the mobility of the thoracoscope.
- Optional: Once the parietal pleura is opened the index finger should examine the pleural cavity and confirm an adequate pleural space.
- Alternatively, the adequate size of the pleural space (and the presence of possible adhesions) can be confirmed by fluoroscopy during the pneumothorax induction (**Fig. 11.14**).
- Once the trocar is in the pleural cavity (**Fig. 11.23b**), the operator can hear the movement of air into and out of the pleural cavity synchronously with the patient's breathing.
- Pressure equilibrium with the atmosphere is established quickly.
- The cannula should lie 1–3 cm within the pleural cavity and be held in position by the assistant. If the trocar is not handled carefully, it might injure the lung.
- If the patient coughs, the assistant will withdraw the cannula within the chest wall, since the cough may have been induced by touching the lung.
- After removal of the trocar, the thoracoscope with a 0° angle is placed in the cannula (**Fig. 11.24**). After removal of the optic, the valve closes and this again results in a closed pneumothorax. This is particularly important in patients with effusion since otherwise pleural fluid

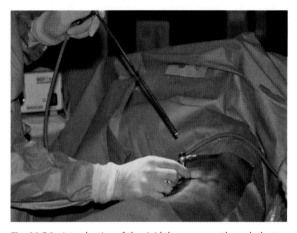

**Fig. 11.24** Introduction of the rigid thoracoscope through the trocar.

may be coughed out. In the absence of pleural effusion, the valve is not needed, but without it there is no protection against cough.
- The thoracoscope (**Fig. 11.25**) is advanced into the pleural cavity under direct vision through the trocar (**Fig. 11.24**).
- The pleural space can be inspected through the thoracoscope/pleuroscope, either directly (**Fig. 11.25**) or indirectly by video (**Fig. 11.26**).
- The pleural fluid is removed with a suction catheter placed through the working channel (or with a larger catheter directly introduced through the cannula).
- The thoracoscope is advanced toward the back and directed toward the diaphragm and the costophrenic angle.
- After completely removing the fluid, a systematic exploration of the chest cavity is performed by maneuvering the thoracoscope. In difficult cases, oblique telescopes are valuable to ensure adequate pleural inspection.

- The orientation is simple, although fine adhesions resembling spiders' webs may interfere with complete examination of the pleural cavity. These can be mechanically separated.
- However, fibrous bands or vascular adhesions should be avoided and can, if necessary, be cauterized by electrocautery.
- Optional: Air can be cautiously introduced to further collapse the lung and improve the inspection of the pleural cavity, but extreme care must be taken to avoid iatrogenic tension pneumothorax and subcutaneous emphysema when insufflating air into the pleural cavity.

The techniques used for sympathectomy and for pericardial fenestration are described separately in the sections of Chapter 3, pp. 48 ff. and 50.

### Direct and Video-Controlled Inspection

The pleural space can be inspected through the thoracoscope, either directly or indirectly by video. Historically, direct-vision telescopes were used (**Figs. 11.13** and **11.25**). Today, most if not all centers use video assistance (**Figs. 11.1** and **11.26**). This allows for a technically easier and safer (sterility!) procedure, allows others in the room to follow the procedure (didactive purposes), and generally produces images of significantly superior quality. Since video equipment and processors are available in most modern pulmonology departments, direct visualization will become obsolete (the commercially available pleuroscope is already a videoscope).

After induction of a pneumothorax, a 7- or 9-mm trocar is inserted in the pleural cavity. The thoracoscopes are introduced through the trocar (see **Fig. 11.24**). To prevent the lenses from fogging up, immerse the tip of the rigid telescope in warm sterile saline or use a defogging agent.

Once the pleural cavity is entered, almost complete visualization of the pleural cavity and lung is possible, if there are no pleural adhesions present. The 0° optics are best for the initial overview. Most thoracoscopists will use the 0° telescope for the initial overview. It allows inspection of most of the pleural cavity using a "natural," circular movement. Oblique angle telescopes may be used for a more panoramic, "periscope-like" viewing of the pleural cavity, if needed. Visual exploration can be performed in a few minutes. The entire pleural surface should be inspected in a systematic fashion including the parietal pleura of the chest wall, diaphragm, lung, mediastinum, heart, and vascular structures.

Anatomical relationships and intrathoracic structures are usually well recognized:
- The orientation on the right can be achieved by locating the point where the three lobes meet, the junction of the oblique fissure and horizontal fissure.
- On the left, the oblique fissure can be used for orientation.
- The diaphragm can be recognized because of the respiration-related movement.
- Ribs, intercostal muscles, fat, blood vessels, and nerves are usually well distinguished.
- The positions of the large vessels such as on the left the aorta and subclavian, and on the right the vena cava and the innominate vein as well as the subclavian artery, are readily recognized (**Figs. 10.1** and **10.2**).
- The heart and the great vessels are identified due to the pulsation, occasionally transmitted to adjacent parts of the lung.

In case of a large pleural effusion, the fluid should be aspirated completely and not too hastily; without risk of development of immediate reexpansion edema, as long as air is allowed to enter the pleural space to replace the aspirated volume (equal pressure procedure).

A probe or the optical forceps enables the physician to push aside any fibrinous strands interfering with clear view. If necessary, firm adhesions should be divided by electrocautery. In some situations, pleuroscopy with the

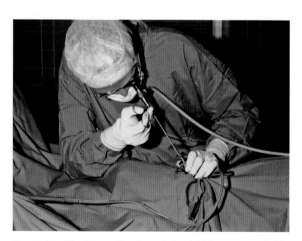

**Fig. 11.25**   Direct inspection through the rigid thoracoscope (while taking a biopsy).

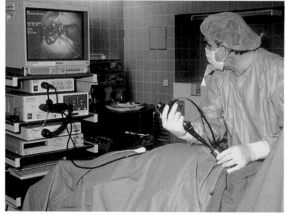

**Fig. 11.26**   Indirect, video-controlled inspection of the pleural cavity through the semiflexible pleuroscope.

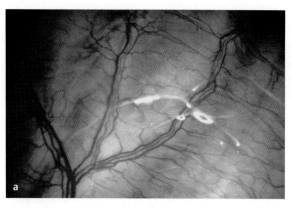 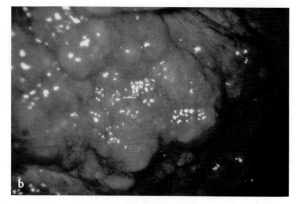

**Fig. 11.27**    **a** In its normal state, the pleura is transparent, allowing the visualization of ribs, fat, and vessels through it. **b** Extensive "mushroom" lesions, typical of malignant pleural invasion.

flexible tip may allow one to look into the area behind the adhesions.

In its normal state the pleura is transparent, allowing visualization of many structures through it. Variable amounts of anthracotic pigment can occasionally be seen within the parietal pleura. Fatty collections are often abundant in the pleura. These are long, yellowish plaques located along the ribs and around the pericardium and diaphragm. Extensive pleural disease is easily recognized, but localized disease or small, isolated nodules may be overlooked.

One of the hardest tasks for the endoscopist is to distinguish between innocuous inflammation and malignancy. It is almost impossible to tell the difference merely by visual observation. Certain patterns of pleural lesions can be seen: lymphangitis appears as a fine reticular pattern, covering part of the pleura; granulomata are 1–3 mm in diameter, seen with tuberculosis or sarcoidosis; and malignant nodules are variable in size and shape (fluorescent light [Chrysanthidis and Janssen 2005] or narrow-band imaging [Schönfeld et al. 2009; Ishida et al. 2009; Froudarakis and Noppen 2009] might improve the identification of suspicious areas).

The lung looks like a cone, narrowing at the apex. Variable adhesions between the visceral and parietal pleura may be seen. When the lung is normal, the surface is pink and soft, with a reticular pattern demarcating the pulmonary lobules, and black anthracotic pigment is scattered over the surface. The visceral pleural surface is transparent. Areas of atelectasis are purplish red with a clear edge. Malignant nodules and other typical pathologies are quite easily seen, as are emphysematous blebs/bullae protruding from the surface (see *Atlas* section).

The observation should be performed from a distance to obtain a panoramic view and then from distance of 1–2 cm for inspection of the cavity very carefully to select the best biopsy sites. Suspicious areas are biopsied through the working channel of the thoracoscope using either a 3- or 5-mm biopsy forceps (see "Biopsy Techniques" below). All abnormalities are systematically recorded.

## Biopsy Techniques

Biopsies of the parietal pleura will be performed in most MT/Ps performed for the diagnosis of unexplained pleural effusions. In its normal state, the pleura is transparent, allowing the visualization of ribs, fat, and vessels through it (**Fig. 11.27a**). Chronic pleural inflammation may lead to a thickened, nontransparent pleura. Malignant lesions often have a characteristic "mushroom" appearance (**Fig. 11.27b**), but it may be impossible to differentiate thickened pleura from malignant invasion, e.g., in case of mesothelioma (**Fig. 15.9** in the *Atlas* section). Multiple biopsies are therefore often necessary. If lesions are present on the parietal pleura, rather than visceral pleural lesions, these should be biopsied, thus avoiding the risk for prolonged air leak.

Before pleural biopsy, the rib and intercostal space should be identified with a blunt probe. If the pleura is thick, the rib will feel hard compared with the spongy intercostal space. If possible, biopsies should always be taken against a rib, minimizing the risk of vessel or nerve injury. However, when the pleura is thick, taking the biopsy is simple with minimal risk of injuring the intercostal arteries. By contrast, when the pleura is thin, the biopsy should certainly be performed against one of the ribs.

Parietal pleural biopsies can be taken with the single-port single-instrument rigid technique, using an optical biopsy forceps with an attached 4-mm telescope (**Fig. 11.28**) or through the pleuroscope (**Fig. 11.29**). Using an optical biopsy forceps, the parietal pleura is grasped and gently pulled toward the operator. It is then pulled sideways, and in a shearing motion a "strip" of pleura can be isolated. Sometimes, large specimens several centimeters long can be obtained in this way.

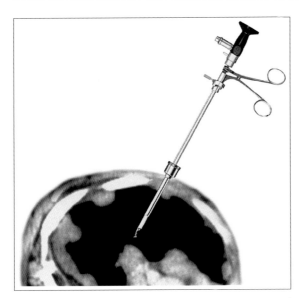

**Fig. 11.28**  Diagram superimposed on a CT image showing several malignant lesions of the parietal pleura from which biopsies can be taken under visual control through the thoracoscope.

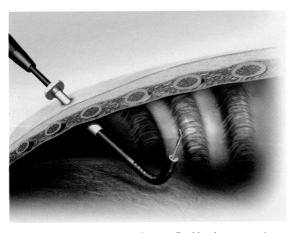

**Fig. 11.29**  Drawing showing the semiflexible pleuroscope introduced through the trocar shaft into the pleural cavity. The flexible forceps is introduced through the pleuroscope and directed toward the parietal pleura for taking a biopsy. (Reprinted with kind permission from Olympus Corporation.)

Typically two to six biopsies of a suspicious pleural lesion will establish a diagnosis. Sufficient quantities of tissue must be obtained, especially if hormonal receptor studies are required for tumors such as carcinoma of the breast. In the presence of undiagnosed pleural effusions, biopsies should be taken at a minimum from macroscopically suspicious lesions at the anterior and posterior chest wall and the diaphragm for histological evaluation, and, if suspicious for tuberculosis, also for mycobacterial culture.

When malignancy is suspected but the endoscopic findings are nonspecific, the total number of biopsies should be increased to up to 10–12 from a variety of areas

on the pleural surface (in the future, autofluorescence as well as narrow-band imaging might be helpful in identifying suspicious areas). Attention should be paid to fibrinous tissue/nodules that may mask malignant pleural lesions. These should be removed with the forceps, and the biopsy taken from the base of the lesion. Biopsies of suspicious lesions and of parietal pleura may cause some oozing of blood, which usually can be controlled by applying local pressure with the tip of the forceps, with epinephrine-soaked gauze, or by coagulation using an electrocautery forceps.

The principal danger for a beginner thoracoscopist/pleuroscopist is hemorrhage from the inadvertent biopsy of an intercostal vessel. This is an extremely rare event when using rigid instruments, and it is even less likely with smaller flexible forceps. If bleeding occurs, immediate external finger pressure should be applied to the intercostal space while preparation is made either for local pressure with epinephrine-soaked gauze or for cauterization of bleeding vessels and tissues with the coagulating forceps or probe.

Contraindications for pulmonary biopsy are suspicion of arteriovenous pulmonary aneurysm, vascular tumors, and hydatid cysts. Taking biopsy samples of honeycomb lung from end-stage pulmonary fibrosis should also be avoided as it contributes to high incidence of bronchopleural fistulae.

To aspirate cysts, we use the operating bayonet optics attached to an adequately calibrated needle and stylet. Cysts are evacuated by means of a suction pump. Evacuation of pericardial cysts is undertaken using a syringe, with which one must proceed with a very steady hand and avoid certain movements.

Biopsies from the lung can be taken without difficulties with the single-port technique. Hemorrhage can be controlled by means of electrocautery, although in practice, this is rarely necessary since only minimal bleeding occurs from the small peripheral vessels, especially if the biopsies are taken from the edge of the lung lobes. The advantage is that the lung shrinks around the biopsy hole, ensuring both hemostasis and aerostasis.

However, some thoracoscopists prefer the two-port technique for lung biopsy. One (or two) additional points of entry can be made under direct thoracoscopic guidance as needed (**Fig. 11.30**). This may be the case when extensive adhesions are present (see **Fig. 11.14** and **Figs. 19.5** and **19.6** in the *Atlas* section), when the single entry site does not allow for complete inspection or does not allow one to reach a suspect lesion for biopsy, when more elaborate procedures are indicated (e.g., extensive adhesiolysis, visceral pleura/lung biopsies, sympathicolysis) (Lee and Colt 2003 b), or when it is necessary to control hemorrhage after biopsy. The position of the second point of entry is determined by viewing through the oblique scope while depressing the possible entry site with the index finger. It is sometimes helpful to insert a needle through the same site while viewing its precise location through

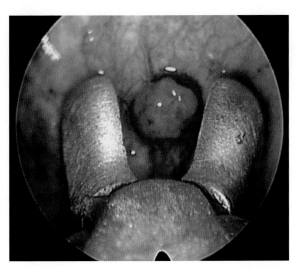

**Fig. 11.30** Parietal pleural biopsy using a two-port technique. The cups of the 5-mm forceps are opened on top of a rib; the pleura is grasped and gently pulled sideways.

the thoracoscope. After administering a local anesthetic, a 5-mm incision is made and the 5-mm trocar is inserted directly.

When MT/P is performed under general anesthesia, the two-port technique is most often used. The accessory instrumentation is usually passed through a 5- or 7-mm insulated trocar. Its cannula will accommodate many instruments designed for its smaller bore. The principles of biopsy of the parietal pleura are the same as described above. Usually, a 5-mm double-spoon insulated coagulation forceps is used. This two-port thoracoscopy may be preferred when pleural metastases are located on the visceral pleura (usually with similar "mushroom" appearance), when isolated or multiple lung parenchymal nodules are present (usually identifiable by umbilication of the visceral surface, or by gentle palpation), or in case of diffuse interstitial lung disease.

The coagulation forceps is positioned perpendicular to the lung; the lung is grasped, the forceps is closed and pulled toward the 5-mm trocar. As the forceps is pulled into the trocar, electrocautery (set at 60–100 W) is applied, with a foot pedal, for about three seconds. The pulling through the sharp end of the trocar "guillotines" the lung, and the electric current provides coagulation and closure of the lung surface. Leaks, when present, are usually small and close spontaneously. Bleeding is rare, as long as the fissures are avoided. Also, biopsies should be avoided in case of bullous lung disease and in case of end-stage lung fibrosis. In cases where diffuse infiltrates are evident on a CT scan, samples should be taken from healthy as well as abnormal areas. An average of 3–4 (range 1–8) biopsy specimens are obtained during any given session. The histological features of biopsy specimens are preserved sufficiently with this technique (Lee and Colt 2003a).

Boutin's group has described the use of a YAG laser after lung biopsy to ensure airtightness. After removing samples of pulmonary parenchyma, the laser fiber is introduced and the pulmonary orifice is closed with 3 to 5 pulses (Boutin 1989; Boutin et al. 1991). The laser was also successfully applied for lysis of adhesions, for cauterization of emphysematous bullae in spontaneous pneumothorax, for coagulation of traumatic bleeding, and for the closure of pleuropulmonary fistulae.

### Stapled Wedge Resection

Lung biopsies can alternatively be performed by experienced thoracoscopists using 3-cm reloads and an endoscopic stapler. Endoscopic staplers cut and staple lung parenchyma, preventing air leaks and bleeding. Stapling makes it easier to obtain vessels and also results in less air leakage. The procedure is usually performed in an operating theater, with the patient under general anesthesia and selectively intubated. Nezu and colleagues describe a technique that allows wedge resection of blebs with the patient under local anesthesia (Nezu et al. 1997). The patient is premedicated with meperidine, 50 mg, and atropine sulfate, 0.5 mg, given intramuscularly. Thirty minutes before surgery, 0.5% lidocaine is instilled into the pleural cavity and 5 mg of diazepam is administered intravenously for pain and anxiety. Thoracoscopic wedge resection of the pulmonary parenchyma at the base of the bleb is performed through two 5-mm ports, which accommodate a rigid telescope and grasping forceps and a 12-mm port for the stapler. This is followed by pleural drainage with a 24 F chest tube. Nezu's procedure was successful in all but two patients, and morbidity was minimal. Aside from minor discomfort at the portal sites, local anesthesia and sedation were adequate in all cases.

*Caution:* Biopsies in perihilar areas must be performed with extra care because of the presence of the pulmonary vessels crossing through the lobes. Fissures themselves, particularly in a peripheral aspect, pose no more danger than working on a flat surface of the lung periphery. Similarly, it is prudent to avoid biopsy of an emphysematous bulla, cyst, or cavity because of significant potential for a prolonged air leak from a bronchopleural fistula. In a patient with honeycomb lungs, any necessary random biopsy specimens should be taken from the mid and upper lung, where emphysematous bullae and cysts are relatively sparse. The average dry weight of lung biopsy specimens ranges from 4 to 37 mg. Cup forceps biopsy is probably best avoided in these patients. When using a stapler device, special care is necessary to avoid tearing the fragile lung parenchyma with either the stapler or the grasping forceps.

If malignant disease is obvious, and if all fluid has been removed, the biopsy procedure can be followed immediately by insufflation of talc for pleurodesis.

# Performance of Semirigid (Semiflexible) Pleuroscopy

The principles of trocar introduction and pleural cavity inspection are similar to those for the rigid instrument. **Figure 11.1** shows it being performed. The semirigid pleuroscope has the "look and feel" of a flexible bronchoscope, and thus may "lower the threshold" for thoracoscopy for the pulmonologist, and may even become more popular than the classical rigid instrumentation.

The semirigid pleuroscope (model LTF 160, Olympus, Japan) has been described in detail earlier. The design, including the handle, is similar to that of a standard flexible bronchoscope and thus the skills involved in operating the instrument are already familiar to the practicing bronchoscopist. Furthermore, it is compatible with the existing video-processors and light sources. The optical quality allows excellent visual exploration as well as good video or photographic documentation. The flexible tip will allow various angles of vision, including straight-ahead and oblique angle of view (see **Fig. 11.6b** and **11.29**). As with a bronchoscope, one very quickly becomes accustomed to the movement of the tip by simply rotating the pleuroscope and manipulating the tip to afford a superb panoramic view of the entire pleural cavity.

Otherwise, the step-by-step performance is similar to the already described technique of rigid medical thoracoscopy via a single entry.

## Comparison of the Rigid and Semirigid Techniques

### Advantages of the Rigid Thoracoscopic Instruments
- Specimens obtained with the rigid forceps are significantly larger than those with the semirigid pleuroscope as they are limited by the size of the flexible forceps (**Fig. 11.31a–c**), which in turn depends on the diameter of the working channel (McLean et al. 1998; Lee and Colt 2005; Lee et al. 2007a). However, this technical limitation can be overcome by taking multiple biopsies of the abnormal areas as well as several "samples" of the same area to obtain tissue of sufficient depth (Lee and Colt 2005; Lee et al. 2007a).
- Besides larger biopsy sizes, the rigid forceps allows taking of biopsies from very dense lesions as well (although the coagulation forceps, or a diathermic knife [Kawahara et al. 2008], used with the semirigid pleuroscope may solve this problem in part).
- The rigid instruments are more suitable when more elaborate procedures are indicated (e.g., extensive adhesiolysis, visceral pleural/lung biopsies, sympathicolysis), or when it is necessary to control hemorrhage after biopsy.

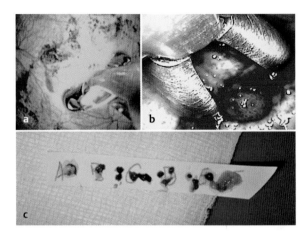

**Fig. 11.31**  Comparison of biopsies obtained with a flexible biopsy of the parietal pleural (**a**) and rigid optical forceps (**b**). **c** Specimens taken with the flexible forceps (A–E) are smaller.

- Rigid instruments are less expensive, more robust, have a longer endurance and may need maintenance and repair less often.

### Advantages of the Semirigid Pleuroscope
- The semirigid thoracoscope has the "look and feel" of a flexible bronchoscope, and thus may "lower the threshold" for medical thoracoscopy for the pulmonologist. It may also be helpful psychologically in overcoming fear of using the rigid (and therefore often regarded as more dangerous) instruments.
- It interfaces easily with existing processors (CV-160, CLV-U40,) and light sources (CV-240, EVIS-100 or 140, EVIS EXERA-145 or 160) made by the manufacturer for flexible bronchoscopy or GI endoscopy, which are available in most endoscopy units without additional cost.
- It helps maintain a clear optical field by allowing concurrent suctioning, which is analogous to the suction techniques used during flexible bronchoscopy.
- It may allow one to overcome a limited view by maneuvering its flexible tip in different directions and around adhesions (Lee and Colt 2005; Lee et al. 2007a).
- Its flexible tip facilitates the homogeneous insufflation of talc (via a catheter, introduced through the working channel) into all areas of the parietal and visceral pleura (see **Fig. 11.11a**).

The ideal is certainly the combination of both techniques, in which rigid medical thoracoscopy can be complemented by the semiflexible pleuroscope in the above-mentioned advantageous situations, which is comparable to the combined use of rigid and flexible bronchoscopy in complex therapeutic endobronchial indications.

## Evaluation of Specimens

The pleural fluid should be sent for the customary chemistry, cytology, possibly tumor markers, and infectious cultures. The cytological examination of pleural effusions should be undertaken by experienced cytologists (biopsies and smears are easier to evaluate and provide a more reliable opinion). The best biopsy specimens should be sent to pathology for processing. If TB or other infections are suspected, biopsies of the parietal pleura as well as fibrinous tissue should be sent for TB bacteriology and fungi and/or anaerobic organisms. Material for electron microscopy should be put in cooled glutaraldehyde.

## Technique of Thoracoscopic Talc Pleurodesis

Thoracoscopic talc pleurodesis is the most widely reported method of instillation of talc into the pleural cavity (talc poudrage). It is mainly used for treatment of malignant or chronic recurrent nonmalignant pleural effusions, but is also used in persistent or recurrent spontaneous pneumothorax (for details see "Thoracoscopic Talc Pleurodesis," Chapter 3, p. 38 ff. and p. 44).

Several technical details should be taken into account to achieve good pleurodesis and avoid complications: All pleural fluid should be removed before the spraying of talc. The fluid can easily be removed during thoracoscopy/pleuroscopy, as air is passively entering the pleural cavity, thus creating a desirable equilibrium in pressures. Complete collapse of the lung is also important, affording a good view of the pleural cavity and the opportunity to biopsy suspicious lesions and also permitting wide distribution of the talc. Another important prerequisite for a successful pleurodesis is that the lung is able to expand completely after the performance of talc poudrage, which may be not achievable in case of a trapped lung (**Fig. 11.32**). Both the visceral and the parietal pleura have to come into close apposition to achieve a lasting pleural symphysis. Furthermore, the success of pleurodesis depends on the presence of mesothelial cells, since they are actively involved in the creation of the symphysis (Jantz and Antony 2008).

Talc is hydrated magnesium silicate ($Mg_3Si_4O_{10}(OH)_2$). Talc composition can vary in the amount of calcium, aluminum and iron, according to its origin. Several mineral contaminants may be present but medicinal talc is asbestos free and is supplied by various chemical supply houses, with a variable particle size generally < 50 μm. In clinical practice, it is the proportion of talc particles < 5 μm in diameter that relates to the severity of local and systemic inflammatory responses, and to safety.

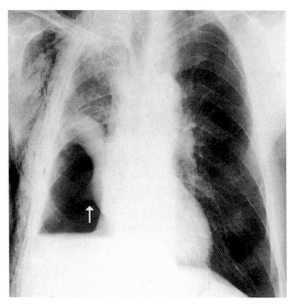

**Fig. 11.32** Chest radiograph showing a partial pneumothorax with a trapped lung (→) that did not expand completely under drainage suction.

In the United States, talc approved by the Food and Drug Administration is provided by the Bryan Corporation (Woburn, MA) in two forms: sterile talc powder (packaged as single dose of 5 g in a 100 mL glass bottle) and as talc aerosol (Sclerosol, a single-dose [4-g] canister with two delivery tubes and using dichlorofluoromethane [CFC-12, 26 g per canister] as propellant). In Europe, commercial talc for pleurodesis is manufactured by Novatech (La Ciotat, France), and is available in four forms: Steritalc F2 (2 g of sterile talc powder in a glass vial), Steritalc F4 (4 g of sterile talc powder in a glass vial), Steritalc Spray (3 g in a spray canister with propellant gas), and Steritalc PF4 spray (4 g in a hand/air-driven pump). The particle size distribution is not stated by Bryan for the FDA-approved talc; the French Novatech talc (not approved for use in the United Sates) is size-calibrated, with a median particle diameter of 31.3 μm.

Although an optimal dose of talc for poudrage in pleural effusions has not been established, usually a dose of approximately 5 g (4–6 g or approx. 8–12 mL) of sterile talc is recommended, whereas for pneumothorax patients 2 (to 3) grams of talc is sufficient. The talc is insufflated into the pleural space through a catheter placed in the working channel of the thoracoscope/pleuroscope (**Fig. 11.33**) or through a cannula (**Figs. 11.3j** and **11.34**). Uniform distribution of the talc on all pleural surfaces is confirmed by direct vision (see Cases 1, 2 and 8 on DVD). For this purpose, one can use a rigid thoracoscope with an angled optical device (see **Figs. 11.3e** and **11.33**) or a bayonet optic (see **Fig. 11.3f** and **11.4b**). The flexible catheter is connected to a small bottle containing talc and to a pneumatic atomizer and is introduced through the working channel of the

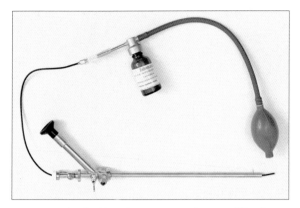

**Fig. 11.33** The flexible catheter, connected to a small bottle containing talc and to a pneumatic atomizer (manual insufflator), is introduced through the working channel of the rigid thoracoscope.

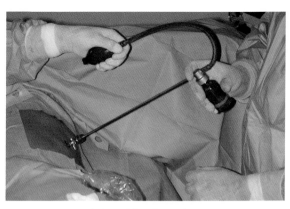

**Fig. 11.34** A cannula is used for talc poudrage.

thoracoscope (**Fig. 11.33**) or of the semirigid pleuroscope. An alternative is the administration as talc aerosol (Sclerosol in the United States, Steritalc Spray or Steritalc PF4 spray in Europe, see above). Care must be taken to avoid talc abrasion of the glass lens of the thoracoscope.

Talc application may be painful, although in malignant pleural effusions usually less so than in pneumothorax where the normal parietal pleura is much more algesic. Accordingly, additional analgesics should be given directly before beginning the talc poudrage (see "Anesthesia for Medical Thoracoscopy/Pleuroscopy," p. 84). Alternatively or additionally, 25 mL of 1% lidocaine (250 mg) can be administered via spray catheter, introduced through the working channel of the thoracoscope/pleuroscope, directly to the parietal chest wall pleura (Lee and Colt 2007b).

After talc insufflation, a chest tube (16–24 F) is left in place, and negative pressure is applied (5–20 cm H$_2$O). The chest tube should be left in place until the fluid drainage is less than 100–150 mL per day and no air leak is present, which is usually 3–6 days. A daily chest radiograph is obtained while the chest tube is in place to assess chest tube position, fluid accumulation, and lung reexpansion. Patients requiring talc pleurodesis remain hospitalized for an average of 3–6 days.

Some authors (P.M.) recommend that before insufflating talc, a chest tube should be placed in the lowest possible intercostal space through a second incision. Since drainage must be complete, it is good to use a large-bore chest tubes, between 24 and 32 F. The chest tube will cause local discomfort, which generally responds to simple analgesics. Before insufflation of talc, the thoracoscope is directed toward the diaphragm; the assistant indents the intercostal spaces or puts a small needle in the chest cavity while the physician documents the lowest intercostal space for entry of the chest tube. Before inserting the chest tube, extra holes are created along the radiopaque line to permit drainage of the entire hemithorax. The chest tube is pushed through the point of entry perpendicular to the skin at first, then pointed in the desired direction until it meets the chest wall. The chest tube is directed posteriorly and then as close to the apex as possible, under pleuroscopic guidance. A second chest tube is directed toward the costocardiac angle, inserted from the pleuroscope entry site. When the chest tube is left in place for drainage, sutures are applied to secure the tube to the skin (**Fig. 11.35a, b**). A purse-string suture usually helps in closing the chest tube wound tightly.

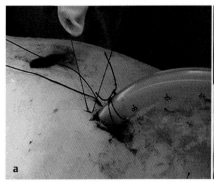
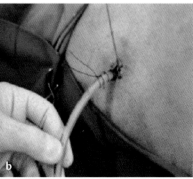

**Fig. 11.35** Chest tube securely sutured in place. **a** Vertical mattress sutures. **b** Double purse-string sutures.

# Chest Tube Care

At the conclusion of the procedure, a chest tube is inserted to drain residual air and fluid from the pleural cavity, allowing the lung to reexpand. Safe placement and ideal orientation can be achieved by indirect thoracoscopic control. For direct optical control of chest tube placement a technique has been proposed by which a rigid telescope is introduced through the chest tube (Zgoda et al. 2005). Since chest tubes can migrate externally, particularly in patients who are obese, debilitated, or restless, it is important that they are securely sutured in place (**Fig. 11.35a, b**), and fixed with an adhesive dressing (**Fig. 11.36**).

Special care should be taken if there is a risk of reexpansion pulmonary edema after the chest tube has been placed and negative pressure is applied by suction. This possibility arises, in particular, when a large amount of pleural fluid has compressed the lung, in case of lung entrapment or trapped lung, in case of endobronchial obstruction, or when a complete pneumothorax has existed already for some time. In all these situations, negative pressure should be applied very cautiously, and the patient should be observed closely (see "Knowledge of the Pathophysiology of the Pleura," Chapter 10, p. 67 and Chapter 9 "Complications and Their Prevention").

Following a diagnostic procedure, when only parietal pleural biopsies are taken, a chest tube may be required for only a few hours. The chest tube (24–28 F) is placed through the same incision (or through the cannula) as the thoracoscope. It is directed cranially to evacuate the pneumothorax created for the procedure. In most cases, there is total resolution of the pneumothorax as indicated by the cessation of "bubbling" through the water seal.

The lung reexpansion should be confirmed radiographically. If there are no air leaks and if the daily fluid production has decreased to about 100–150 mL, the chest tube is removed. The patient can commonly leave the hospital the following day after spending no more than 24 hours in hospital. If pleural drainage requires more than 24 hours, a Heimlich valve may be used in place of the water seal, allowing the patient to move about freely during the day.

As mentioned above, when talc pleurodesis has been performed, the chest tube will usually be left in place until the fluid drainage is less than 100–150 mL per day.

However, it has been questioned whether this drainage duration is needed. In a study comparing the tube removal after 24 h with removal after 72 h in patients with talc slurry pleurodesis, no difference in recurrence of pleural effusion was seen, but the length of hospitalization was significantly reduced when the chest drain was removed after 24 h (4 d versus 8 d) (Goodman and Davies 2006).

It is essential for optimal patient outcome that well-trained nurses are responsible for wound care, maintenance of the chest drainage system, pain management, and vigilant assessment of the cardiorespiratory system following MT/P (Davidson and Colt 1997).

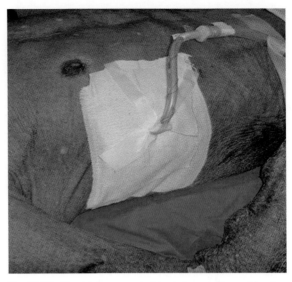

**Fig. 11.36** Chest tube connected to drainage system with adhesive dressing after medical thoracoscopy/pleuroscopy.

## Drainage Systems

Multiple drainage systems have been used to maintain the integrity of the pleural space. The goals have been to collect the fluids drained from the chest tube and at the same time either to prevent the negative inspiratory intrathoracic pressures from causing air flow through the tube into the pleural space or to apply an external negative pressure to the pleural space. The early collection systems were of glass and consisted of one to three bottles in series. A fluid collection chamber, present in all of the systems, allowed for the fluid drained from the tube to be collected. In the single-bottle system, the collection bottle also acted as a water seal to prevent influx of air into the pleural space. The water seal principle includes a chamber vented to the atmosphere with a long tube extending below the surface of a small amount of water in the chamber. This long tube is then attached to the chest tube. When drainage of air or fluid occurs, the substance passes freely into the chamber with little resistance. However, when negative pressure is generated in the thorax, the water is then siphoned up into the tube in the chamber until the height of the water column is equal to the negative intrathoracic pressure, thus preventing influx of air into the pleural space. Of note, the small magnitude of the negative pressures generated in the thorax is not sufficient to aspirate the water column into the chest unless the chamber is at or near the level of the chest. The water seal should thus be kept at a level below that of the patient's chest. The single-bottle system is adequate for drainage of a simple pneumothorax, but if fluid drainage is excessive, the fluid collects in the single bottle and thus the water seal pressure increases as the fluid level in the bottle rises. A higher positive pressure is then necessary to generate flow of air or fluid from the chest and into the bottle.

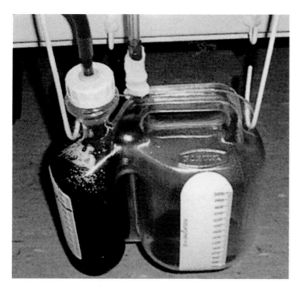

**Fig. 11.37**  Two-bottle systems include separate bottles for collection of the drained fluid and for regulation of the water seal.

The two-bottle system includes separate bottles for collection of the drained fluid and for regulation of the water seal (**Fig. 11.37**). This system corrects the problem of alteration of water seal pressure by accumulation of the drained fluids. The collection chamber is simply a bottle that is not vented to the atmosphere but has two small tubes just entering through the lid of the chamber and not protruding below the fluid level. The collection chamber is connected to the system between the water seal and the thoracostomy tube itself. The two-bottle system works sufficiently well for the drainage of simple air and fluid collections. However, occasionally a negative pressure placed on the thoracostomy tube is needed to either forcefully remove collections of air or fluid or expand a partially collapsed lung.

A suction pump can be placed on either the one- or the two-bottle systems if the pump allows for a regulated negative pressure, as is the case with the Emerson pump. However, this pump is then dedicated to use on only a single patient at any time and is relatively clumsy and expensive. Most hospitals have installed a large-scale suction system throughout the hospital that is accessed through a specialized outlet. The difficulty in this situation is that this form of suction is at a much higher negative pressure than is appropriate for the pleural space and is highly variable. To correct for the high level and variability of all suction, a third bottle is then added to the system and acts as a suction regulator (**Fig. 11.38**). This bottle is a manometer, which uses a water or mercury column with an immersed tube exposed to the outside air. The regulator chamber lies between the wall suction and the water seal chamber. There are two short tubes protruding through the top of the chamber and not below the water level in the chamber. These are connected to the wall suction and

the water seal. A third tube then is left open to the atmosphere and protrudes down into the fluid in the regulator chamber. When the suction is then turned on, the air above the fluid in the regulator chamber is placed at a negative pressure. The suction is then increased to generate a flow of bubbles from outside the bottle, down the third tube and up into the air chamber. The depth of the longer tube within the fluid then corresponds to the negative pressure generated above the fluid level and transmitted to the water-seal chamber and the collection chamber. The level of the fluid in the regulator chamber then is adjustable, thus adjusting the negative pressure applied to the pleural space. The wall suction in the system must be adjusted to high enough levels to generate a steady flow of bubbles through the regulator chamber. Higher levels of wall suction above this point will not generate higher system vacuum, but will promote faster evaporation of the water in the regulator chamber.

A seldom-used variation on this system is to use mercury in the regulation chamber to more easily generate high negative pressures to be applied to the pleural space. Understandably, with the environmental hazards of mercury exposure and the limited usefulness of these excessive negative pressures, this practice has fallen into disfavor.

Many commercially prepared chest-drainage systems are available. Most of these are a variation on the three-chamber system made as single-use devices. The use of plastics has made these systems more durable. The majority of the system is as described above and is graduated to allow for easy measurement of fluid drained. Use is relatively easy with the only necessary preparation being the filling of the water-seal and pressure-regulation chambers. One important variation on these systems is the replacement of the regulator chamber with a vacuum regulation valve. The valve allows fewer gradations of negative pressure, but does allow for higher negative pressures without the use of mercury, typically to 40 cm $H_2O$.

Decisions regarding the type of the apparatus preferred depends on availability, physician bias, need for hospitalization, amount of daily fluid, and patients' desire for autonomy and ambulation.

## Assessment of Chest Tube Function

Once the thoracostomy is placed, proper placement within the thoracic cavity is verified either by fluid flow or by the development of condensation within the tube as air freely flows into and out of the tube from the thorax. Assessment of placement with plain chest radiography is also essential. Ideally, posteroanterior and lateral films would be checked to verify the tube's course within the thorax and verify that all of the holes in the tube lie within the chest cavity. These are marked by interruptions in the radiopaque line, which makes the tube visible on radiographs. Progression of treatment for the pathological pro-

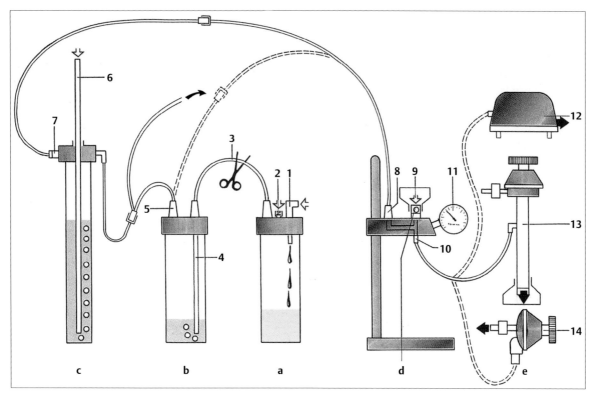

**Fig. 11.38** Constant-suction drainage apparatus (three-bottle system). (From Brandt et al. 1985.)

**a** *Secretions collection bottle* with connectors (**1**) for connecting tubing from the pleural drain (→), pressure release valve (**2**), connecting hose (**3**), and clamp for transport purposes.

**b** Water-seal *bottle* (**4**) for control of fistula, connector (**5**) to negative pressure regulator (**c** or **d**).

**c** *Alternative negative pressure regulator A* (water seal) with adjustable pressure tube (**6**) and connector to the negative pressure regulator (**7**).

**d** *Alternative negative pressure regulator B* (ball valve): connector (**8**) for hose from the bottle (**b**) or the water seal (**c**), dust filter for the ball valve (**9**), connector and hose for the negative pressure generator (**10**), pressure manometer 0–100 mbar (**11**).

**e** Various *negative pressure generators:* electric membrane pump (**12**), Venturi pump (**13**), vacuum regulator (**14**).

cess and tube placement is then assessed on a daily basis with serial films. In certain clinical circumstances, computed tomography may be beneficial for assessment of the pathological process, especially in the case of complicated parapneumonic effusions.

An essential part of the therapy for processes requiring thoracostomy placement is the diligent serial assessment of tube function. This is done by a serial assessment of clinical parameters (a fever curve, level of leukocytosis, assessment of dyspnea, assessment of oxygenation and ventilation) and also by assessment of the functioning of the tube and drainage system. The clinician must evaluate for air bubbling in the water-seal chamber, tidal movements in the water seal chamber, absence of large fluid collections in the tubing itself, and the description and amount of drainage. Chest radiography can also be very helpful.

Bubbling within the water-seal chamber is a very important initial observation. This bubbling indicates one of several things: that the intrathoracic air collection has not yet fully been removed by the tube; that there exists a persistent communication between the tracheobronchial tree and the pleural space (bronchopleural fistula); or that there is an air leak outside of the patient and within the drainage system or associated tubing. Of note, if suction is not applied, an air leak in the system, external to the patient, will cause incomplete evacuation of air from the chest but will not necessarily manifest as bubbling in the water-seal chamber.

Provided the patient's clinical situation has stabilized, air leaks within the drainage systems may be ruled out by clamping the tube at the level of the skin with a forceps. If the bubbling in the water-seal chamber stops, then the air is coming from within the patient. If it does not, the drainage system should be evaluated for leaks. Chest radiography is of benefit at this time; if there is no visible pneumothorax, then a bronchopleural fistula exists. If pneumothorax is present within the patient on water seal, the system should be set to suction in an attempt to reexpand the lung. If the chest tube has been on suction and the pneumothorax has not been reexpanded, then a bronchopleural fistula exists.

In general, the management of bronchopleural fistula would include titration to both maximize expansion of the underlying lung and minimize the air flow across the bronchopleural communication. In some patients, the flow is minimized while on water seal; other patients have decreased flow on the application of either an intermediate or a high level of suction, as much as −25 cm $H_2O$. The clinician must also observe the movements of the water column in the water-seal chamber. This may be difficult if the tube has been set to suction. The suction may be temporarily removed to assess "tidaling" (swinging/fluctuating motion). Tidal movements in the water-seal chamber are indicative of transmission of the intrapleural pressures through the tube, similarly to a manometer. During inspiration in typical negative-pressure breathing, the fluid level is elevated and the opposite occurs for expiration. In contrast, if the patient is on positive-pressure breathing, i.e., mechanical ventilation, the inspiratory phase will result in depression of the fluid level and expiration will cause elevation. Cough in either situation will depress the fluid level. The presence of tidal motion guarantees proper tube function, while absence of tidal motion indicates tube occlusion or kinking.

Clearance of debris occluding a thoracostomy tube can be accomplished by "stripping" or "milking." The connecting tubing is grasped and occluded near the thoracostomy tube with one hand, while the other hand is used to grasp the tube proximal to the first hand. The second hand then occludes the tube and is withdrawn in the direction of the drainage system. Then the two hands are separated by 30–60 cm, the initial occlusion is released, and the first hand again occludes the tube beside the second hand. This motion is then repeated several times with the goal of creating suction within the tube and hopefully dislodging and clearing fibrin clots or other debris that were occluding the tube. In addition, some would advocate the instillation of streptokinase into the tube to dissolve any fibrin clot present. The usual protocol uses 250 000 units in 100 mL of normal saline, which is left in the tube for several hours with the system clamped; after unclamping, the tube is then reassessed.

In any case, a nonfunctioning chest tube is of no benefit to the patient and presents a significant cumulative risk of infection. Nonfunctioning tubes should be removed promptly. The decision must then be made whether another chest tube placement is indicated at another site.

Recording the amount and description of fluid drainage is another matter of daily concern. The disposable drainage systems have a convenient method of measurement as the collection chambers are graduated; however, the fluid level must be marked on at least a daily basis to more easily measure the daily output. For most indications, the thoracostomy tube may be removed after the drainage is less than 100–150 mL, but this must be assessed in conjunction with plain chest radiography or computed tomography to ensure that the fluid collection is actually drained rather than loculated.

## Chest Tube Removal

The indications for removal of chest tubes placed for various pathological processes are as varied as the indications for tube placement. In general, absence of air leakage and cessation of fluid flow are reasonable guidelines. The sterile occlusive dressing is placed on a small stack of gauze. The sutures are then removed (or retained in the case of purse string suture). The tube is then removed while the patient performs a Valsalva maneuver to create positive pleural pressure and minimize the risk of air entry into the site during removal. The tube is removed with a steady tug, quickly. The occlusive dressing is held over the site as the tube is removed so that pressure may be applied over the site as the end of the tube is removed. If the purse string suture technique was used, the sutures are then re-tied. The occlusive dressing with gauze pad is taped into place and a plain chest radiograph is checked to verify absence of pneumothorax.

# 12 Documentation

Documentation of the procedure is essential since it not only provides the information to colleagues—chest physicians, oncologists, pathologists, thoracic surgeons, and others—but it is also a permanent part of the patient's medical history. It consists of a handwritten or (better) typed report in which details of the procedure as well as of the abnormal findings should be included. These should be supplemented, if possible, by endoscopic photographs and/or video recordings. Newer systems most often allow both photographs and video. The use of a computerized documentation program is the ideal; these are available not only for bronchoscopy but also for medical thoracoscopy/pleuroscopy.

# 13 Teaching Methods

Thoracoscopy skills should be developed over an extended period during which physicians acquire expertise in pleural diseases and procedures (see Chapter 10, "Knowledge and Skills Required"). Technical skills are best learned under the direct supervision of an experienced thoracoscopist. Because manual dexterity, confidence, and expertise may vary from one physician to another, it is difficult to specify a minimum number of procedures necessary to obtain the skill or to maintain competence. It is unlikely that any specific number of procedures will guarantee competence. However, a minimum number of 20 procedures is desirable to achieve sufficient familiarity with the instrumentation and interpretation of normal and pathological thoracoscopic findings. Procedural competence can probably be maintained if about 10–12 thoracoscopies are performed yearly.

Physicians acquiring skills in thoracoscopy should be experienced in the diagnosis and management of diverse pleural and pulmonary disorders. Familiarity with endoscopic and video instrumentation and techniques is mandatory. Physicians should be proficient at pleural procedures, including thoracentesis and closed needle pleural biopsy; competence in both procedures is required in the United States by the American Board of Internal Medicine for Pulmonary Diseases Board Certification. In addition, physicians should be proficient at tube insertion and management, a procedure required for Critical Care Board Certification in the United States.

Adequate training in both the cognitive and technical aspects of thoracoscopy is essential. This is unlikely to be provided by a single two-day course. Training courses should be encouraged and may be extremely beneficial if they follow, for example, Accreditation Council for Graduate Medical Education (ACGME) guidelines for full Continuing Medical Education (CME) accreditation and include didactic lectures as well as laboratory sessions. By attending hands-on training seminars, lectures, and symposia, physicians can learn basic concepts and acquire greater understanding of the appropriate indications, risks, benefits, and limitations of thoracoscopic/pleuroscopic interventions. These sessions should allow physicians to achieve familiarity and comfort with basic thoracoscopic/pleuroscopic techniques and instrumentation. Physicians should be encouraged to work with a mentor within their community until the necessary criteria are met for medical thoracoscopy/pleuroscopy privileges within their own institutions. This form of a mini-fellowship may be ideal for training physicians in procedures not learned during formal subspecialty training. Physicians in training should maintain records of their experience during the training process.

A competent medical thoracoscopist/pleuroscopist, therefore, should be more than a master of the instrument within the pleural space, but should be a complete consultant for pleuropulmonary disorders ("window to the pleural space").

## Suggestions for Learning the Technique

- There are currently no good simulation or inanimate models on the market with which to learn medical thoracoscopy/pleuroscopy (R.L. uses one phantom produced for Olympus).
- A variety of animal models have been used (see Chapter 5 "MT/P in Animals", p. 54 ff.) in training courses along with didactic lectures including videos.
- The learning is best done by being an assistant to a physician who is well versed in the art of medical thoracoscopy/pleuroscopy.
- A good opportunity to learn the inspection of the pleural space and its pathological situations is given by the observation of procedures on the video screen or live transmission to a bigger group.
- Physicians performing this procedure should have ample experience, excellent knowledge of pleural and thoracic anatomy, mature judgment in interpreting radiographic images related to pleural disease, and sufficient endoscopic skill. The American College of Chest Physicians (ACCP) suggests that the trainees should perform at least 20 procedures in a supervised setting to establish basic competency (Ernst et al. 2003).
- After such training, mentoring with a thoracic surgeon by participation during VATS procedures would certainly complement the training.
- Start with easy situations such as large pleural effusion or pneumothorax when the placement of a chest tube is indicated.
- As with all technical procedures there is a learning curve before full competence in medical thoracoscopy/pleuroscopy is achieved (Boutin et al. 1981a; Rodriguez-Panadero 1995).
- To maintain competency, dedicated operators should perform at least 10 procedures per year (Ernst et al. 2003).

# Section B: Atlas

# 14 Malignant Pleural Effusions due to Lung Cancer

**Fig. 14.1**

**a  Malignant pleural effusion due to small-cell lung cancer.**
After drainage of 4200 mL of serous effusion, the view toward
the apex of the right thoracic cavity. Upper lobe (**1**) completely
infiltrated by tumor. Lower lobe (**2**) partially infiltrated (→).
Parietal pleura with the first three ribs and the intercostal spaces
appear normal.

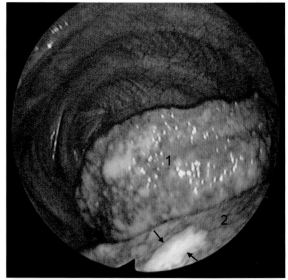

**b  Malignant pleural effusion due to small-cell lung cancer.**
Same patient as in **a**: several small to middle-sized tumor
nodules (→) on the anterior chest wall and in the fatty tissue (↦).

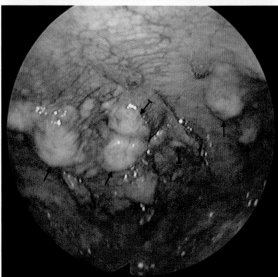

**Fig. 14.2**

**Malignant pleural effusion due to small-cell lung cancer**
(recurrent under second-line chemotherapy). After drainage of
2300 mL of serous effusion, there is ubiquitous tumor growth on
the right visceral and parietal pleura; here middle-sized nodules (→)
and flat infiltrations (↦) on the posterior chest-wall pleura.

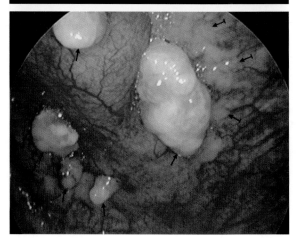

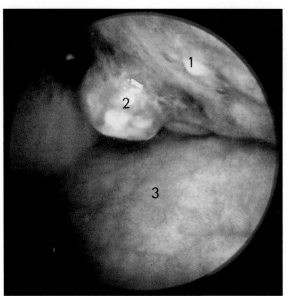

**Fig. 14.3**
**Malignant pleural effusion due to small-cell lung cancer invading into the pleural space.** After drainage of 500 mL of clear serous effusion, the base of the right lower lobe (**1**) is retracted cranially. One sees the hazelnut-sized, yellowish necrotic tumor nodule breaking through into the pleural cavity (**2**). The diaphragm (**3**) shows numerous dilated vessels and very discreet, barely visible, small nodules.

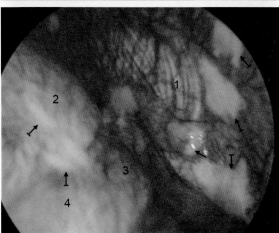

**Fig. 14.4**
**Malignant pleural effusion due to adenocarcinoma of the right lower lobe (recurrent).** After drainage of 800 mL of serous effusion: whitish nodular (→) and flat (↦) tumor growth on the anterior chest-wall pleura (**1**). Flat tumor infiltrations (↦) on the visceral pleura between the upper lobe (**2**), middle lobe (**3**), and lower lobe (**4**).

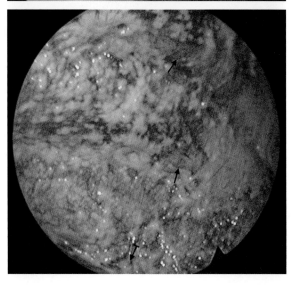

**Fig. 14.5**
**Progressive malignant pleural effusion due to adenocarcinoma of the middle lobe.** After drainage of 1300 mL of effusion: diffuse patchy whitish nodular tumor infiltrations, here on the posterior chest wall, and only small areas of normal fatty pleura surface (→). One spot with anthracotic pigmentation (↦).

**Fig. 14.6**
**Malignant pleural effusion due to adenocarcinoma of the left lower lobe (recurrent under chemotherapy).** After drainage of 2800 mL of serous effusion: a thickened and red chest-wall tumor with tumor nodules of different sizes (→) and a few fibrinous bands (↦).

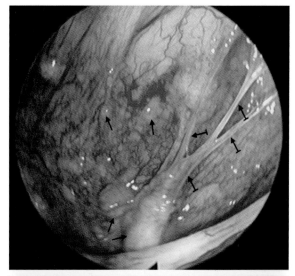

**Fig. 14.7**
**Malignant pleural effusion due to squamous cell carcinoma of the right lung.** After drainage of 1600 mL of cloudy serous effusion, the lung is retracted and bound down by thick opalescent pleura (**1**). Adhesions from the base of the lung (→), which previously attached the lung to the chest wall. Thickening and opacification of the parietal pleura (**2**).

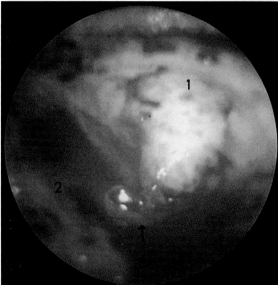

**Fig. 14.8**
**Paramalignant pleural effusion due to hemorrhagic pulmonary infarction in squamous cell lung carcinoma of the left lower lobe.** After drainage of 450 mL of effusion, the lung is seen from the back: the upper lobe (**1**) is distended, with a delicate pattern typical of emphysema. The posterior mediastinum with delicate, well vascularized adhesions (**2**). The lower lobe (**3**) is infiltrated with tumor showing a geographic, white, fibrous pleural thickening (**4**) with, in the mediastinal area, distended pleural vessels (→), having the appearance of capillary obstruction. Adjacent to the widened lobar fissure, there is a hyperemic edematous area of lung (**5**).

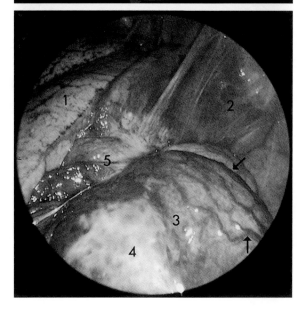

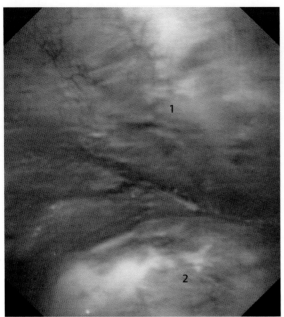

**Fig. 14.9**
**a Malignant pleural effusion due to adenocarcinoma.**
After drainage of 1200 mL of serous effusion: larger tumor nodules on the chest wall pleura. Here, an area with chronic inflammatory changes on the chest-wall pleura (**1**) and the lung (**2**). The photograph was taken during white-light thoracoscopy.

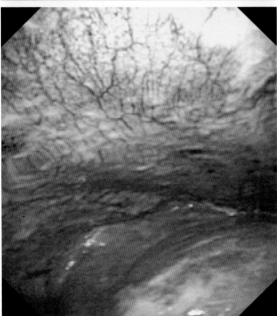

**b Same patient using narrow band imaging (NBI).** This photograph taken with NBI thoracoscopy shows distinctly more and better-delineated vessels.

(From Schönfeld N, Schwarz C, Kollmeier J, Blum T, Bauer TT, Ott S. Narrow band imaging (NBI) during medical thoracoscopy: first impressions. J Occup Med Toxicol 2009; 4: 24, reprinted with kind permission from the authors.)

# 15 Pleural Effusions due to Diffuse Malignant Mesothelioma and Asbestos-related Pleural Diseases

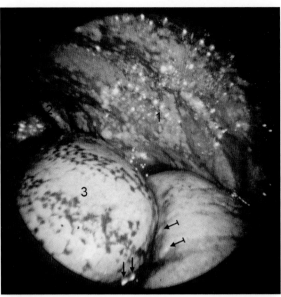

**Fig. 15.1**
**Diffuse malignant mesothelioma (biphasic).** After drainage of 3000 mL of hemorrhagic effusion, view toward the apex of the left thoracic cavity. Patchy nodular tumor growth on the left anterior chest-wall pleura (**1**), larger nodule in the apex (**2**). Normal-appearing upper lobe (**3**) with some anthracotic pigmentation and a few tumor nodules at the base (→), small tumor nodules also on the lower lobe close to the fissure (↦).

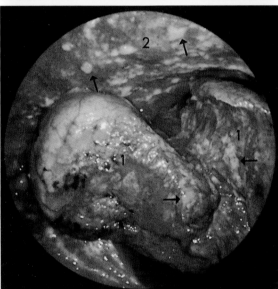

**Fig. 15.2**
**Diffuse malignant mesothelioma (biphasic).** After drainage of 3700 mL of hemorrhagic effusion, view toward the apex of the right thoracic cavity. The lung (**1**) is retracted and compressed; air-containing parenchyma is seen in only a few places. On the visceral pleura (**1**), the parietal pleura (**2**), and the diaphragm are numerous white nodules (→).

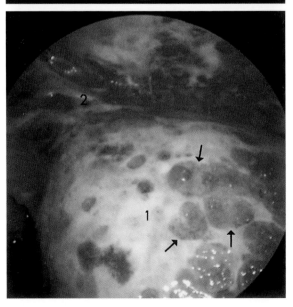

**Fig. 15.3**
**Diffuse malignant mesothelioma (undifferentiated).** After drainage of 1500 mL of hemorrhagic effusion, the lung is retracted and covered by a thick pleural peel. The left upper lobe (**1**) is infiltrated by numerous disklike hyperemic nodules (→) as well as thick adhesions to the chest wall (**2**), which also contains small hemorrhagic nodules.

**Fig. 15.4**
**Diffuse malignant mesothelioma (epithelioid).** After drainage of
350 mL of gelatinous fluid (**1**), both pleural surfaces were covered
with coarse, irregular grapelike nodules, here on the chest-wall
pleura (→).

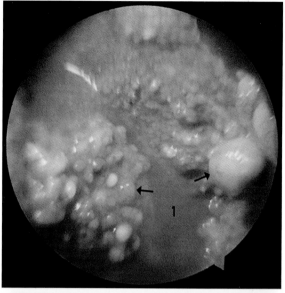

**Fig. 15.5**
**Diffuse malignant mesothelioma (biphasic) with pleural plaque.**
After drainage of 2000 mL of dark serous fluid, the entire parietal
pleura was completely covered by a reddish, irregular layer of tumor
from which protruded regular, cauliflower-like whitish tumor nodules (**1**). In addition, an irregular pleural plaque is seen (**2**).

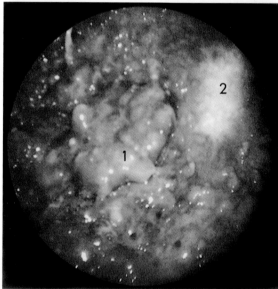

**Fig. 15.6**
**Diffuse malignant mesothelioma (biphasic) with bilateral pleu-
ral plaques.** After drainage of 1350 mL of hemorrhagic effusion:
adhesions between the right upper lobe (**1**) and the chest wall (**2**),
along the ribs coarse hyaline plaques (→) and, nearby, distinct
tumor nodules (↦).

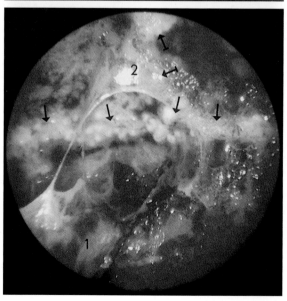

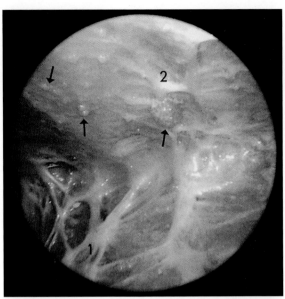

**Fig. 15.7**
**Diffuse malignant mesothelioma (biphasic).** After drainage of 2200 mL of brownish, cloudy serous effusion, the lung (**1**), covered with numerous fibrous strands, obscured chest-wall demarcation (**2**) because it was also covered with greatly thickened pleura; numerous nodules (→) can be identified.

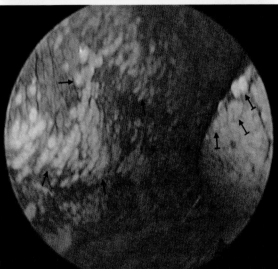

**Fig. 15.8**
**Diffuse malignant mesothelioma (epithelioid).** After drainage of 1200 mL of serous effusion: patchy tumor growth on the posterior chest wall (→) and few small nodules on the surface of the lower lobe (↦).

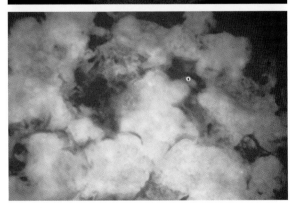

**Fig. 15.9**
**Diffuse malignant mesothelioma (biphasic).** After drainage of 800 mL of serous effusion: thickened parietal pleura with signs of lymphangiosis.

**Fig. 15.10**
**Diffuse malignant mesothelioma (sarcomatoid).**
After drainage of 3300 mL of slightly hemorrhagic pleural
effusion: larger tumor nodules on the right anterior chest wall (→)
and large and flat plaquelike areas (↦).

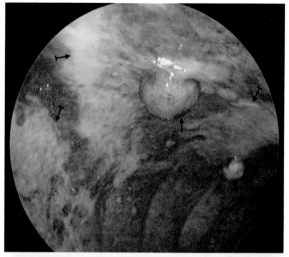

**Fig. 15.11**
**Diffuse malignant mesothelioma (sarcomatoid).**
After drainage of 1800 mL of hemorrhagic pleural effusion (**1**),
large tumor nodules on the right anterior chest-wall pleura (→).

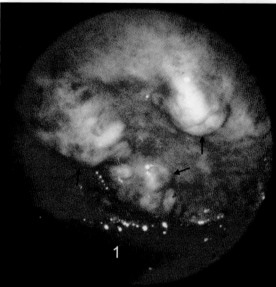

**Fig. 15.12**
**Diffuse malignant mesothelioma (sarcomatoid).**
After drainage of 2200 mL of slightly hemorrhagic effusion:
middle-sized to large tumor nodules on the right posterior chest-
wall pleura (→) as well as plaques in-between (**1**); a few small
tumor nodules on the surface of the lower lobe (↦).

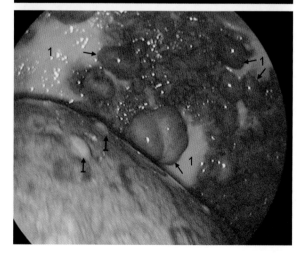

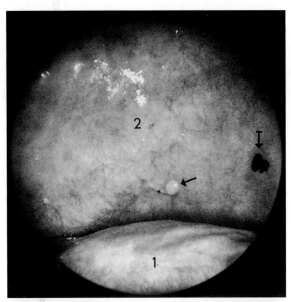

**Fig. 15.13**
**Benign asbestos pleural effusion.** After removal of a small amount of fluid: thickened pleura on the diaphragm (**1**) and on the posterior chest wall (**2**), with increased vascular injection. On the chest wall, an island of anthracotic pigment (↦) as well as a small whitish hyaline plaque (→).

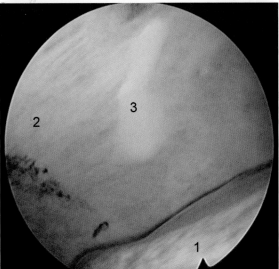

**Fig. 15.14**
**a  Benign asbestos pleural effusion.** After removal of 600 mL of turbid fluid: thickened pleura on the right lung (**1**) and the chest wall (**2**), here covering an elongated plaque (**3**).

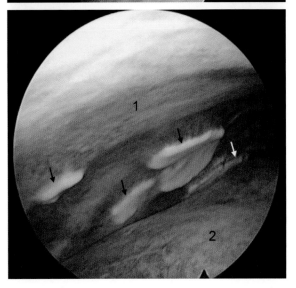

**b  Benign asbestos pleural effusion.** Same patient with pleural plaques (↑) on the posterior chest wall (**1**). Thickened visceral pleura (**2**).

**Fig. 15.15**
**Bilateral hyaline pleural plaques with fibrinous pleuritis**
**(no effusion).** After pneumothorax induction, the junction of horizontal and oblique fissures is seen between the right upper lobe (**1**), lower lobe (**2**), and middle lobe (**3**). The visceral pleura is markedly injected at the lobar margin (↦). Adjacent lobes are fused together. The anterior chest wall (**4**) shows firm, irregular hyaline plaques (→) with raised, vascularized margins. The visceral pleura shows fibrinous change beneath one of these plaques (↦).

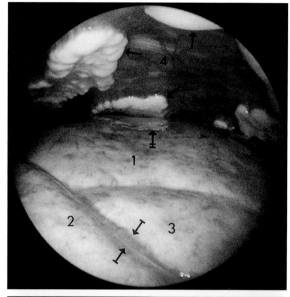

**Fig. 15.16**
**Hyaline pleural plaques (no effusion).** After pneumothorax induction: a right paravertebral 2 cm × 1 cm white, smooth plaque (**1**) along the fourth rib and a second plaque on the fifth rib (→); right upper lobe (**2**) and chest wall (**3**) (additional plaque on the diaphragm).

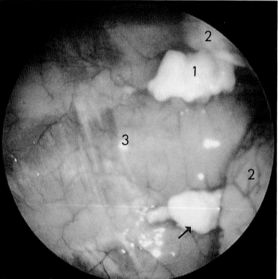

**Fig. 15.17**
**Bilateral hyaline pleural plaques (no effusion).** After pneumothorax induction: on the parietal pleura white, irregular, thickened hyaline plaques (like sugar frosting) with notable vascular injection on its edge.

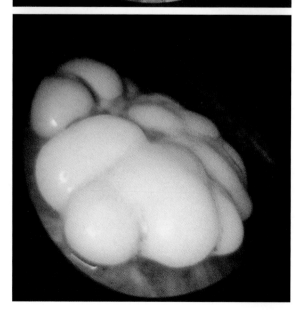

# 16 Malignant Pleural Effusions Secondary to Metastatic Neoplasms

**Fig. 16.1**
**Malignant pleural effusion from metastatic uterine carcinoma.**
After drainage of 800 mL of serous effusion, numerous, whitish nodules on both visceral and parietal pleura. The photograph shows a section of the chest wall with marked hyperemia. The horizontally oriented ribs and intercostal spaces are noted as well as numerous pale tumor nodules (→) which in part infiltrate the surrounding pleura in a radial fashion.

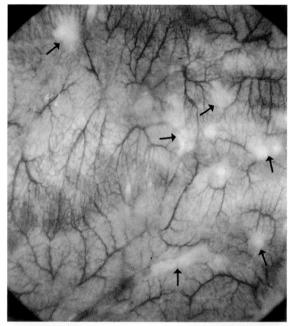

**Fig. 16.2**
**Malignant pleural effusion from metastatic cancer of unknown origin.** After drainage of 1800 mL of serous effusion, normal surface of the right lower lobe (**1**) with anthracotic pigmentation (→). Whitish small tumor nodules (↦) on the posterior chest wall (**2**).

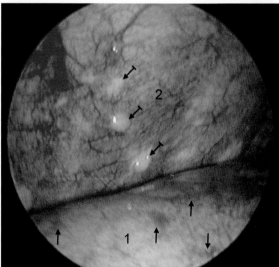

**Fig. 16.3**
**Malignant pleural effusion from metastatic breast cancer.**
After drainage of 900 mL of serous effusion: small tumor nodules on the surface of the left lower lobe (→) and slightly larger nodules (↦) on the posterior chest wall (**1**) close to the diaphragm (**2**).

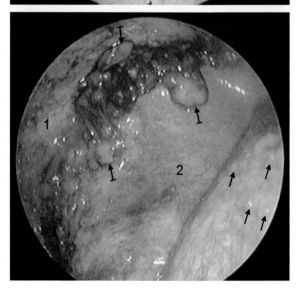

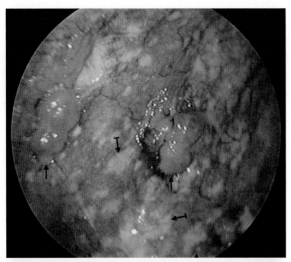

**Fig. 16.4**
**Bilateral pleural effusions from metastatic breast cancer.**
After drainage of 1700 mL of serous effusion: nodular (→) and flat, whitish (↦) tumor lesions on the posterior chest wall (and on the diaphragm).

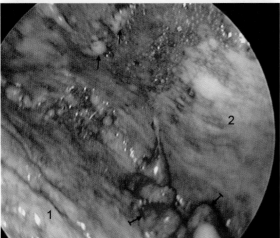

**Fig. 16.5**
**Malignant pleural effusion from metastatic breast cancer.**
After drainage of 2800 mL of serous effusion: small and middle-sized tumor nodules on the diaphragm (**1**) and the chest wall (**2**), in part anthracotically pigmented (→). Fatty tissue with tumor infiltration (↦).

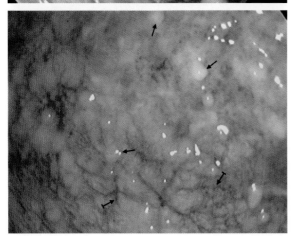

**Fig. 16.6**
**Malignant pleural effusion from metastatic breast cancer.**
After drainage of 500 mL of hemorrhagic effusion: nodular (→) and lymphangiotic (↦) tumor growth on the left posterior chest wall.

**Fig. 16.7**
**Malignant pleural effusion from metastatic breast cancer.**
After drainage of 2450 mL of serous effusion: tumor nodules (→)
on firm adhesions between lung (**1**) and chest wall (**2**).

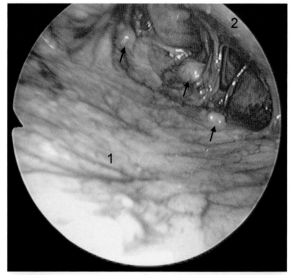

**Fig. 16.8**
**a  Malignant pleural effusion from unknown metastatic cancer.**
After drainage of 4000 mL of serous effusion: atelectatic middle and
lower lobes; flat, whitish meadow-like tumor nodules (→) on the
posterior chest wall.

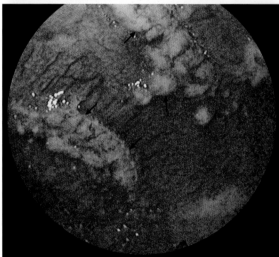

**b  Malignant pleural effusion from unknown metastatic cancer.**
The same patient with tumor nodule on the diaphragm (→) and
on the chest wall (↦).

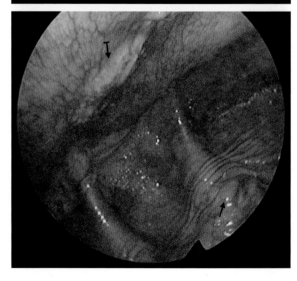

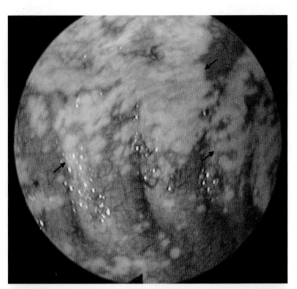

**Fig. 16.9**
**Malignant pleural effusion from metastatic gastric cancer.**
After drainage of 2000 mL of serous effusion: patchy whitish tumor growth ( ↑ ) on the posterior chest wall.

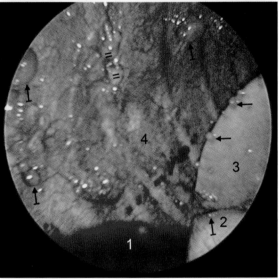

**Fig. 16.10**
**a Malignant pleural effusion from metastatic Ewing sarcoma.**
After drainage of 2500 mL of hemorrhagic effusion (**1**): small tumor nodules ( ↑ ) on the edge of the middle lobe (**2**) and lower lobe (**3**) and small to middle-sized nodules (↦) on the posterior chest wall (**4**), partially growing on intercostal fat (=).

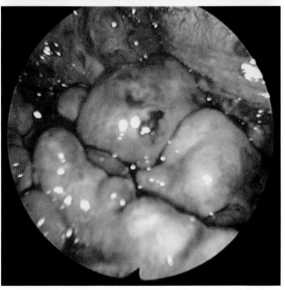

**b Malignant pleural effusion from metastatic Ewing sarcoma.**
The same patient with large nodules in the phrenicocostal sinus, originating from the diaphragmatic pleura.

**Fig. 16.11**
**Pleural effusion from metastatic renal carcinoma.** After drainage of 2000 mL of hemorrhagic effusion small nodules on the chest wall, and on the diaphragm (**1**) plum-sized, white tumor nodules (**2**) with tortuous vessels extending to the chest wall (**3**), which were very friable on contact.

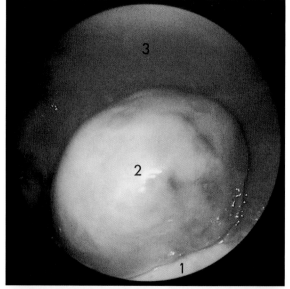

**Fig. 16.12**
**Malignant pleural effusion from metastatic adenocarcinoma of unknown origin.** After drainage of 1200 mL of very thick mucoid gel, the collapsed lung was seen lying free in the thoracic cavity, with coarse nodular, irregular green and white, glairy surface (with similar changes on the parietal pleura).

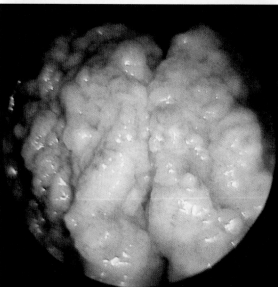

**Fig. 16.13**
**Malignant pleural effusion from metastatic ovarian carcinoma.** After drainage of 900 mL of slightly hemorrhagic effusion, the parietal pleura looks completely normal. Only the visceral pleura of the left lower lobe shows patchy nodular and lymphangitic tumor growth.

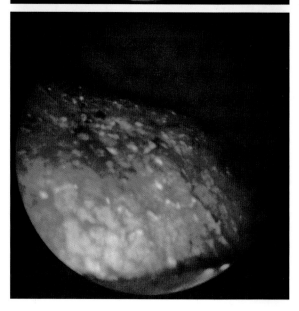

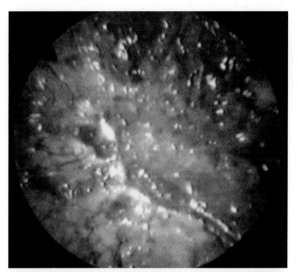

**Fig. 16.14**
**a Malignant pleural effusion from metastatic breast cancer.**
Patchy tumor growth on the chest-wall pleura. Photograph taken during white-light thoracoscopy (WLT).

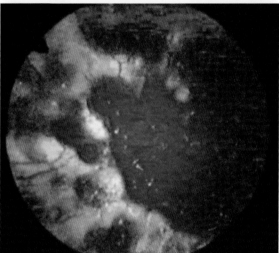

**b Same patient using autofluorescence (AF).** The color of the malignant tissue was light pink during WLT, but appears deep red during autofluorescence thoracoscopy, whereas the nonmalignant fibrous tissue has turned white. The line between the normal and malignant tissue is well demarcated.

(From Chrysanthidis and Janssen 2005, reprinted with kind permission from ERS Journals Ltd.)

# 17 Pleural Effusions due to Malignant Lymphoma/Myeloproliferative Neoplasm

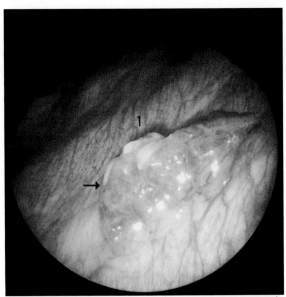

**Fig. 17.1**
**Malignant pleural effusion due to lymphoplasmocytic lymphoma (immunocytoma).** After drainage of 2500 mL of cloudy serous effusion: cauliflower-like tumor (→) on the anterior chest wall (**1**); otherwise normal lung and pleura.

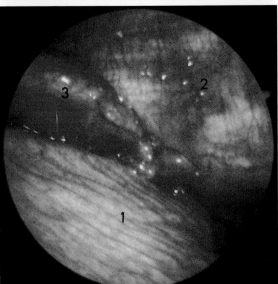

**Fig. 17.2**
**Malignant pleural effusion due to follicular lymphoma.**
After drainage of 1600 mL of serous effusion: a view of the right costocardiophrenic angle with the diaphragm (**1**), chest wall (**2**) injected with many vessels in the parietal pleura, and firm hyperemic fat pad (**3**) from which a biopsy was taken showing a follicular lymphoma.

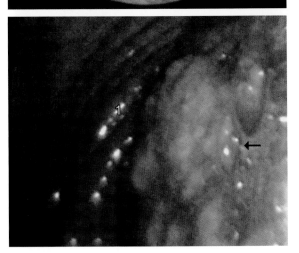

**Fig. 17.3**
**Bilateral pleural effusion due to primary myelofibrosis with extramedullary (pleura and lung) hematopoiesis.** After drainage of 1200 mL of serous exudate: dense middle-sized tumorous nodules, mainly on the left posterior chest wall (←), but also on the diaphragm (**1**), the anterior chest wall and on the visceral pleura. Forceps biopsies from the lesions without bleeding problems.

(From Schwarz C, Bittner R, Kirsch A, et al. A 62-year-old woman with bilateral pleural effusions and pulmonary infiltrates caused by extramedullary hematopoiesis. Respiration 2009; 78 (1): 110–113, with permission from Karger AG.)

# 18 Tuberculous Pleural Effusions

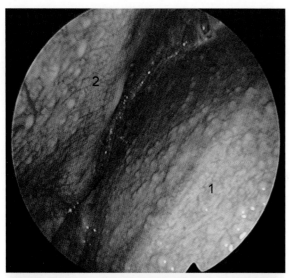

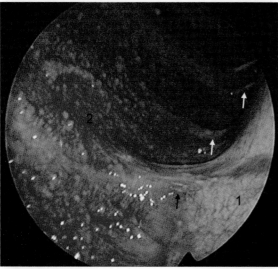

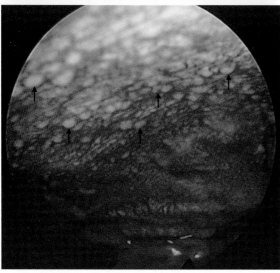

**Fig. 18.1**

**a  Tuberculous pleural effusion.** After drainage of 800 mL of serous effusion: typical miliary sagolike nodules in all parts of the right parietal pleura, here on the diaphragm (**1**) and the anterior chest wall (**2**).

**b  Tuberculous pleural effusion.** Same patient with firm adhesions (→) between the right lower lobe (**1**) and reddened, inflamed posterior chest wall (**2**), covered with sagolike miliary nodules.

**c  Tuberculous pleural effusion.** Same patient with white miliary, sagolike nodules (→) on the anterior chest wall, which is highly inflamed.

**Fig. 18.2**
**Tuberculous pleural effusion.** After drainage of 350 mL of serous effusion: small, miliary yellow-whitish nodules and patches of organized fibrin (→) on the pleural surface of the chest wall (**1**) and the lung (**2**).

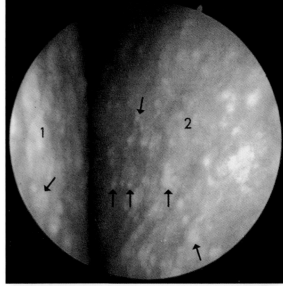

**Fig. 18.3**
**Tuberculous pleural effusion.** After drainage of 2500 mL of serous effusion: numerous small discrete nodules on all parts of the pleura. Here is seen a section of the chest wall with patchy granular surface consisting of nodules of different sizes (→). The vessels of the inflamed pleura are clearly dilated. Intercostal vessels and ribs (↦) show through the thickened parietal pleura.

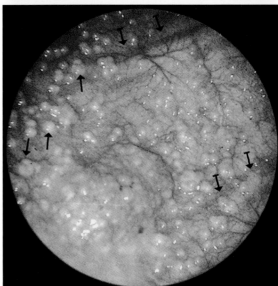

**Fig. 18.4**
**Tuberculous pleural effusion.** After drainage of 400 mL of opaque serous effusion, the visceral and parietal pleura show hyperemia and several fibrin patches. The photograph shows a magnification of a section of the chest wall, revealing serpiginous, partially distended, parallel vessels between which are relatively hyperemic, partially necrotic or fibrin-covered, millet-sized lesions (→).

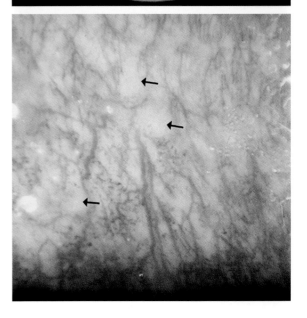

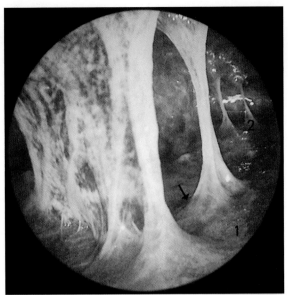

**Fig. 18.5**
**Tuberculous pleural effusion.** After drainage of 2000 mL of serous effusion: inflamed and hyperemic visceral and parietal pleura, covered with fibrinous patches. The posterior costovertebral region is shown with the diaphragm (**1**) and the chest wall (**2**). The lung cannot be visualized because it is fibrin-covered. The fibrinous adhesions pull the diaphragm cranially, producing tenting, and show vascularization at their base (→).

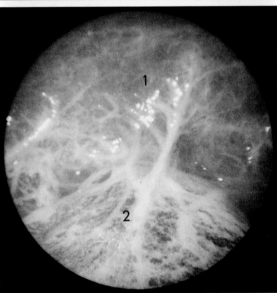

**Fig. 18.6**
**Tuberculous pleural effusion.** After drainage of 1400 mL of serous effusion, the lung (**1**) is covered with fibrin. The parenchyma can be seen as a slight reddish blush through the weblike dense fibrin (**2**) extending to the chest wall which is also covered by dense fibrin. Loculated cavities were opened, and biopsies were taken from the chest wall and adhesions.

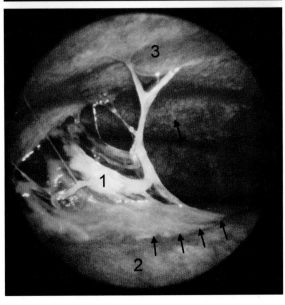

**Fig. 18.7**
**Tuberculous pleural effusion.** After drainage of 600 mL of serous effusion: fibrinous adhesions (**1**) between right lung (**2**) at the horizontal fissure ( ↑ ) and the anterior chest wall (**3**). A few small nodules (↦).

**Fig. 18.8**
**Tuberculous pleural effusion.** After drainage of 750 mL of serous effusion: multiple loculations with tender, partly translucent fibrinous membranes (**1**) and thickened chest-wall pleura (**2**).

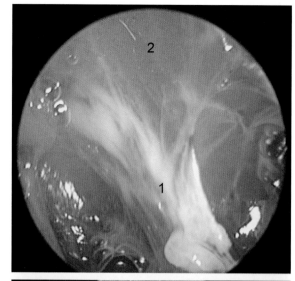

**Fig. 18.9**
**Tuberculous pleural effusion.** After drainage of 300 mL of slightly hemorrhagic effusion: reddened, inflamed, and thickened visceral and parietal pleura. The right lower lobe (**1**) is pulled toward the chest wall (**2**) by fibrinous adhesions. On the upper lobe (**3**), a few fibrinous patches (→).

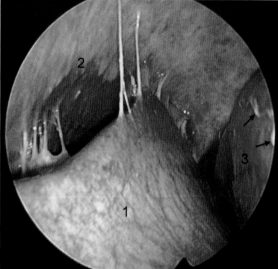

**Fig. 18.10**
**Tuberculous pleural effusion.** After drainage of 400 mL of serous effusion, the lung appeared adherent and was covered by translucent pleura. The base of the lower lobe (**1**) shows anthracotic pigment hardly recognizable through the thickened fibrinous pleura. The edges of the lung are rounded and furrowed. A dense, fibrinous strand (**2**) is seen arising from the visceral pleura (**3**) at an iatrogenic hemorrhagic effusion. The chest wall (**4**) shows inflammatory changes.

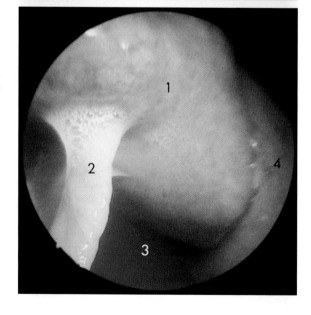

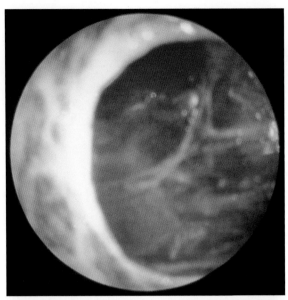

**Fig. 18.11**
**Tuberculous pleural effusion.** After drainage of 650 mL of serous effusion: reddened chest-wall pleura, fibrinous adhesions and multiple loculations.

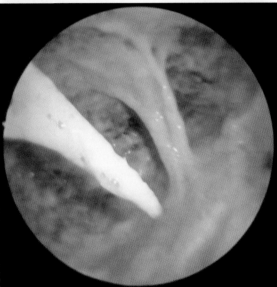

**Fig. 18.12**
**Tuberculous empyema.** After drainage of 300 mL of thick, putrid, and odorless pleural fluid: multiple adhesions and thickened visceral pleura.

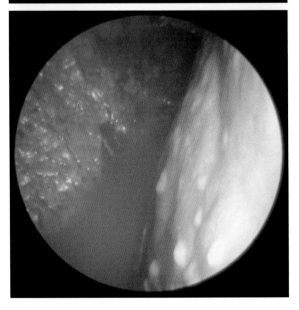

**Fig. 18.13**
**Tuberculous empyema.** After drainage of 800 mL of putrid, odorless pleural fluid: thickened visceral and parietal pleura with small nodules.

# 19 Pleural Effusions of Other Origin

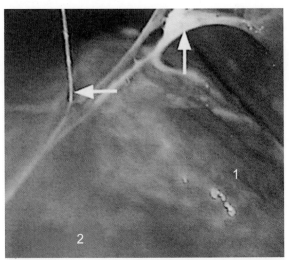

**Fig. 19.1**
**Complicated parapneumonic effusion.**
The lung (**1**) is bathed in turbid fluid (**2**) and fibrinous adhesions (→).

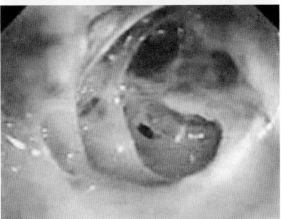

**Fig. 19.2**
**Fibrinopurulent stage of empyema.** The photograph shows
the fluid collection and fibrin, creating adhesions and loculations.

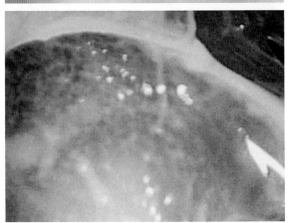

**Fig. 19.3**
**Fibrinopurulent stage of empyema.** The photograph shows
fibrin adhesions and the formation of a loculation, filled with
empyema fluid.

**Fig. 19.4**
**Nonspecific pleural effusion with adenovirus infection.**
After pneumothorax induction, there was only minimal effusion.
The right upper lobe was adherent dorsally. The lower lobe (**1**) and
middle lobe (**2**) look normal; the interlobar septum was displaced
by a flat, nonvascularized wide adhesion. Additional adhesions are
present between the lower lobe and the diaphragm (**3**), which
appears brownish through the remaining effusion.

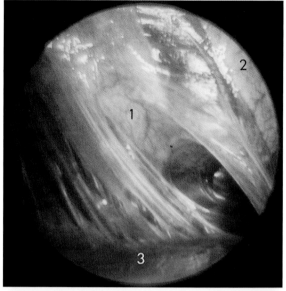

**Fig. 19.5**
**Nonspecific pleuritis with pleuropulmonary adhesions.**
The picture shows the right lower lobe (**1**) attached to the chest wall
by a broad adhesion and the base of the middle lobe (**2**) with an
adhesion toward the diaphragm.

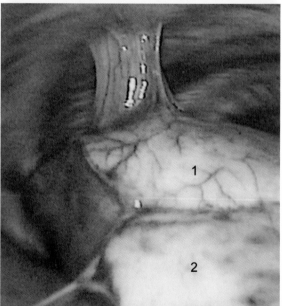

**Fig. 19.6**
**Nonspecific pleuritis with pleuropulmonary adhesion.**
The picture shows a broad adhesion between lung and chest wall.

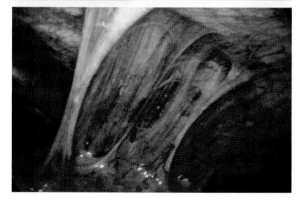

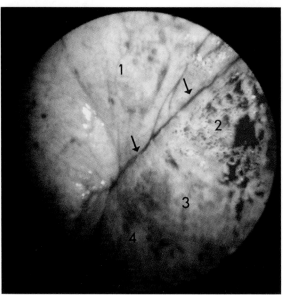

**Fig. 19.7**
**Pleural effusion associated with pulmonary infarct.** After drainage of 300 mL of amber effusion: a normal left upper lobe (**1**). The edge of the lower lobe (**2**) shows some bloody effusion on its surface. In the underlying, subapical lower lobe segment is seen a bandlike, firm hemorrhagic infarct (**3**) adjacent to the somewhat hyperemic lateral basal segment (**4**). Intersegmental septum (→).

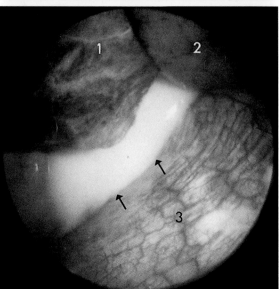

**Fig. 19.8**
**Idiopathic chylothorax.** After drainage of 2100 mL of chylous pleural effusion, the upper lobe and lower lobe (**1**) are atelectatic; the middle lobe (**2**) is well ventilated. Parietal pleura and diaphragm (**3**) are not inflamed and have normal vascularity. From the interlobar septum, a chylous stream flows (→).

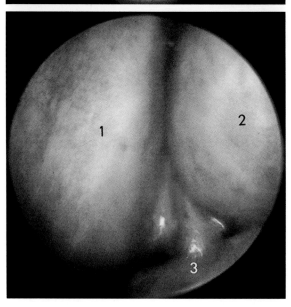

**Fig. 19.9**
**Pleural effusion associated with systemic lupus erythematosus.** After drainage of 150 mL of serous pleural effusion, the left upper lobe (**1**) and the lower lobe (**2**) are covered with markedly thickened pleura. Above the diaphragm (**3**) is a bluish area of atelectasis at the edge of the upper lobe. The lung structure is poorly identified; the lobar edges are rounded; the visceral pleura is hyperemic.

**Fig. 19.10**
**Rheumatoid pleuritis and pulmonary fibrosis.** After drainage
of 250 mL of serous effusion, the lung (**1**) is adherent to the chest
wall (**2**). On the right side of the picture, on the visceral pleura (**3**)
are white fibrin deposits (→). The parietal pleura (**2**) appears gray.
(Courtesy of P. Faurschou and K. Viskum.)

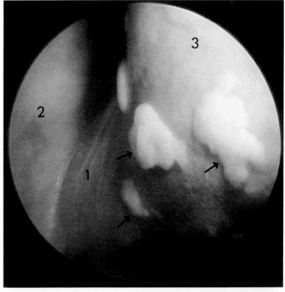

**Fig. 19.11**
**Rheumatoid pleural effusion.** After drainage of 1500 mL of
serous effusion: inflamed and thickened chest-wall pleura (**1**)
and visceral pleura (**2**). The lung structure is poorly recognizable.
White fibrin deposits (→) on both pleural layers.

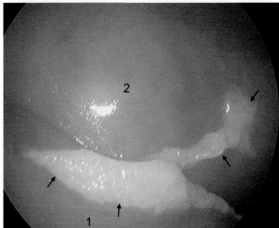

**Fig. 19.12**
**Loculated rheumatoid pleural effusion.** After drainage of 100 mL
of cloudy, fibrinous effusion, the walls of the loculated cavity are
covered by extremely dense fibrin so that neither lung nor parietal
pleura is recognizable.

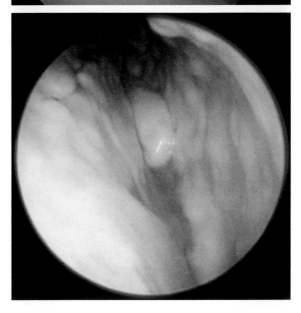

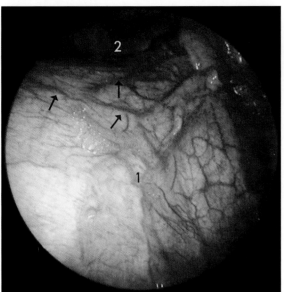

**Fig. 19.13**
**Hydrothorax associated with hepatic cirrhosis.** After drainage of 500 mL of icteric effusion, the entire lung is collapsed, the visceral parietal pleura is shiny and unremarkable. On the diaphragm (**1**), are tortuous, greatly distended veins (→) that can be followed to the mediastinum. The lung is seen at the upper edge of the picture (**2**).

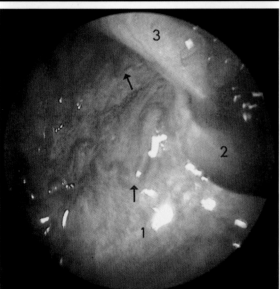

**Fig. 19.14**
**Hemothorax with hepatic cirrhosis.** After drainage of 3100 mL of hemorrhagic effusion, the anterior mediastinum (**1**), the pericardium (**2**), and the fat pad (**3**) are seen in the picture. On the mediastinal pleura are tortuous venous varices (→) and between these marked capillary hyperemia.

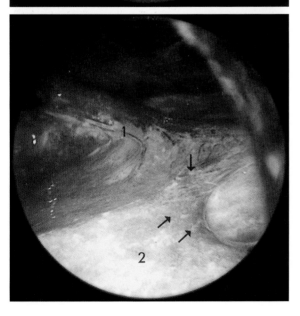

**Fig. 19.15**
**Pleural effusion due to pancreatitis.** After drainage of 2000 mL of cloudy serous effusion, the right upper and lower lobes are partially fused with the chest wall. The middle lobe (**1**) is markedly vascularized, compressed, and bound to the diaphragm by adhesions (**2**). The diaphragm as well as the remaining parietal pleura are thickened by whitish fibrin. Numerous small calcific areas are present (→).

**Fig. 19.16**
**Chronic congestive pleural effusion due to mitral stenosis.**
After drainage of 1800 mL of clear exudate, the picture gives a view of the paravertebral region (**1**), the upper lobe (**2**), and the middle lobe (**3**). The upper lobe particularly is covered and surrounded by gelatinous effusion. Blue pigment in the lung can barely be seen. In the interlobar septum is a gelatinous mass (→) of firm consistency.

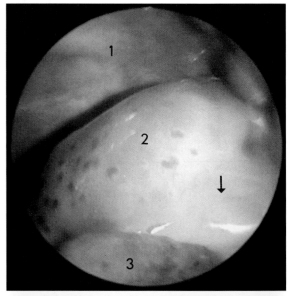

**Fig. 19.17**
**Chronic congestive pleural effusion due to left-ventricular failure.** After drainage of 140 mL of effusion: between the right upper lobe (**1**) and the lower lobe (**2**) in the interlobar septum, some effusion (→) and a dense fibrous strand (↦) tethering the lung to the dorsal chest wall (**3**). The visceral and parietal pleura is thickened, and the lung can be seen through these only with difficulty.

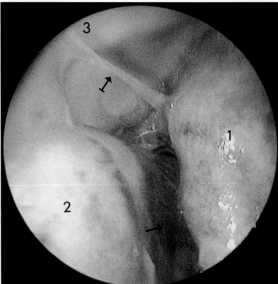

**Fig. 19.18**
**Pleural effusion associated with postmyocardial infarction syndrome.** After drainage of 200 mL of cloudy serous effusion, the entire visceral pleura of the right lower lobe (**1**), upper lobe (**2**), and the parietal pleura show hyaline thickening and a reticular network of dilated vessels. Behind a broad fibrinous membrane (**3**) is the middle lobe that cannot be visualized.

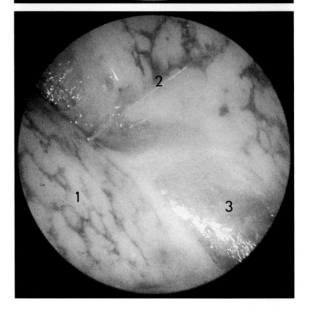

# 20 Pneumothorax

## Fig. 20.1
**Primary spontaneous pneumothorax.** After introduction of the thoracoscope into the sixth intercostal space in the mid-axillary line, the lung is retracted. Visceral and parietal pleura are normal. The view toward the apex of the thoracic cavity shows the upper lobe (**1**), which appears pinkish at its apex and is air-containing, at its base bluish and atelectatic; between these is a pigmented area and a whitish spot (**2**) which represents a small ruptured bleb. Subclavian artery (**3**), phrenic nerve (**4**), subclavian vein (**5**), internal thoracic artery (**6**), first rib (**7**), superior intercostal artery (**8**), stellate ganglion at the head of the first rib (**9**), head of the second rib (**10**), sympathetic trunk (**11**), anterior longitudinal ligament (**12**), intercostal artery (**13**), intercostal vein (**14**).

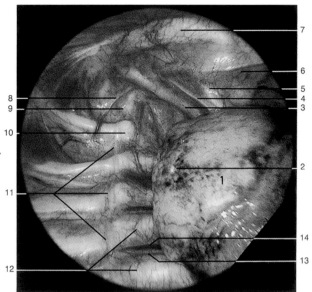

## Fig. 20.2
**Primary spontaneous pneumothorax.** The right upper lobe (**1**) is bluish and atelectatic, at its apex is an egg-sized bleb (**4**) and a smaller whitish hemorrhagic strand (**2**) that is one end of the torn adhesion. At the thoracic apex on the first rib (**3**), a blackish hemorrhagic area represents the point on the parietal pleura at which the adhesion was attached. The lung has meanwhile separated from the apex of the thoracic cavity. Phrenic nerve (**5**), subclavian vein (**6**), subclavian artery (**7**), chest wall with ribs and intercostal vessels (**8**).

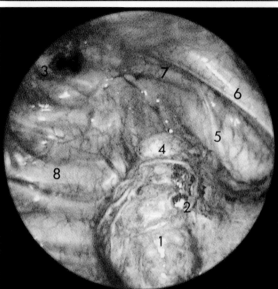

## Fig. 20.3
**Primary spontaneous pneumothorax.** The photograph shows a small apical bleb in a patient with recurrences of pneumothorax. The bleb is not deflated, hence not leaking.

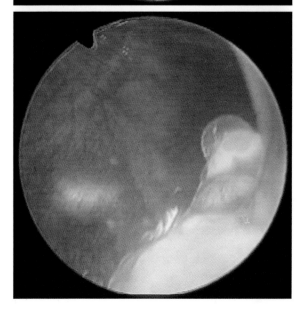

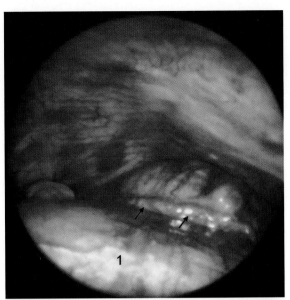

**Fig. 20.4**
**Primary spontaneous pneumothorax.**
Small bleb (→) at the apex of the left upper lobe (**1**).

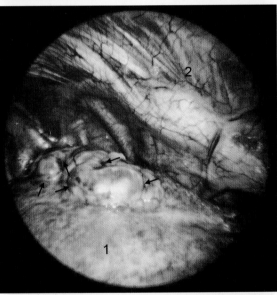

**Fig. 20.5**
**Primary spontaneous pneumothorax.** Multiple blebs ( ↑ )
at the apex of the left upper lobe, which is covered with fibrin (**1**).
Normal chest-wall pleura (**2**).

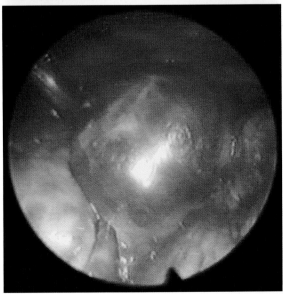

**Fig. 20.6**
**Primary spontaneous pneumothorax.** The photograph shows
a large bulla in a 35-year-old smoker with primary spontaneous
pneumothorax, located at the left lower lobe. The bulla is not
leaking at the time of thoracoscopy.

**Fig. 20.7**
**Primary spontaneous pneumothorax.** The photograph shows the atelectatic right upper lobe (**1**) with pleural thickening and beneath this, in the open fissure, the whitish pericardium (**2**) covered with delicate vessels. The median segment of the middle lobe (**3**) is atelectatic; the visceral pleura is cloudy; the lateral middle lobe segment (**4**) is pinkish, and on its leading edge one sees grapelike small emphysematous blebs (→) lying on the diaphragm (**5**).

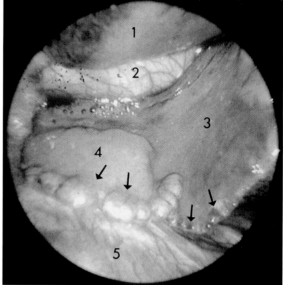

**Fig. 20.8**
**a  Primary spontaneous pneumothorax.** The photograph shows a deformation at the left upper lobe in a patient with recurrence of pneumothorax. There is marked systemic vascularization of the malformation.

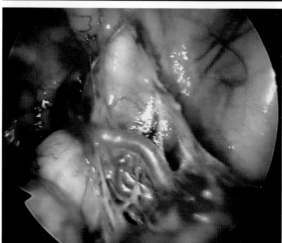

**b  Primary spontaneous pneumothorax.** Same patient. Situation after fluorescein inhalation, and during blue light thoracoscopy. The air leak is clearly visible at the base of the malformation.

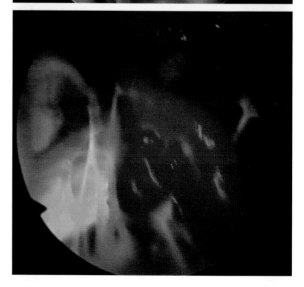

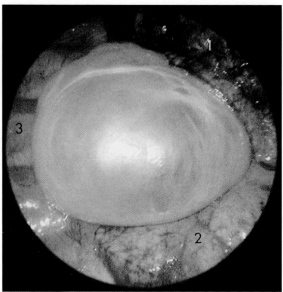

**Fig. 20.9**
**Secondary spontaneous pneumothorax (bullous emphysema).**
The base of the right upper lobe (**1**) is blackened and atelectatic with numerous emphysematous blebs not shown in the picture. From the tip of the lower lobe (**2**) a large bulla, the size of a goose egg, extends downwards; it is delicate and distended. In the background, the posterior chest wall and ribs (**3**) can be seen.

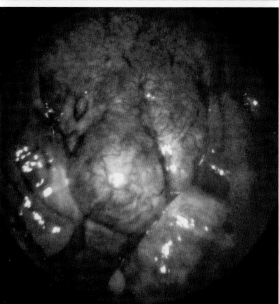

**Fig. 20.10**
**Secondary spontaneous pneumothorax with bullous emphysema.** The left lower lobe is destroyed by several bullae.

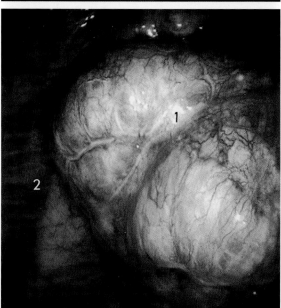

**Fig. 20.11**
**Secondary spontaneous pneumothorax with bullous emphysema.** The upper lobe (**1**) is destroyed by innumerable bullae. The surface of the lung is replaced by a network of vascularized connective tissue. A bronchopleural fistula is not evident. In the background is the dorsal chest wall (**2**).

(Courtesy of C. Boutin.)

**Fig. 20.12**
**Secondary spontaneous pneumothorax.** Several blebs in the apex of the left upper lobe in a patient with emphysema.

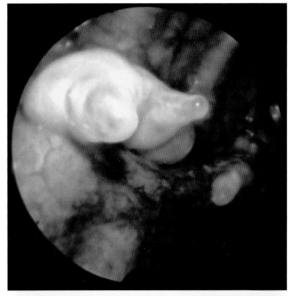

**Fig. 20.13**
**Secondary spontaneous pneumothorax.** An adhesion is attached to the apex (→). Ruptured emphysematous bleb, through which the lung parenchyma gapes. Chest wall (**1**) with ribs and the apical segment of the upper lobe (**2**).

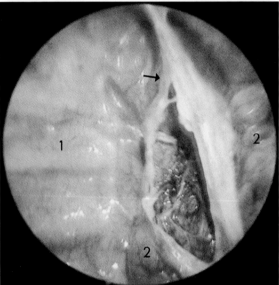

**Fig. 20.14**
**Large emphysematous bulla.** Unintended introduction of the thoracoscope into a left-sided bulla, which had been interpreted wrongly as pneumothorax ("bulloscopy"). The vascularized walls of the bulla moved inward during expiration; at the base of the bulla is some slightly hemorrhagic fluid.

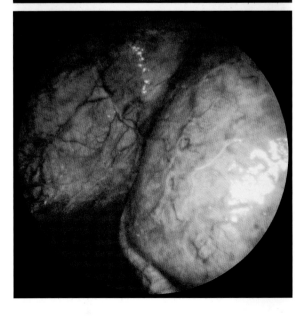

# 21 Diffuse Lung Diseases

**Fig. 21.1**
**Sarcoidosis stage II.** After induction of a right-sided pneumothorax, in the interlobular septae, anthracotic pigment is seen outlining subpleural lymphatics. Upper lobe (**1**). In the middle lobe (**2**) there is whitish thickening of the interstitium, in part stellate and in part geographic (→).

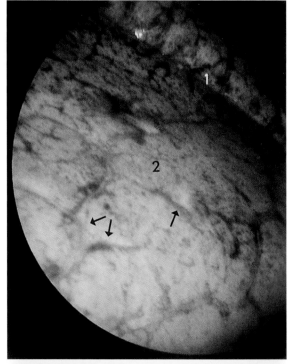

**Fig. 21.2**
**Sarcoidosis stage II with pleural lesion.** After induction of a left-sided pneumothorax, the lung (**1**) shows nodular lesions (→) on the surface of the left lower lobe (**1**) and upper lobe (**2**); on the chest wall is one typical sarcoid nodule (↦).

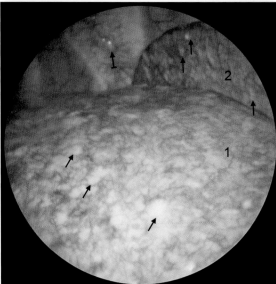

**Fig. 21.3**
**Sarcoidosis stage II with pleural lesions.** After induction of a left pneumothorax, the parietal pleura shows increased numbers of dilated vessels. In some places (→), whitish nodules, surrounded by a hyperemic zone protrude into the pleural space.

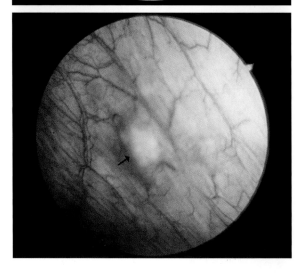

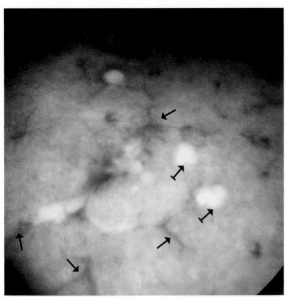

**Fig. 21.4**
**Sarcoidosis stage III.** After induction of a right pneumothorax, the interlobar regions are hyperemic (→). In all lobes there are small whitish nodules of 2–3 mm diameter without pigmented edge (↦).

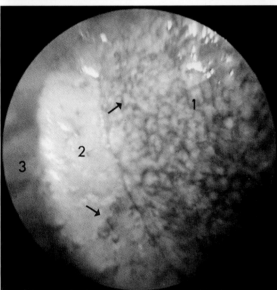

**Fig. 21.5**
**Sarcoidosis stage III.** After induction of a right pneumothorax, the lung is seeded with whitish nodules containing anthracotic pigment (→). Right upper lobe (**1**), interlobar pleura of the lower lobe (**2**), chest wall and ribs (**3**).

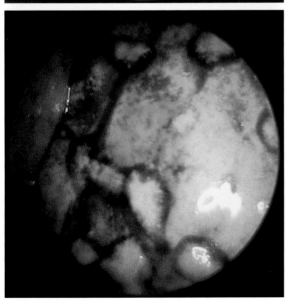

**Fig. 21.6**
**Sarcoidosis stage III.** After induction of a right pneumothorax, scattered over all lung lobes are lentil- to pea-sized, firm, whitish nodules containing bluish pigment.

**Fig. 21.7**
**Langerhans cell histiocytosis.** After induction of a right pneumothorax, all lobes show distinct thickening of the interlobar septae (→) interspersed with small pale blebs (↦) covered with vessels. Upper lobe (**1**), middle lobe (**2**), lower lobe (**3**). Interlobar fissures clear.

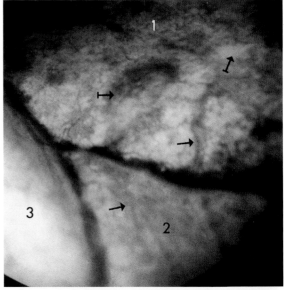

**Fig. 21.8**
**Desquamative interstitial pneumonia (DIP).** After induction of a pneumothorax, the lung retracted well but appeared stiff. Widened fissure between the upper lobe (**1**), lower lobe (**2**), and middle lobe (**3**). The parietal pleura of the chest wall (**4**) is shiny. In the upper lobe were firm, whitish deposits arranged around the interlobular septae (→). The bluish-green pigmented areas were retracted. Between these are well-ventilated pale areas of lung parenchyma.

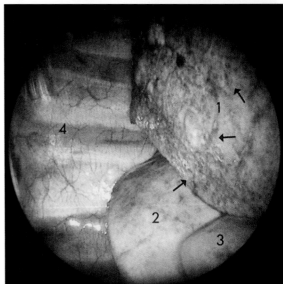

**Fig. 21.9**
**Idiopathic pulmonary fibrosis (IPF).** After induction of a right-sided pneumothorax, the interlobular septae of the middle lobe (**1**) and lower lobe (**3**) are brownish, clearly thickened, and in part retracted (→). Parenchymal lymph node in the middle lobe (↦). Mediastinum (**2**). Histology of the biopsies was consistent with UIP (usual interstitial pneumonia).

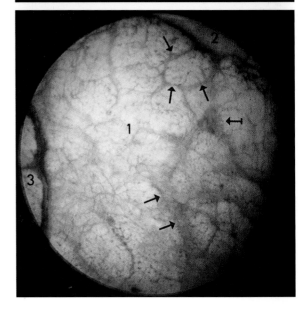

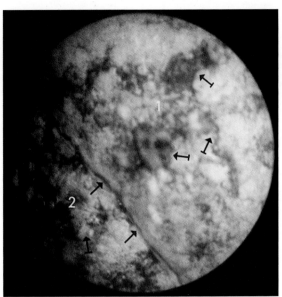

**Fig. 21.10**
**Idiopathic pulmonary fibrosis (IPF).** After induction of a right pneumothorax, the lung is retracted, the oblique fissure is visualized (→) between the upper lobe (**1**) and lower lobe (**2**). The lung has an irregular pigmented surface. In all lobes, there are areas of whitish nodules with peripherally thickened pigmented zones (↦).

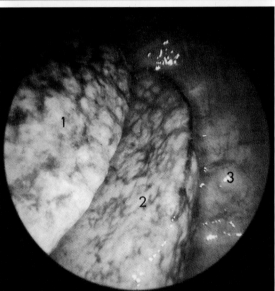

**Fig. 21.11**
**Respiratory bronchiolitis-associated interstitial lung disease (RBILD).** The lung is markedly retracted and stiff and shows a widened, interlobar septum between the upper lobe (**1**) and lower lobe (**2**). The surface is irregular and wrinkled, and the interlobar septa are retracted and thickened. In several places there are small emphysematous blebs. Chest wall (**3**).

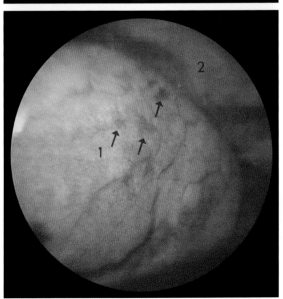

**Fig. 21.12**
**Alveolar proteinosis.** After induction of a right-sided pneumothorax, increased vascularity and slight brownish pigmentation in the upper lobe (**1**) as in the rest of the lung (**2**). In some places there are reddish-brown spots (→) of 2–3 cm diameter (alveolar filling).

**Fig. 21.13**
**Silicosis.** After induction of a right-sided pneumothorax, the lung is retracted and somewhat firm. In the upper lobe (**1**) and lower lobe (**2**), 1–2-mm grayish nodules with anthracotic pigment (→), partially confluent. The middle lobe (**3**) is unremarkable, between the lobes the oblique and horizontal fissures.

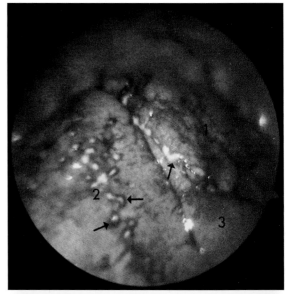

**Fig. 21.14**
**Anthracosilicosis.** After induction of a left-sided pneumothorax, originating from the upper lobe (**1**): white, vascularized adhesions (**2**) to the anterior chest wall, radiating whitish scars (→) in the markedly anthracotic-pigmented lung.

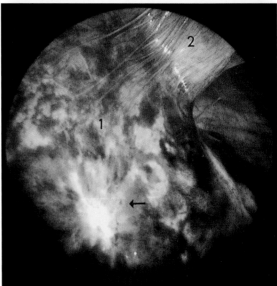

**Fig. 21.15**
**Anthracosis.** After induction of a pneumothorax: complete retraction of the lung. Upper lobe (**1**) with blackish pigmentation; reddish interlobar region of the lower lobe (**2**). Carbon pigmentation of the middle lobe (**3**) and diaphragm (**4**) with anthracotic pigmentation (→).

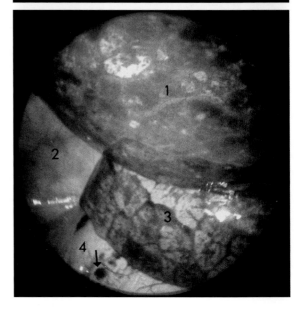

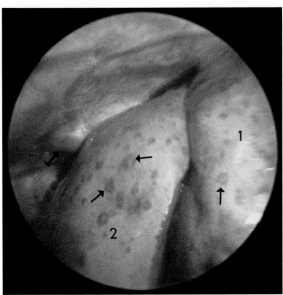

**Fig. 21.16**
**Lung metastases from thyroid carcinoma.** After induction of a right-sided pneumothorax: numerous foci between 1 and 3 mm with hemorrhagic surface (→) in the upper lobe (**1**) and lower lobe (**2**). In the apical portion of the thorax, the subclavian vein (↦) can be seen.

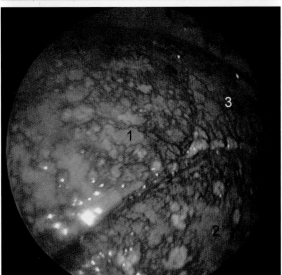

**Fig. 21.17**
**Lung metastases from ovarian carcinoma.** After iatrogenic pneumothorax due to transbronchial biopsy: multiple whitish tumor nodules in all lobes; upper lobe (**1**), lower lobe (**2**), middle lobe (**3**); multiple pulmonary metastases of an ovarian cancer.

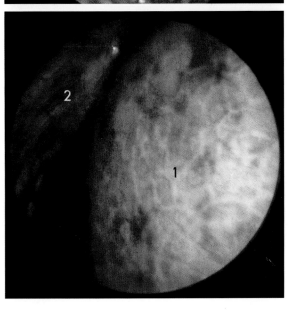

**Fig. 21.18**
**Lymphangiosis carcinomatosa of the lung in association with an ovarian carcinoma.** After induction of a left-sided pneumothorax: view from posterior toward the lower lobe (**1**) and the anterior chest wall (**2**). The lung shows a whitish reticular surface pattern; the lobules are somewhat reddened by dilated vessels and are somewhat congested.

# 22 Other Indications

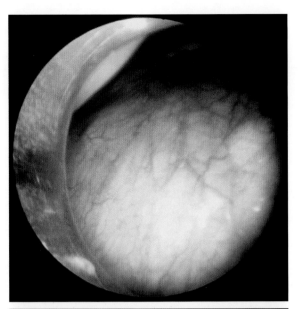

**Fig. 22.1**
**a  Malignant pericardial effusion.** View of the pericardium from the left side.

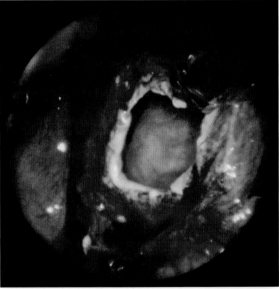

**b  Thoracoscopic pericardial fenestration.** Same case, showing the fenestration of the pericardium created by laser coagulation.

(Courtesy of B. Vogel and W. Mall.)

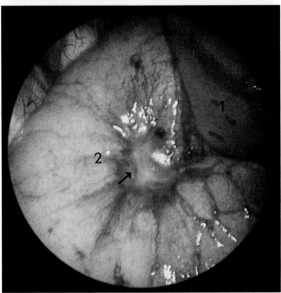

**Fig. 22.2**
**Adenocarcinoma of the lung with malignant retraction.**
After induction of a right-sided pneumothorax, the upper lobe (**1**) is unremarkable. In the apex of the lower lobe (**2**) there is typical carcinomatous retraction (→) with radiating scars particularly on the interlobar fissure. In the center, covered with shiny pleura, the tumor is seen as a yellowish-gray mass.

**Fig. 22.3**
**Hamartochondroma.** After iatrogenic pneumothorax due to fine-needle aspiration, the pneumothorax was utilized for thoracoscopy. The apex of the right lower lobe (**1**) is congested as a result of the needle aspiration; the laterobasal segment (**2**) is separated by the intersegmental septum. The posterobasal segment (**3**) shows, on its leading edge, an irregular gray-brown lesion (→) which is also somewhat hemorrhagic as a result of the previous puncture.

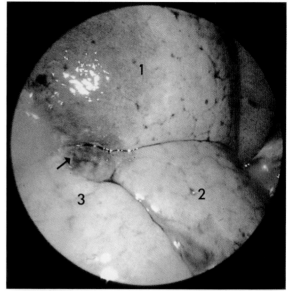

**Fig. 22.4**
**Leiomyofibroma of the middle lobe.** After iatrogenic right-sided pneumothorax due to transthoracic needle aspiration: a yellowish-gray irregular tumor, 2 cm × 3 cm (**1**), between the middle lobe (**2**) and lower lobe (**3**), covered with fresh blood. The upper lobe (**4**) is covered by delicate pleura, the anterior chest wall (**5**), and the diaphragm (**6**). Surgery revealed that the leiomyofibroma originated from the middle lobe.

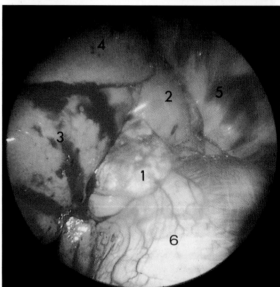

**Fig. 22.5**
**Multiple bilateral tuberculomas.** After induction of a right-sided pneumothorax, the lung shows spotty pigmentation. In several areas are whitish-gray foci extending to 1 cm diameter, infiltrated with vessels and with a pigmented border. Atypical focus (**1**) on the periphery of the upper lobe; histologically scarred tuberculoma with fresh epitheloid cell satellite lesions.

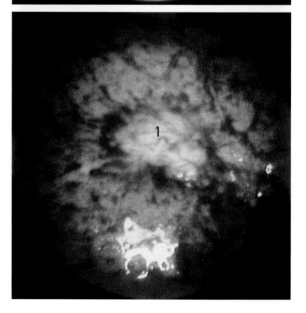

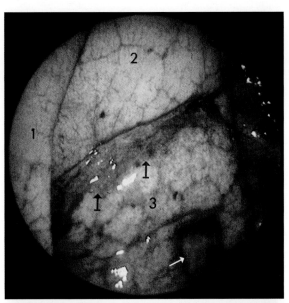

**Fig. 22.6**
**Hemorrhagic pulmonary infarct.** After induction of a left-sided pneumothorax, the edge of the upper lobe (**1**), like the segmented lower lobe (**2**), is unremarkable. The base of the lower lobe (**3**) shows in the lower portion (→) a rhomboid blue-red region with a hemorrhagic edge of a pulmonary infarct. The surrounding area of lung also shows hemorrhagic congestion. On the upper edge of the base of the lower lobe, there is a bandlike area of atelectasis (↦) with several pinhead-sized petechiae. Chest wall and ribs (**4**).

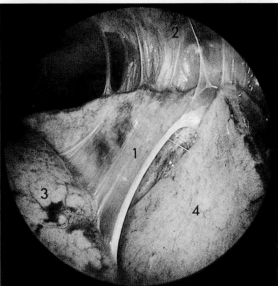

**Fig. 22.7**
**Old pulmonary infarct with fibrous pleuritis.** After induction of a right pneumothorax, the base of the upper lobe (**1**) shows adhesions to the chest wall (**2**), to the lower lobe (**3**), and to the middle lobe (**4**). Through the adhesions, one sees a bluish area of pneumonic consolidation in the base of the upper lobe.

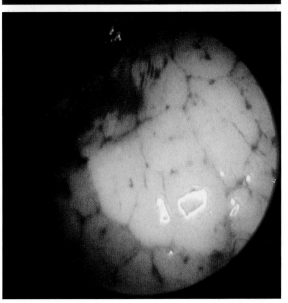

**Fig. 22.8**
**Anemic pulmonary infarct associated with recurrent pulmonary emboli.** After induction of a right-sided pneumothorax, the lung showed delicate surface lining. The lateral segment of the right lower lobe showed a white, sharply defined lobular area of 3 cm diameter.

**Fig. 22.9**
**Atelectasis of the lateral segment of the middle lobe.** After induction of a right pneumothorax, the junction of oblique and horizontal fissures is seen. Between the aerated upper lobe (**1**), lower lobe (**2**), and the medial segment of the middle lobe (**3**) is the lateral middle lobe segment (**4**). This is sharply delineated, blue, and atelectatic. The atelectasis resulted from a bronchial obstruction by a metastasizing pancreas carcinoma.

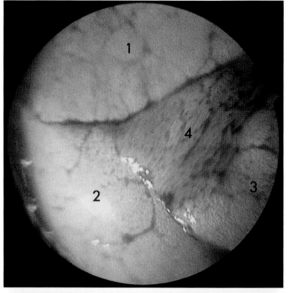

**Fig. 22.10**
**Arteriovenous aneurysm of the lung.** After induction of a right pneumothorax, one sees the upper lobe (**1**) and the lower lobe (**2**). In the middle lobe (**3**), ventrolaterally is a serpentine, blue, distended blood vessel the size of a large bean (→), lying on a clearly delineated, pale, subsegmental zone (↦).

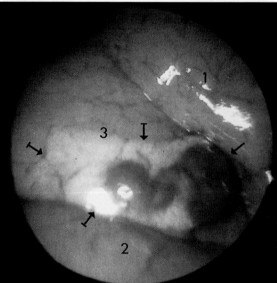

**Fig. 22.11**
**Lipoma of the right chest wall.** After induction of a right pneumothorax, the lung was well retracted. On the chest wall, a smooth, well-defined, yellow lipoma was seen.

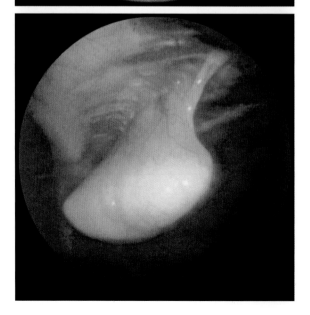

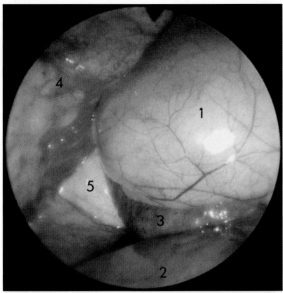

**Fig. 22.12**
**Lipoma in the right cardiophrenic angle.** After induction of a right-sided pneumothorax, a smooth, well-defined yellow lipoma (**1**) above the diaphragm (**2**) was seen. The middle lobe (**3**), upper lobe (**4**) and the white pericardium (**5**) can be recognized.

(Courtesy of P. Faurschou and K. Viskum.)

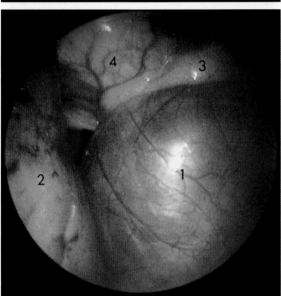

**Fig. 22.13**
**Right pleuropericardial cyst.** After induction of a right-sided pneumothorax, the lung (**2**) is completely retracted. In the anterior cardiophrenic angle, a distended cyst covered by delicate vessels (**1**) on top of which is a small lipoma (**3**). Pericardium (**4**). Aspiration revealed watery fluid and subsequently the flaccid cyst wall was seen to be attached to the pericardium by a narrow stem.

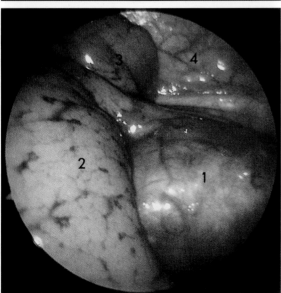

**Fig. 22.14**
**Solitary pleural fibroma of the middle lobe.** After pneumothorax induction, the unremarkable lower lobe is identified (**2**). On the caudal edge of the middle lobe (**3**) is a polypoid, violet, lobulated tumor (**1**) which can be separated from the pericardium (**4**) and from the diaphragm. Surgical removal confirmed a pedunculated solitary fibrous tumor originating from the middle-lobe pleura.

# References

Aelony Y, King R, Boutin C. Thoracoscopic talc poudrage pleurodesis for chronic recurrent pleural effusions. Ann Intern Med 1991; 115 (10): 778–782

Aelony Y, King RR, Boutin C. Thoracoscopic talc poudrage in malignant pleural effusions: effective pleurodesis despite low pleural pH. Chest 1998; 113 (4): 1007–1012

Aelony Y, Yao JF. Prolonged survival after talc poudrage for malignant pleural mesothelioma: case series. Respirology 2005; 10 (5): 649–655

Aelony Y. Talc pleurodesis and acute respiratory distress syndrome. Lancet 2007; 369 (9572): 1494–1496

Akçay S, Pinelli V, Marchetti GP, Tassi GF. The diagnosis of sarcoidosis pleurisy by medical thoracoscopy: report of three cases. Tuberk Toraks 2008; 56 (4): 429–433

Al-Kattan KM, Kaplan DK, Goldstraw P. The non-functioning pleuro-peritoneal shunt: revise or replace? Thorac Cardiovasc Surg 1994; 42: 310–312

Al-Muffarej F, Margolis M, Tempesta B, et al. From Jacobaeus to da Vinci: thoracoscopic applications of the robot. Surg Laparosc Endosc Tech 2010; 20: 1–9

Alcozer G, Dorigoni A. La toracoscopia diagnostica. Florence: Nardini; 1984

Alexander J. Closed intrapleural pneumolysis. In: Alexander J. The Collapse Therapy of Pulmonary Tuberculosis (Chapter XII). London: Baillière, Tindall; 1937: 314–315

Alifano M, Roth T, Broët SC, Schussler O, Magdeleinat P, Regnard JF. Catamenial pneumothorax: a prospective study. Chest 2003; 124 (3): 1004–1008

Alifano M, Jablonski C, Kadiri H, et al. Catamenial and noncatamenial, endometriosis-related or nonendometriosis-related pneumothorax referred for surgery. Am J Respir Crit Care Med 2007; 176 (10): 1048–1053

American Thoracic Society; European Respiratory Society. American Thoracic Society/European Respiratory Society International Multidisciplinary Consensus Classification of the Idiopathic Interstitial Pneumonias. This joint statement of the American Thoracic Society (ATS), and the European Respiratory Society (ERS) was adopted by the ATS board of directors, June 2001 and by the ERS Executive Committee, June 2001. Am J Respir Crit Care Med 2002; 165 (2): 277–304

Amjadi K, Alvarez GG, Vanderhelst E, Velkeniers B, Lam M, Noppen M. The prevalence of blebs or bullae among young healthy adults: a thoracoscopic investigation. Chest 2007; 132 (4): 1140–1145

Andrivet P, Djedaini K, Teboul JL, Brochard L, Dreyfuss D. Spontaneous pneumothorax. Comparison of thoracic drainage vs immediate or delayed needle aspiration. Chest 1995; 108 (2): 335–339

Angelillo-Mackinlay T, Lyons GA, Piedras MB, Angelillo-Mackinlay D. Surgical treatment of postpneumonic empyema. World J Surg 1999; 23 (11): 1110–1113

Antony VB, Loddenkemper R, Astoul P, et al. Management of malignant pleural effusions. [ATS/ERS Statement] Am J Respir Crit Care Med 2000; 162: 1987–2001 [and Eur Respir J 2001; 18: 402–419]

Antony VB, Nasreen N, Mohammed KA, et al. Talc pleurodesis: basic fibroblast growth factor mediates pleural fibrosis. Chest 2004; 126 (5): 1522–1528

Ash SR, Manfredi F. Directed biopsy using a small endoscope: thoracoscopy and peritoneoscopy simplified. N Engl J Med 1974; 291 (26): 1398–1399

Astoul P, Cheikh R, Cabanot C, Vialette JP, Vestri R, Boutin C. [Pleural amyloidosis: thoracoscopic diagnosis and physiopathological approach]. Rev Mal Respir 1992; 9 (6): 629–631

Astoul P, Viallat JR, Laurent JC, Brandely M, Boutin C. Intrapleural recombinant IL-2 in passive immunotherapy for malignant pleural effusion. Chest 1993; 103 (1): 209–213

Atkinson JL, Fealey RD. Sympathotomy instead of sympathectomy for palmar hyperhidrosis: minimizing postoperative compensatory hyperhidrosis. Mayo Clin Proc 2003; 78 (2): 167–172

Audier M, Boutin C, Arnaud A, D'Journo J. [Case of cardiac effusion treated by pleuroscopic talc spray]. Mars Med 1967; 104 (10): 866–869

Augoulea A, Lambrinoudaki I, Christodoulakos G. Thoracic endometriosis syndrome. Respiration 2008; 75 (1): 113–119

Avrahami R, Watemberg S, Hiss Y. Thoracoscopy vs conventional autopsy of the thorax. A promising perspective. Arch Surg 1995; 130: 956–958

Ayed AK. Video-assisted thoracoscopic lung biopsy in the diagnosis of diffuse interstitial lung disease. A prospective study. J Cardiovasc Surg (Torino) 2003; 44 (1): 115–118

Ayed AK, Chandrasekaran C, Sukumar M. Video-assisted thoracoscopic surgery for primary spontaneous pneumothorax: clinicopathological correlation. Eur J Cardiothorac Surg 2006; 29 (2): 221–225

Baas P, Triesscheijn M, Burgers S, van Pel R, Stewart F, Aalders M. Fluorescence detection of pleural malignancies using 5-aminolaevulinic acid. Chest 2006; 129 (3): 718–724

Balderson SS, D'Amico TA. Thoracoscopic lobectomy for the management of non-small cell lung cancer. Curr Oncol Rep 2008; 10 (4): 283–286

Balduyck B, Hendriks J, Lauwers P, Van Schil P. Quality of life evolution after surgery for primary or secondary spontaneous pneumothorax: a prospective study comparing different surgical techniques. Interact Cardiovasc Thorac Surg 2008; 7 (1): 45–49

Barker A, Maratos EC, Edmonds L, Lim E. Recurrence rates of video-assisted thoracoscopic versus open surgery in the prevention of recurrent pneumothoraces: a systematic review of randomised and non-randomised trials. Lancet 2007; 370 (9584): 329–335

Baumann MH, Strange C, Heffner JE, et al; AACP Pneumothorax Consensus Group. Management of spontaneous pneumothorax: an American College of Chest Physicians Delphi consensus statement. Chest 2001; 119 (2): 590–602

Baumann MH, Noppen M. Pneumothorax. Respirology 2004; 9 (2): 157–164

Baumann MH, Nolan R, Petrini M, Lee YC, Light RW, Schneider E. Pleural tuberculosis in the United States: incidence and drug resistance. Chest 2007; 131 (4): 1125–1132

Bayle JY, Pirollet B, Guérin JC. [Thoracoscopy in pulmonary histiocytosis X]. Rev Pneumol Clin 1988; 44 (6): 292–296

Beamis JF Jr, Mathur PN, eds. Interventional pulmonology. New York: McGraw-Hill; 1999

Beamis JF, Mathur PN, Mehta AC, eds. Interventional pulmonary medicine. In: Lung biology in health and disease. Vol. 189. New York: Marcel Dekker; 2004: 483–502

Beauchamp HD, Kundra NK, Aranson R, Chong F, MacDonnell KF. The role of closed pleural needle biopsy in the diagnosis of malignant mesothelioma of the pleura. Chest 1992; 102 (4): 1110–1112

Ben-Isaac FE, Simmons DH. Flexible fiberoptic pleuroscopy: pleural and lung biopsy. Chest 1975; 67 (5): 573–576

Bensard DD, McIntyre RC Jr, Waring BJ, Simon JS. Comparison of video thoracoscopic lung biopsy to open lung biopsy in the diagnosis of interstitial lung disease. Chest 1993; 103 (3): 765–770

Bense L, Eklund G, Wiman LG. Smoking and the increased risk of contracting spontaneous pneumothorax. Chest 1987; 92 (6): 1009–1012

Bense L, Lewander R, Eklund G, Hedenstierna G, Wiman LG. Nonsmoking, non-alpha 1-antitrypsin deficiency-induced emphysema in nonsmokers with healed spontaneous pneumothorax, identified by computed tomography of the lungs. Chest 1993; 103 (2): 433–438

Bethune N. Pleural poudrage: new technique for the deliberate production of pleural adhesion as preliminary to lobectomy. J Thorac Surg 1935; 4: 251–255

Bielsa S, Martín-Juan J, Porcel JM, Rodríguez-Panadero F. Diagnostic and prognostic implications of pleural adhesions in malignant effusions. J Thorac Oncol 2008; 3 (11): 1251–1256

Blanc FX, Atassi K, Bignon J, Housset B. Diagnostic value of medical thoracoscopy in pleural disease: a 6-year retrospective study. Chest 2002; 121 (5): 1677–1683

Bloomberg AE. Thoracoscopy in perspective. Surg Gynecol Obstet 1978; 147 (3): 433–443

Boley TM, Belangee KN, Markwell S, Hazelrigg SR. The effect of thoracoscopic sympathectomy on quality of life and symptom management of hyperhidrosis. J Am Coll Surg 2007; 204 (3): 435–438

Bouros D, Pneumatikos I, Tzouvelekis A. Pleural involvement in systemic autoimmune disorders. Respiration 2008; 75 (4): 361–371

Boutin C, Arnaud A, Farisse P, et al. [Pleural biopsies: complications and current value of Abram's needle biopsy. Apropos of 1,000 samples. Value of pleuroscopic biopsy]. Poumon Coeur 1975; 31 (6): 317–321

Boutin C, Cargnino P, Viallat JR. Thoracoscopy in the early diagnosis of malignant pleural effusions. Endoscopy 1980; 12 (4): 155–160

Boutin C, ed. [Symposium on thoracoscopy in pleuro-pulmonary diseases]. Poumon Coeur 1981; 37: 3–77

Boutin C, Viallat JR, Cargnino P, Farisse P. Thoracoscopy in malignant pleural effusions. Am Rev Respir Dis 1981a; 124 (5): 588–592

Boutin C, Jullian H, Viallat JR, Sébastien P, Cargnino P. [Lung biopsy by thoracoscopy (author's transl)]. Rev Fr Mal Respir 1981b; 9 (4): 337–344

Boutin C, Viallat JR, Cargnino P, Rey F. Thoracoscopic lung biopsy. Experimental and clinical preliminary study. Chest 1982; 82 (1): 44–48

Boutin C, Viallat JR, Cargnino P. Thoracoscopy. In: Chrétien J, ed. The pleura in health and disease. New York: Marcel Dekker; 1985a: 587–621

Boutin C, Rey F, Viallat JR. Etude randomisée de l'efficacité du talcage thoracoscopique et de l'instillation de tétracycline dans le traitement des pleurésies cancéreuses récidivantes. Rev Mal Resp 1985b; 2: 374–379

Boutin C. The laser in thoracoscopy. Pneumologie 1989; 43 (2): 96–97

Boutin C, Viallat JR, Aelony Y. Practical thoracoscopy. Berlin, Heidelberg, New York: Springer; 1991

Boutin C, Rey F. Thoracoscopy in pleural malignant mesothelioma: a prospective study of 188 consecutive patients. Part 1: Diagnosis. Cancer 1993; 72 (2): 389–393

Boutin C, Loddenkemper R, Astoul P. Diagnostic and therapeutic thoracoscopy: techniques and indications in pulmonary medicine. Tuber Lung Dis 1993a; 74 (4): 225–239

Boutin C, Rey F, Gouvernet J, Viallat JR, Astoul P, Ledoray V. Thoracoscopy in pleural malignant mesothelioma: a prospective study of 188 consecutive patients. Part 2: Prognosis and staging. Cancer 1993b; 72 (2): 394–404

Boutin C, Nussbaum E, Monnet I, et al. Intrapleural treatment with recombinant gamma-interferon in early stage malignant pleural mesothelioma. Cancer 1994; 74 (9): 2460–2467

Boutin C, Astoul P, Rey F, Mathur PN. Thoracoscopy in the diagnosis and treatment of spontaneous pneumothorax. Clin Chest Med 1995a; 16 (3): 497–503

Boutin C, Rey F, Viallat JR. Prevention of malignant seeding after invasive diagnostic procedures in patients with pleural mesothelioma. A randomized trial of local radiotherapy. Chest 1995b; 108 (3): 754–758

Boutin C, Dumortier P, Rey F, Viallat JR, De Vuyst P. Black spots concentrate oncogenic asbestos fibers in the parietal pleura. Thoracoscopic and mineralogic study. Am J Respir Crit Care Med 1996; 153 (1): 444–449

Boutin C, Schlesser M, Frenay C, Astoul P. Malignant pleural mesothelioma. Eur Respir J 1998; 12 (4): 972–981

Brandt HJ. Technik der Hilus- und Mediastinalpunktion während der Thorakoskopie. In: Grunze H. Klinische Zytologie der Thoraxkrankheiten. Stuttgart: Enke; 1955: 154–156

Brandt HJ. [Thoracoscopy in diseases of the pleura and mediastinum.]. Internist (Berl) 1964a; 5: 391–395

Brandt HJ. [Bronchoscopy and thoracoscopy]. Dtsch Med J 1964b; 15: 233–234

Brandt HJ, Kund H. [The efficiency of diagnostic thoracoscopy]. Prax Pneumol 1964; 18: 304–332

Brandt HJ, Mai J. [Differential diagnosis of pleural effusion using thoracoscopy]. Pneumonologie 1971; 145: 192–203

Brandt HJ. [Pulmonary biopsy under visual control (author's transl)]. Poumon Coeur 1981; 37 (5): 307–311

Brandt HJ, Loddenkemper R, Mai J. Atlas der diagnostischen Thorakoskopie. Indikationen – Technik. Stuttgart: Thieme; 1983

Brandt HJ, Loddenkemper R, Mai J. Atlas of diagnostic thoracoscopy. Indications—Technique. New York: Thieme; 1985

Brandt HJ. A message from one of the last veterans in thoracoscopy. Int Surg 1997; 82: 20–21

Brazinsky SA, Colt HG. Thoracoscopic diagnosis of pleurolithiasis after laparoscopic cholecystectomy. Chest 1993; 104 (4): 1273–1274

Breen D, Fraticelli A, Greillier L, Mallawathantri S, Astoul P. Redo medical thoracoscopy is feasible in patients with pleural diseases—a series. Interact Cardiovasc Thorac Surg 2009; 8 (3): 330–333

Bresticker MA, Oba J, LoCicero J III, Greene R. Optimal pleurodesis: a comparison study. Ann Thorac Surg 1993; 55 (2): 364–366; discussion 367

Breuer GS, Deeb M, Fisher D, Nesher G. Therapeutic options for refractory massive pleural effusion in systemic lupus erythematosus: a case study and review of the literature. Semin Arthritis Rheum 2005; 34 (5): 744–749

Brezler M, Abeles H. Differentiation between hydropneumothorax and destroyed lung by thoracoscopy with a fiberoptic bronchoscope. Chest 1975; 68 (2): 267–268

Bridges KG, Welch G, Silver M, Schinco MA, Esposito B. CT detection of occult pneumothorax in multiple trauma patients. J Emerg Med 1993; 11 (2): 179–186

Brown KT, Brody LA, Getrajdman GI, Napp TE. Outpatient treatment of iatrogenic pneumothorax after needle biopsy. Radiology 1997; 205 (1): 249–252

Brutsche MH, Tassi GF, Györik S, et al. Treatment of sonographically stratified multiloculated thoracic empyema by medical thoracoscopy. Chest 2005; 128 (5): 3303–3309

Buchanan DR, Neville E. Thoracoscopy for physicians: A practical guide. London: Arnold; 2004

Bülau G. Für die Heber-Drainage bei Behandlung des Empyems. Z Klin Med 1891; 18: 31–45

Bueno R, Reblando J, Glickman J, Jaklitsch MT, Lukanich JM, Sugarbaker DJ. Pleural biopsy: a reliable method for determining the diagnosis but not subtype in mesothelioma. Ann Thorac Surg 2004; 78 (5): 1774–1776

Burdine J, Joyce LD, Plunkett MB, Inampudi S, Kaye MG, Dunn DH. Feasibility and value of video-assisted thoracoscopic surgery wedge excision of small pulmonary nodules in patients with malignancy. Chest 2002; 122 (4): 1467–1470

Burgers JA, Kunst PW, Koolen MG, Willems LN, Burgers JS, van den Heuvel M. Pleural drainage and pleurodesis: implementation of guidelines in four hospitals. Eur Respir J 2008; 32 (5): 1321–1327

Burrows CM, Mathews WC, Colt HG. Predicting survival in patients with recurrent symptomatic malignant pleural effusions: an assessment of the prognostic values of physiologic, morphologic, and quality of life measures of extent of disease. Chest 2000; 117 (1): 73–78

Burrows NJ, Ali NJ, Cox GM. The use and development of medical thoracoscopy in the United Kingdom over the past 5 years. Respir Med 2006; 100 (7): 1234–1238

Bydder S, Phillips M, Joseph DJ, et al. A randomised trial of single-dose radiotherapy to prevent procedure tract metastasis by malignant mesothelioma. Br J Cancer 2004; 91 (1): 9–10

Cameron RJ. Management of complicated parapneumonic effusions and thoracic empyema. Intern Med J 2002; 32 (8): 408–414

Campos JR, Werebe EC, Vargas FS, Jatene FB, Light RW. Respiratory failure due to insufflated talc. Lancet 1997; 349 (9047): 251–252

Camuset J, Laganier J, Brugière O, et al. Needle aspiration as first-line management of primary spontaneous pneumothorax. Presse Med 2006; 35 (5 Pt 1): 765–768

Cantó A, Blasco E, Casillas M, et al. Thoracoscopy in the diagnosis of pleural effusion. Thorax 1977; 32 (5): 550–554

Cantó A, Rivas J, Saumench J, Morera R, Moya J. Points to consider when choosing a biopsy method in cases of pleurisy of unknown origin. Chest 1983; 84 (2): 176–179

Cantó A, Ferrer G, Romagosa V, Moya J, Bernat R. Lung cancer and pleural effusion. Clinical significance and study of pleural metastatic locations. Chest 1985; 87 (5): 649–652

Cantó A, Arnau A, Galbis J, et al. [The so-called malignant pleural effusion: a new review of direct data obtained with diagnostic pleuroscopy]. Arch Bronconeumol 1996; 32 (9): 453–458

Cardillo G, Carleo F, Carbone L, et al. Long-term lung function following videothoracoscopic talc poudrage for primary spontaneous recurrent pneumothorax. Eur J Cardiothorac Surg 2007; 31 (5): 802–805

Carnochan FM, Walker WS, Cameron EW. Efficacy of video assisted thoracoscopic lung biopsy: an historical comparison with open lung biopsy. Thorax 1994; 49 (4): 361–363

Celikoglu F, Teirstein AS, Krellenstein DJ, Strauchen JA. Pleural effusion in non-Hodgkin's lymphoma. Chest 1992; 101 (5): 1357–1360

Chan SS, Rainer TH. Primary spontaneous pneumothorax: 1-year recurrence rate after simple aspiration. Eur J Emerg Med 2006; 13 (2): 88–91

Chan SS. The role of simple aspiration in the management of primary spontaneous pneumothorax. J Emerg Med 2008; 34 (2): 131–138

Chang DB, Yang PC, Luh KT, Kuo SH, Yu CJ. Ultrasound-guided pleural biopsy with Tru-Cut needle. Chest 1991; 100 (5): 1328–1333

Chang YT, Chou SH, Kao EL, et al. Video-assisted extrathoracic bleb excision: an ultra-minithoracotomy for primary spontaneous pneumothorax. Minim Invasive Ther Allied Technol 2007; 16 (6): 323–327

Chegou NN, Walzl G, Bolliger CT, Diacon AH, van den Heuvel MM. Evaluation of adapted whole-blood interferon-gamma release assays for the diagnosis of pleural tuberculosis. Respiration 2008; 76 (2): 131–138

Chen D, Barber C, McLoughlin P, Thavaneswaran P, Jamieson GG, Maddern GJ. Systematic review of endoscopic treatments for gastro-oesophageal reflux disease. Br J Surg 2009; 96 (2): 128–136

Chen LE, Langer JC, Dillon PA, et al. Management of late-stage parapneumonic empyema. J Pediatr Surg 2002; 37 (3): 371–374

Chernow B, Sahn SA. Carcinomatous involvement of the pleura: an analysis of 96 patients. Am J Med 1977; 63 (5): 695–702

Chhajed PN, Kaegi B, Rajasekaran R, Tamm M. Detection of hypoventilation during thoracoscopy: combined cutaneous carbon dioxide tension and oximetry monitoring with a new digital sensor. Chest 2005; 127 (2): 585–588

Cho K, Ozawa S, Kuzihara M, et al. Cardiorespiratory changes in thoracoscopy under local anesthesia. J Bronchol 2000; 7: 215–220

Choi SH, Lee SW, Hong YS, Kim SJ, Moon JD, Moon SW. Can spontaneous pneumothorax patients be treated by ambulatory care management? Eur J Cardiothorac Surg 2007; 31 (3): 491–495

Chrysanthidis MG, Janssen JP. Autofluorescence videothoracoscopy in exudative pleural effusions: preliminary results. Eur Respir J 2005; 26 (6): 989–992

Chung CL, Chen CH, Yeh CY, Sheu JR, Chang SC. Early effective drainage in the treatment of loculated tuberculous pleurisy. Eur Respir J 2008; 31 (6): 1261–1267

Clark G, Licker M, Younossian AB, et al. Titrated sedation with propofol or midazolam for flexible bronchoscopy: a randomized trial. Eur Respir J 2009; 4: 1277–1283

Clarkson K, Power CK, O'Connell F, Pathmakanthan S, Burke CM. A comparative evaluation of propofol and midazolam as sedative agents in fiberoptic bronchoscopy. Chest 1993; 104 (4): 1029–1031

Cohen RG, Shely WW, Thompson SE, et al. Talc pleurodesis: talc slurry versus thoracoscopic talc insufflation in a porcine model. Ann Thorac Surg 1996; 62 (4): 1000–1002, discussion 1003–1004

Colice GL, Curtis A, Deslauriers J, et al. Medical and surgical treatment of parapneumonic effusions: an evidence-based guideline. Chest 2000; 118 (4): 1158–1171

Collins TR, Sahn SA. Thoracocentesis. Clinical value, complications, technical problems, and patient experience. Chest 1987; 91 (6): 817–822

Colt HG. Thoracoscopy: new frontiers. Pulmon Perspect 1992; 9: 1–4

Colt HG. Thoracoscopy. A prospective study of safety and outcome. Chest 1995a; 108 (2): 324–329

Colt HG. Thoracoscopic management of malignant pleural effusions. Clin Chest Med 1995b; 16 (3): 505–518

Colt HG, Russack V, Shanks TG, Moser KM. Comparison of wedge to forceps videothoracoscopic lung biopsy. Gross and histologic findings. Chest 1995; 107 (2): 546–550

Colt HG, Russack V, Chiu Y, et al. A comparison of thoracoscopic talc insufflation, slurry, and mechanical abrasion pleurodesis. Chest 1997; 111 (2): 442–448

Colt HG. Thoracoscopy: window to the pleural space. Chest 1999; 116: 1409–1415

Congregado M, Merchan RJ, Gallardo G, Ayarra J, Loscertales J. Video-assisted thoracic surgery (VATS) lobectomy: 13 years' experience. Surg Endosc 2008; 22 (8): 1852–1857

Council of Society of Thoracic Surgeons. Video-assisted thoracic surgery pleural disease. Ann Thorac Surg 1994; 58 (2): 597–598

Cova F. Toracoscopia, Operazione di Jacobaeus. Milan: Sperling & Kupfer; 1927

Cova F. Atlas thoracoscopicon. Milan: Sperling & Kupfer; 1928

Cruise FR. The endoscope as an aid to the diagnosis and treatment of disease. BMJ 1865; 8: 345–347

Cuschieri A. The laparoscopic revolution—walk carefully, before we run. J R Coll Surg Edinb 1990; 35: 200

Cuschieri A, Buess G, Perissat J, eds. Operative manual of endoscopic surgery. Berlin: Springer; 1992

Das DK. Serous effusions in malignant lymphomas: a review. Diagn Cytopathol 2006; 34: 335–347

Davidson AC, George RJ, Sheldon CD, Sinha G, Corrin B, Geddes DM. Thoracoscopy: assessment of a physician service and comparison of a flexible bronchoscope used as a thoracoscope with a rigid thoracoscope. Thorax 1988; 43 (4): 327–332

Davidson JE, Colt HG. Thoracoscopy: nursing implications for optimal patient outcomes. Dimens Crit Care Nurs 1997; 16 (1): 20–28

Davies HE, Nicholson JE, Rahman et al. Outcome of patients with nonspecific pleuritis/fibrosis on thoracoscopic pleural biopsies. Eur J Cardiothorac Surg 2010, March 8 (Epub ahead of print)

Davies HE, Musk AW, Lee YC. Prophylactic radiotherapy for pleural puncture sites in mesothelioma: the controversy continues. Curr Opin Pulm Med 2008; 14 (4): 326–330

De Leyn P, Lismonde M, Ninane V, et al. Guidelines Belgian Society of Pneumology. Guidelines on the management of spontaneous pneumothorax. Acta Chir Belg 2005; 105 (3): 265–267

De Smedt A, Vanderlinden E, Demanet C, De Waele M, Goossens A, Noppen M. Characterisation of pleural inflammation occurring after primary spontaneous pneumothorax. Eur Respir J 2004; 23 (6): 896–900

De Weerdt S, Noppen M, Everaert H, Vincken W. Positron emission tomography scintigraphy after thoracoscopic talcage. Respiration 2004; 71 (3): 284

Diacon AH, Van de Wal BW, Wyser C, et al. Diagnostic tools in tuberculous pleurisy: a direct comparative study. Eur Respir J 2003; 22 (4): 589–591

DiBonito L, Falconieri G, Colautti I, Bonifacio D, Dudine S. The positive pleural effusion. A retrospective study of cytopathologic diagnoses with autopsy confirmation. Acta Cytol 1992; 36 (3): 329–332

Diehl K, Kremer W. Thorakoskopie und Thorakokaustik. Berlin: Springer; 1929

Dijkman JH, van der Meer JW, Bakker W, Wever AM, van der Broek PJ. Transpleural lung biopsy by the thoracoscopic route in patients with diffuse interstitial pulmonary disease. Chest 1982; 82 (1): 76–83

Dijkman JH. [Thoracoscopy in the immunosuppressed patient]. Pneumologie 1989; 43 (2): 116–118

Dijkman JH, Martinez Gonzales del Rio J, Loddenkemper R, Prowse K, Siafakas N. Report of the working party of the "UEMS Monospeciality Section on Pneumology" on training requirements and facilities in Europe. Eur Respir J 1994; 7 (5): 1019–1022

Dikensoy O, Light RW. Alternative widely available, inexpensive agents for pleurodesis. Curr Opin Pulm Med 2005; 11 (4): 340–344

Diwok K, Platz S, Seipt G. [Analysis of sarcoidosis cases at a university clinical center from the years 1957-1971]. Z Gesamte Inn Med 1974; 29 (15): 621–627

Donnelly RJ, Page RD, Berrisford RG, Dedeilias PG. Videothoracoscopic surgery. Eur J Cardiothorac Surg 1993; 7 (6): 281–285, discussion 285–286

Doolabh N, Horswell S, Williams M, et al. Thoracoscopic sympathectomy for hyperhidrosis: indications and results. Ann Thorac Surg 2004; 77 (2): 410–414, discussion 414

Dresler CM, Olak J, Herndon JE II, et al; Cooperative Groups Cancer and Leukemia Group B; Eastern Cooperative Oncology Group; North Central Cooperative Oncology Group; Radiation Therapy Oncology Group. Phase III intergroup study of talc poudrage vs talc slurry sclerosis for malignant pleural effusion. Chest 2005; 127 (3): 909–915

Edenborough FP, Hussain I, Stableforth DE. Use of a Heimlich flutter valve for pneumothorax in cystic fibrosis. Thorax 1994; 49 (11): 1178–1179

Edmondstone WM. Investigation of pleural effusion: comparison between fibreoptic thoracoscopy, needle biopsy, and cytology. Respir Med 1990; 84: 23–26

Elis A, Blickstein D, Mulchanov I, et al. Pleural effusion in patients with non-Hodgkin's lymphoma: a case-controlled study. Cancer 1998; 83 (8): 1607–1611

Enerson DM, McIntyre J. A comparative study of the physiology and physics of pleural drainage systems. J Thorac Cardiovasc Surg 1966; 52 (1): 40–46

Enk B, Viskum K. Diagnostic thoracoscopy. Eur J Respir Dis 1981; 62 (5): 344–351

Ernst A, Hersh CP, Herth F, et al. A novel instrument for the evaluation of the pleural space: an experience in 34 patients. Chest 2002; 122 (5): 1530–1534

Ernst A, Silvestri GA, Johnstone D; American College of Chest Physicians. Interventional pulmonary procedures: Guidelines from the American College of Chest Physicians. Chest 2003; 123 (5): 1693–1717

Faber LP. Thoracoscopy: A surgeon's or a pulmonologist's domain. Pro surgeon. J Bronchol 1994; 1: 155–159

Faruqi S, Gupta D, Aggarwal AN, Jindal SK. Role of simple needle aspiration in the management of pneumothorax. Indian J Chest Dis Allied Sci 2004; 46 (3): 183–190

Faurschou P. Rheumatoid pleuritis and thoracoscopy. Scand J Respir Dis 1974; 55 (5): 277–283

Faurschou P, Madsen F, Viskum K. Thoracoscopy: influence of the procedure on some respiratory and cardiac values. Thorax 1983; 38 (5): 341–343

Faurschou P. Diagnostic thoracoscopy in pleuro-pulmonary infiltrations without pleural effusion. Endoscopy 1985a; 17: 21–25

Faurschou P, Francis D, Faarup P. Thoracoscopic, histological, and clinical findings in nine case of rheumatoid pleural effusion. Thorax 1985b; 40 (5): 371–375

Faurschou P. Thoracoscopy in rheumatoid pleural effusion. Pneumologie 1989; 43 (2): 69–71

Faurschou P, Viskum K. Artificial pneumothorax by the Veress cannula: efficacy and safety. Respir Med 1997; 91 (7): 402–405

Feller-Kopman D, Parker MJ, Schwartzstein RM. Assessment of pleural pressure in the evaluation of pleural effusions. Chest 2009; 135 (1): 201–209

Ferguson GC. Cholesterol pleural effusion in rheumatoid lung disease. Thorax 1966; 21 (6): 577–582

Ferrer JS, Muñoz XG, Orriols RM, Light RW, Morell FB. Evolution of idiopathic pleural effusion: a prospective, long-term follow-up study. Chest 1996; 109 (6): 1508–1513

Fishbein MC. Diagnosis: to biopsy or not to biopsy: assessing the role of surgical lung biopsy in the diagnosis of idiopathic pulmonary fibrosis. Chest 2005; 128 (5, Suppl 1): 520S–525S

Fishman A, Martinez F, Neuheim K, et al. National Emphysema Treatment Trial Research Group. A randomized trial comparing lung-volume-reduction surgery with medical therapy for severe emphysema. N Engl J Med 2003; 348: 2059–2073

Fletcher SV, Clark RJ. The Portsmouth thoracoscopy experience, an evaluation of service by retrospective case note analysis. Respir Med 2007; 101 (5): 1021–1025

Forlanini C. A contribuzione della terapia chirurgica della tisi. Ablazione del polmone? Pneumothorace arteficiale? Gazzetta degli Ospitali 1882; 3: 537–539

Forssbohm M, Zwahlen M, Loddenkemper R, Rieder HL. Demographic characteristics of patients with extrapulmonary tuberculosis in Germany. Eur Respir J 2008; 31 (1): 99–105

Froudarakis ME. Diagnostic work-up of pleural effusions. Respiration 2008; 75: 4–13

Froudarakis ME, Klimathianaki M, Pougounias M. Systemic inflammatory reaction after thoracoscopic talc poudrage. Chest 2006; 129 (2): 356–361

Froudarakis ME, Noppen M. Medical thoracoscopy: New tricks for an old trade (editorial). Respiration 2009; 78: 373–374

Furrer M, Rechsteiner R, Eigenmann V, et al. Thoracotomy and thoracoscopy: postoperative pulmonary function, pain, and chest wall complaints. Eur J Cardiothorac Surg 1997; 12: 82–87

Gaensler EA, Carrington CB. Open biopsy for chronic diffuse infiltrative lung disease: clinical, roentgenographic, and physiological correlations in 502 patients. Ann Thorac Surg 1980; 30 (5): 411–426

Genc O, Petrou M, Ladas G, Goldstraw P. The long-term morbidity of pleuroperitoneal shunts in the management of recurrent malignant effusions. Eur J Cardiothorac Surg 2000; 18 (2): 143–146

Georghiou GP, Stamler A, Sharoni E, et al. Video-assisted thoracoscopic pericardial window for diagnosis and management of pericardial effusions. Ann Thorac Surg 2005; 80 (2): 607–610

Gibbon N. The laparoscopic revolution—walk carefully before we run. J R Coll Surg Edinb 1990; 35 (3): 200

Goh PM, Cheah WK, De Costa M, Sim EK. Needlescopic thoracic sympathectomy: treatment for palmar hyperhidrosis. Ann Thorac Surg 2000; 70 (1): 240–242

Goldstraw P, Crowley J, Chansky K, et al; International Association for the Study of Lung Cancer International Staging Committee; Participating Institutions. The IASLC Lung Cancer Staging Project: proposals for the revision of the TNM stage groupings in the forthcoming (seventh) edition of the TNM Classification of malignant tumours. J Thorac Oncol 2007; 2 (8): 706–714

Gonfiotti A, Davini F, Vaggelli L, et al. Thoracoscopic localization techniques for patients with solitary pulmonary nodule: hookwire versus radio-guided surgery. Eur J Cardiothorac Surg 2007; 32 (6): 843–847

Goodman A, Davies CW. Efficacy of short-term versus long-term chest tube drainage following talc slurry pleurodesis in patients with malignant pleural effusions: a randomised trial. Lung Cancer 2006; 54 (1): 51–55

Gopi A, Madhavan SM, Sharma SK, Sahn SA. Diagnosis and treatment of tuberculous pleural effusion in 2006. Chest 2007; 131 (3): 880–889

Gordon P. Clinical reports of rare cases, occurring in the Whitworth and Hartwicke Hospitals: most extensive pleuritic effusion rapidly becoming purulent, paracentesis, introduction of a drainage tube, recovery, examination of interior of pleura by the endoscope. Dublin Quarterly Journal of Medical Science 1866; 41: 83–90

Gotoh M, Yamamoto Y, Igai H, Chang S, Huang C, Yokomise H. Clinical application of infrared thoracoscopy to detect bullous or emphysematous lesions of the lung. J Thorac Cardiovasc Surg 2007; 134 (6): 1498–1501

Grant A, Wileman S, Ramsay C, et al; REFLUX Trial Group. The effectiveness and cost-effectiveness of minimal access surgery amongst people with gastro-oesophageal reflux disease—a UK collaborative study. The REFLUX trial. Health Technol Assess 2008; 12 (31): 1–181, iii–iv

Greillier L, Cavailles A, Fraticelli A, et al. Accuracy of pleural biopsy using thoracoscopy for the diagnosis of histologic subtype in patients with malignant pleural mesothelioma. Cancer 2007; 110 (10): 2248–2252

Greillier L, Astoul P. Mesothelioma and asbestos-related pleural diseases. Respiration 2008; 76 (1): 1–15

Guy P, Kasparian P, Guibout P. Biopsies pulmonaires par thoracoscopie. Poumon Coeur 1983; 39: 179–181

Gwin E, Pierce G, Boggan M, Kerby G, Ruth W. Pleuroscopy and pleural biopsy with the flexible fiberoptic bronchoscope. Chest 1975; 67 (5): 527–531

Györik S, Erni S, Studler U, Hodek-Wuerz R, Tamm M, Chhajed PN. Long-term follow-up of thoracoscopic talc pleurodesis for primary spontaneous pneumothorax. Eur Respir J 2007; 29 (4): 757–760

Haas AR, Sterman DH, Musani AI. Malignant pleural effusions: management options with consideration of coding, billing, and a decision approach. Chest 2007; 132 (3): 1036–1041

Hampson C, Lemos JA, Klein JS. Diagnosis and management of parapneumonic effusions. Semin Respir Crit Care Med 2008; 29 (4): 414–426

Harris RJ, Kavuru MS, Rice TW, Kirby TJ. The diagnostic and therapeutic utility of thoracoscopy. A review. Chest 1995; 108 (3): 828–841

Hartman DL, Gaither JM, Kesler KA, Mylet DM, Brown JW, Mathur PN. Comparison of insufflated talc under thoracoscopic guidance with standard tetracycline and bleomycin pleurodesis for control of malignant pleural effusions. J Thorac Cardiovasc Surg 1993; 105 (4): 743–747, discussion 747–748

Hartman DL, Antony VB. Thoraocscopy: the pulmonologist's role. Semin Respir Crit Care Med 1995; 16: 354–360

Hartmann J, Menenakos C, Ordemann J, Nocon M, Raue W, Braumann C. Long-term results of quality of life after standard laparoscopic vs. robot-assisted laparoscopic fundoplications for gastro-oesophageal reflux disease. A comparative clinical trial. Int J Med Robot 2009; 5 (1): 32–37

Hashmonai M, Assalia A, Kopelman D. Thoracoscopic sympathectomy for palmar hyperhidrosis. Ablate or resect? Surg Endosc 2001; 15 (5): 435–441

Hatakenaka R, Ikeda S, Hitomi S, Funatsu T, Kahi T, Nagaishi C. A new method of intrathoracal biopsy using thoracoscope and tissue adhesive. Bronchopneumologie 1976; 26 (2): 161–173

Hatz RA, Kaps MF, Meimarakis G, Loehe F, Müller C, Fürst H. Long-term results after video-assisted thoracoscopic surgery for first-time and recurrent spontaneous pneumothorax. Ann Thorac Surg 2000; 70 (1): 253–257

Heffner JE, Klein JS. Recent advances in the diagnosis and management of malignant pleural effusions. Mayo Clin Proc 2008; 83 (2): 235–250

Heffner JE, Klein JS, Hampson C. Interventional management of pleural infections. Chest 2008; 136: 1148–1159

Heine F. Die Probeexcision aus Veränderungen in Thoraxraum und Lunge unter thorakoskopischer Sicht. [Biopsy from changes of thoracic space & lung under thoracoscopic view]. Beitr Klin Tuberk Spezif Tuberkoloseforsch 1957; 116: 615–627

Heine F. Probeexzisionen aus dem Lungenparenchym. In: Hoppe R, ed. Sarkoidose. Bericht über die Tagung der Rhein-Westf. Tuberk.-Vereinig, Düsseldorf, March 14, 1964. Stuttgart: Schattauer; 1965

Henry M, Arnold T, Harvey J; Pleural Diseases Group, Standards of Care Committee, British Thoracic Society. BTS guidelines for the management of spontaneous pneumothorax. Thorax 2003; 58 (Suppl 2): ii39–ii52

Hersh CP, Feller-Kopman D, Wahidi M, Garland R, Herth F, Ernst A. Ultrasound guidance for medical thoracoscopy: a novel approach. Respiration 2003; 70 (3): 299–301

Herth FJ, Becker HD, Ernst A. Aspirin does not increase bleeding complications after transbronchial biopsy. Chest 2002; 122 (4): 1461–1464

Hewett C. Drainage for empyema. BMJ 1876; I: 317

Hirsch A, Ruffie P, Nebut M, Bignon J, Chrétien J. Pleural effusion: laboratory tests in 300 cases. Thorax 1979; 34 (1): 106–112

Hitomi S, Tamada J, Ikeda S, Funatsu T, Kahi T, Kurata M. Thoracoscopic lung biopsy using tissue adhesive material and/or deep ligator. Chest 1984; 86 (1): 155

Hoffman A, Goetz M, Vieth M, Galle PR, Neurath MF, Kiesslich R. Confocal laser endomicroscopy: technical status and current indications. Endoscopy 2006; 38 (12): 1275–1283

Hoksch B, Birken-Bertsch H, Müller JM. Thoracoscopy before Jacobaeus. Ann Thorac Surg 2002; 74 (4): 1288–1290

Hoksch B, Ablassmaier B, Walter M, Müller JM. [Complication rate after thoracoscopic and conventional lobectomy]. Zentralbl Chir 2003; 128 (2): 106–110

Hooper CE, Lee YC, Maskell NA. Interferon-gamma release assays for the diagnosis of TB pleural effusions: hype or real hope? Curr Opin Pulm Med 2009; 15 (4): 358–365

Horio H, Nomori H, Kobayashi R, Naruke T, Suemasu K. Impact of additional pleurodesis in video-assisted thoracoscopic bullectomy for primary spontaneous pneumothorax. Surg Endosc 2002; 16 (4): 630–634

Howington JA. The role of VATS for staging and diagnosis in patients with non-small cell lung cancer. Semin Thorac Cardiovasc Surg 2007; 19 (3): 212–216

Hsu C. Cytologic detection of malignancy in pleural effusion: a review of 5,255 samples from 3,811 patients. Diagn Cytopathol 1987; 3 (1): 8–12

Hunninghake GW, Zimmerman MB, Schwartz DA, et al. Utility of a lung biopsy for the diagnosis of idiopathic pulmonary fibrosis. Am J Respir Crit Care Med 2001; 164 (2): 193–196

Hunt I, Barber B, Southon R, Treasure T. Is talc pleurodesis safe for young patients following primary spontaneous pneumothorax? Interact Cardiovasc Thorac Surg 2007; 6 (1): 117–120

Inderbitzi R, Molnar J. [Experiences in the diagnostic and surgical video-endoscopy of the thoracic cavity] Schweiz Med Wochenschr 1990; 120: 1965–1970

Inderbitzi R, Althaus U. Therapeutic thoracoscopy, a new surgical technique (abstr.). Thorac Cardiovasc Surg 1991; 39 (Suppl): 35

Inderbitzi R. Chirurgische Thorakoskopie. Berlin: Springer; 1993

Ishida A, Ishikowa F, Nakamura M, et al. Narrow band imaging applied to pleuroscopy for the assessment of vascular patterns of the pleura. Respiration 2009; 78: 432–439

Iwasaki A, Yamamoto S, Shiraishi T, Shirakusa T. How much skill should we need for a VATS lobectomy in stage I lung cancer? An evaluation of surgeon groups. Int Surg 2008; 93 (3): 169–174

Jacobaeus HC. Über die Möglichkeit, die Zystoskopie bei Untersuchung seröser Höhlungen anzuwenden. Munch Med Wochenschr 1910; 57: 2090–2092

Jacobaeus HC. Über Laparo- und Thorakoskopie. Beitr Klin Tuberk 1912; 25: 185–354

Jacobaeus HC. Endopleurale Operationen unter Leitung des Thorakoskops. Beitr Klin Tuberk 1916; 35: 1–35

Jacobaeus HC, Key E. Some experiences of intrathoracic tumors, their diagnosis and their operative treatment. Acta Chir Scand 1921; 53: 573–623

Jacobaeus HC. The cauterization of adhesions in artificial pneumothorax therapy of tuberculosis. Am Rev Tuberc 1922a; 6: 871

Jacobaeus HC. The practical importance of thoracoscopy in surgery of the chest. Surg Gynecol Obstet 1922b; 34: 289–296

Jacobaeus HC. Die Thorakoskopie und ihre praktische Bedeutung. Ergeb Gesamten Med 1925; 7: 112–166

Janik JS, Nagaraj HS, Groff DB. Thoracoscopic evaluation of intrathoracic lesions in children. J Thorac Cardiovasc Surg 1982; 83 (3): 408–413

Janssen JP, Boutin C. Extended thoracoscopy: a biopsy method to be used in case of pleural adhesions. Eur Respir J 1992; 5 (6): 763–766

Janssen JP, Joosten HJ, Postmus PE. Thoracoscopic treatment of postoperative chylothorax after coronary bypass surgery. Thorax 1994a; 49 (12): 1273

Janssen JP, van Mourik J, Cuesta Valentin M, Sutedja G, Gigengack K, Postmus PE. Treatment of patients with spontaneous pneumothorax during videothoracoscopy. Eur Respir J 1994b; 7 (7): 1281–1284

Janssen JP, Thunissen FBJM, Visser FJ. Comparison of the 2.0 mm and 3.5 mm minithoracoscopy set to standard equipment for medical thoracoscopy. Eur Respir J 2003; 22 (Suppl 45): S541

Janssen JP, Ramlal S, Mravunac M. The long-term follow-up of exudative pleural effusion after nondiagnostic thoracoscopy. J Bronchol 2004; 11: 169–174

Janssen JP, Collier G, Astoul P, et al. Safety of pleurodesis with talc poudrage in malignant pleural effusion: a prospective cohort study. Lancet 2007; 369 (9572): 1535–1539

Jantz MA, Antony VB. Pathophysiology of the pleura. Respiration 2008; 75 (2): 121–133

Jimenez CA, Mhatre AD, Martinez CH, Eapen GA, Onn A, Morice RC. Use of an indwelling pleural catheter for the management of recurrent chylothorax in patients with cancer. Chest 2007; 132 (5): 1584–1590

Johnson G. Traumatic pneumothorax: is a chest drain always necessary? J Accid Emerg Med 1996; 13 (3): 173–174

Johnston WW. The malignant pleural effusion. A review of cytopathologic diagnoses of 584 specimens from 472 consecutive patients. Cancer 1985; 56 (4): 905–909

Judson MA, Sahn SA. The pleural space and organ transplantation. Am J Respir Crit Care Med 1996; 153 (3): 1153–1165

Kaiser D. [Indications for thoracoscopy in pleural empyema]. Pneumologie 1989; 43 (2): 76–79

Kaiser D. [Minimally invasive thoracic surgery]. Dtsch Med Wochenschr 1994; 119 (13): 469–472

Kaiser D. Indikation zur chirurgischen Therapie beim Spontanpneumothorax. Chir Praxis 2000; 57: 239–248

Kaiser D, Allica E, Noack F. Behandlung des Pneumothorax. Viszeralchirurgie 2000; 35: 309–315

Kaiser GC. Practice guidelines in cardiothoracic surgery. Ann Thorac Surg 1994; 58: 903–910

Kaiser LR, Daniel TM, eds. Thoracoscopic surgery. Boston, Toronto, London: Little, Brown; 1993

Kapferer R, Sticker G. Die Werke des Hippokrates. Stuttgart: Hippokrates;1933

Kapsenberg PD. Thoracoscopic biopsy under visual control. Poumon Coeur 1981; 37: 313–316

Karfis EA, Roustanis E, Beis J, Kakadellis J. Video-assisted cervical mediastinoscopy: our seven-year experience. Interact Cardiovasc Thorac Surg 2008; 7 (6): 1015–1018

Karmy-Jones R, Sorenson V, Horst HM, Lewis JW Jr, Rubinfeld I. Rigid thorascopic debridement and continuous pleural irrigation in the management of empyema. Chest 1997; 111 (2): 272–274

Kawahara K, Sasada S, Nagano T, et al. Pleural MALT lymphoma diagnosed on thoracoscopic resection under local anesthesia using an insulation-tipped diathermic knife. Pathol Int 2008; 58 (4): 253–256

Keller R, Gutersohn J, Herzog H. [The management of persistent pneumothorax by thoracoscopic procedures (author's transl)] Thoraxchir Vask Chir 1974; 22: 457–460

Kelling G. Über Oesophagoskopie, Gastroskopie und Kölioskopie. Munch Med Wochenschr 1902; 1: 21–24

Kennedy L, Rusch VW, Strange C, Ginsberg RJ, Sahn SA. Pleurodesis using talc slurry. Chest 1994; 106 (2): 342–346

Kennedy L, Sahn SA. Talc pleurodesis for the treatment of pneumothorax and pleural effusion. Chest 1994; 106 (4): 1215–1222

Kennedy L, Vaughan LM, Steed LL, Sahn SA. Sterilization of talc for pleurodesis. Available techniques, efficacy, and cost analysis. Chest 1995; 107 (4): 1032–1034

Kern JA, Rodgers BM. Thoracoscopy in the management of empyema in children. J Pediatr Surg 1993; 28 (9): 1128–1132

Klohnen A, Peroni JF. Thoracoscopy in horses. Vet Clin North Am Equine Pract 2000; 16 (2): 351–362, vii

Koegelenberg CF, Diaconi AH, Bolliger CT. Parapneumonic pleural effusion and empyema. Respiration 2008; 75 (3): 241–250

Koegelenberg CF, Bollinger CT, Theron J et al. A direct comparison of the diagnostic yield of ultrasound-assisted Abrams and Tru-Cut needle biopsies for pleural tuberculosis. Thorax 2009; Dec 8 (epub ahead of print)

Körner H, Andersen KS, Stangeland L, Ellingsen I, Engedal H. Surgical treatment of spontaneous pneumothorax by wedge resection without pleurodesis or pleurectomy. Eur J Cardiothorac Surg 1996; 10 (8): 656–659

Kolschmann S, Ballin A, Gillissen A. Clinical efficacy and safety of thoracoscopic talc pleurodesis in malignant pleural effusions. Chest 2005; 128 (3): 1431–1435

Kovak JR, Ludwig LL, Bergman PJ, Baer KE, Noone KE. Use of thoracoscopy to determine the etiology of pleural effusion in dogs and cats: 18 cases (1998–2001). J Am Vet Med Assoc 2002; 221 (7): 990–994

Krasna MJ. Thoracoscopic sympathectomy: a standardized approach to therapy for hyperhidrosis. Ann Thorac Surg 2008; 85 (2): S764–S767

Kropp R, Loddenkemper R. [Recurring, menstruation-dependent spontaneous pneumothorax—successful treatment with chemical pleurodesis]. Prax Klin Pneumol 1985; 39 (6): 208–209

Kux E. Thorakoskopische Eingriffe am Nervensystem. Stuttgart: Thieme; 1954

Kux M. Thoracic endoscopic sympathectomy in palmar and axillary hyperhidrosis. Arch Surg 1978; 113 (3): 264–266

Lamb CR, Feller-Kopman D, Ernst A, et al. An approach to interventional pulmonary fellowship training. Chest 2010; 137: 195–199

Lamy P, Canet B, Martinet Y, Lamaze R. [Evaluation of diagnostic means in pleural effusions (from two hundred observations) (author's transl)]. Poumon Coeur 1980; 36 (2): 83–94

Landreneau RJ, Mack MJ, Hazelrigg SR, et al. Video-assisted thoracic surgery: basic technical concepts and intercostal approach strategies. Ann Thorac Surg 1992; 54 (4): 800–807

Landreneau RJ, Hazelrigg SR, Mack MJ, et al. Thoracoscopic mediastinal lymph node sampling: useful for mediastinal lymph node stations inaccessible by cervical mediastinoscopy. J Thorac Cardiovasc Surg 1993; 106 (3): 554–558

Landreneau RJ, Keenan RJ, Hazelrigg SR, Mack MJ, Naunheim KS. Thoracoscopy for empyema and hemothorax. Chest 1995; 109: 18–24

Lange P, Mortensen J, Groth S. Lung function 22-35 years after treatment of idiopathic spontaneous pneumothorax with talc poudrage or simple drainage. Thorax 1988; 43 (7): 559–561

Langmack EL, Martin RJ, Pak J, Kraft M. Serum lidocaine concentrations in asthmatics undergoing research bronchoscopy. Chest 2000; 117 (4): 1055–1060

Lee P, Colt HG, eds. Flex-rigid pleuroscopy, step by step. Singapore: CMP Medica; 2005

Lee P, Colt HG. Using diagnostic thoracoscopy to optimal effect. J Respir Dis 2003a; 24: 503–509

Lee P, Colt HG. Thoracoscopy: an update on therapeutic applications. J Respir Dis 2003b; 24: 530–536

Lee P, Lan RS, Colt HG. Survey of pulmonologists' perspectives on thoracoscopy. J Bronchol. 2003; 10: 99–106

Lee P, Mather PN, Colt HG. Advances in thoracoscopy: 100 years since Jacobaeus. Respiration 2010; 79: 177–186

Lee P, Yap WS, Pek WY, Ng AW. An audit of medical thoracoscopy and talc poudrage for pneumothorax prevention in advanced COPD. Chest 2004; 125 (4): 1315–1320

Lee P, Colt HG. Rigid and semirigid pleuroscopy: the future is bright. Respirology 2005; 10 (4): 418–425

Lee P, Colt HG. State of the art: pleuroscopy. J Thorac Oncol 2007; 2 (7): 663–670

Lee P, Hsu A, Lo C, Colt HG. Prospective evaluation of flex-rigid pleuroscopy for indeterminate pleural effusion: accuracy, safety and outcome. Respirology 2007; 12 (6): 881–886

Lee P, Colt HG. A spray catheter technique for pleural anesthesia: a novel method for pain control before talc poudrage. Anesth Analg 2007; 104 (1): 198–200

Lee YC, Baumann MH, Maskell NA, et al. Pleurodesis practice for malignant pleural effusions in five English-speaking countries: survey of pulmonologists. Chest 2003; 124 (6): 2229–2238

Lee YCG, Light RW. Future directions. In: Light RW, Lee YCG, eds. Textbook of pleural diseases. 2nd ed. London: Hodder Arnold; 2008: 621–627

Lenglinger FX, Schwarz CD, Artmann W. Localization of pulmonary nodules before thoracoscopic surgery: value of percutaneous staining with methylene blue. AJR Am J Roentgenol 1994; 163 (2): 297–300

Lesur O, Delorme N, Fromaget JM, Bernadac P, Polu JM. Computed tomography in the etiologic assessment of idiopathic spontaneous pneumothorax. Chest 1990; 98 (2): 341–347

Levine MN, Young JE, Ryan ED, Newhouse MT. Pleural effusion in breast cancer. Thoracoscopy for hormone receptor determination. Cancer 1986; 57 (2): 324–327

Lewis JW Jr. Thoracoscopy: a surgeon's or a pulmonologist's domain. Pro pulmonologist. J Bronchol 1994; 1: 152–154

Lewis RJ, Kunderman PJ, Sisler GE, Mackenzie JW. Direct diagnostic thoracoscopy. Ann Thorac Surg 1976; 21 (6): 536–539

Lewis RJ, Caccavale RJ, Sisler GE, Mackenzie JW. One hundred consecutive patients undergoing video-assisted thoracic operations. Ann Thorac Surg 1992; 54 (3): 421–426

Li WW, Lee RL, Lee TW, et al. The impact of thoracic surgical access on early shoulder function: video-assisted thoracic surgery versus posterolateral thoracotomy. Eur J Cardiothorac Surg 2003; 23 (3): 390–396

Li X, Tu YR, Lin M, Lai FC, Chen JF, Dai ZJ. Endoscopic thoracic sympathectomy for palmar hyperhidrosis: a randomized control trial comparing T3 and T2-4 ablation. Ann Thorac Surg 2008; 85 (5): 1747–1751

Li X, Tu YR, Lin M, Lai FC, Chen JF, Miao HW. Minimizing endoscopic thoracic sympathectomy for primary palmar hyperhidrosis: guided by palmar skin temperature and laser Doppler blood flow. Ann Thorac Surg 2009; 87 (2): 427–431

Li ZG, Chen HZ, Jin H, et al. Surgical treatment of esophageal leiomyoma located near or at the esophagogastric junction via a thoracoscopic approach. Dis Esophagus 2009; 22 (2): 185–189

Licht PB, Pilegaard HK. Severity of compensatory sweating after thoracoscopic sympathectomy. Ann Thorac Surg 2004; 78 (2): 427–431

Liebig S, Freise G. [Indications for pulmonary biopsy with open thorax] Bronchopneumologie 1977; 27: 453–458

Light RW. Management of spontaneous pneumothorax. Am Rev Respir Dis 1993; 148 (1): 245–248

Light RW. Diagnostic principles in pleural disease. Eur Respir J 1997; 10 (2): 476–481

Light RW, Cheng DS, Lee YC, Rogers J, Davidson J, Lane KB. A single intrapleural injection of transforming growth factor-beta (2) produces an excellent pleurodesis in rabbits. Am J Respir Crit Care Med 2000; 162 (1): 98–104

Light RW. Talc should not be used for pleurodesis. Am J Respir Crit Care Med 2000; 162 (6): 2024–2026

Light RW. The undiagnosed pleural effusion. Clin Chest Med 2006; 27 (2): 309–319

Light RW, ed. Pleural diseases. 5th ed. Philadelphia: Lippincott Williams & Wilkins; 2007

Light RW. Update on tuberculous pleural effusion. Respirology 2010; 15: 451–458

Light RW, Lee YC, eds. Textbook of pleural diseases. 2nd ed. London: Hodder Arnold; 2008

Lilienthal H. Thoracoscopy (Letter to the editor). Surg Gynecol Obstet 1922; 35: 123–124

Lin TS. Video-assisted thoracoscopic "resympathicotomy" for palmar hyperhidrosis: analysis of 42 cases. Ann Thorac Surg 2001; 72 (3): 895–898

Lin CC, Telaranta T. Lin-Telaranta classification: the importance of different procedures for different indications in sympathetic surgery. Ann Chir Gynaecol 2001; 90 (3): 161–166

LoCicero J II. Minimally invasive thoracic surgery, video-assisted thoracic surgery and thoracoscopy. [Editorial]. Chest 1992; 102 (2): 330–331

Loddenkemper R, Mai J, Scheffler N, Brandt HJ. Prospective individual comparison of blind needle biopsy and of thoracoscopy in the diagnosis and differential diagnosis of tuberculous pleurisy. Scand J Respir Dis Suppl 1978; 102: 196–198

Loddenkemper R. Thoracoscopy: results in non cancerous and idiopathic pleural effusions. Poumon Coeur 1981; 37 (4): 261–264

Loddenkemper R, Grosser H, Gabler A, et al. Prospective evaluation of biopsy methods in the diagnosis of malignant pleural effusions. Intrapatient comparison between pleural fluid cytology, blind needle biopsy and thoracoscopy. Am Rev Respir Dis 1983a; 128 (Suppl 4): 114

Loddenkemper R, Grosser H, Mai J, Preussler H, Wundschock M, Brandt HJ. [Diagnosis of tuberculous pleural effusion: prospective comparison of laboratory chemical, bacteriologic, cytologic and histologic study results]. Prax Klin Pneumol 1983b; 37 (11): 1153–1156

Loddenkemper R. [Thoracoscopy Symposium 1987]. Pneumologie 1989; 43 (2): 45–125

Loddenkemper R, Boutin C. Thoracoscopy: present diagnostic and therapeutic indications. Eur Respir J 1993; 6 (10): 1544–1555

Loddenkemper R. Thoracoscopy—state of the art. Eur Respir J 1998; 11 (1): 213–221

Loddenkemper R. Thoracoscopy under local anesthesia. Is it safe? [Editorial] J Bronchol 2000; 7: 207–209

Loddenkemper R. Thoracoscopy: what are the perspectives for pulmonologists? [Editorial] J Bronchol 2003; 10: 95–96

Loddenkemper R. Pleural effusion. In: Albert R, St. Spiro J Jett, eds. Clinical respiratory medicine, 2nd ed. Section 15, Chapter 63. Philadelphia: Mosby; 2004a, 723–741

Loddenkemper R. Medical thoracoscopy—historical perspective. In: Beamis JF Jr, Mathur PN, Mehta AC, eds. Interventional pulmonary medicine. New York: Marcel Dekker; 2004b: 411–429

Loddenkemper R, Kaiser D, Frank W. Treatment of parapneumonic pleural effusion and empyema—conservative view. Eur Respir Mon 2004; 29: 199–207

Loddenkemper R, McKenna RJ. Thoracoscopy and other invasive procedures. In: Mason RJ, Broaddus VC, Murray JF, Nadel JA, eds. Textbook of respiratory medicine. 4th ed. Vol. 1. Philadelphia: Elsevier Saunders; 2005: 651–670

Loddenkemper R, Severin T, Eiselé JL, et al. HERMES: a European core syllabus in respiratory medicine. Breathe 2006; 3: 59–69

Loddenkemper R. Medical thoracoscopy. In: Light RW, Lee YCG, eds. Textbook of pleural diseases. 2nd ed. London: Arnold; 2008: 583–597

Loddenkemper R, Haslam PL, Séverin T, et al. European curriculum recommendations for training in adult respiratory medicine: 2nd report of the HERMES task force. In: Loddenkemper R, Haslam P, eds. European standards for training in adult respiratory medicine: syllabus, curriculum and diploma. Lausanne: European Respiratory Society; 2008: 27–66

Loddenkemper R, Noppen M. Pleuroscopy and medical thoracoscopy. In: Mason RJ, Broaddus VC, Martin TR, et al. (eds.). Murray and Nadel's textbook of respiratory medicine, 5th ed. Philadelphia: Elsevier (Saunders), 2010, 506–521

Loubani M, Lynch V. Video assisted thoracoscopic bullectomy and acromycin pleurodesis: an effective treatment for spontaneous pneumothorax. Respir Med 2000; 94 (9): 888–890

Low EM, Khoury GG, Matthews AW, Neville E. Prevention of tumour seeding following thoracoscopy in mesothelioma by prophylactic radiotherapy. Clin Oncol (R Coll Radiol) 1995; 7 (5): 317–318

Luh SP, Hsu GJ, Cheng-Ren C. Complicated parapneumonic effusion and empyema: pleural decortication and video-assisted thoracic surgery. Curr Infect Dis Rep 2008; 10 (3): 236–240

Maassen W. Direkte Thorakoskopie ohne vorherige oder mögliche Pneumothoraxanlage. Zugleich eine neue Methode der chirurgischen Pleura- und Lungenbiopsie. Endoskopie 1972; 4: 95–98

Maassen W. [Thoracoscopy and lung biopsy without initial pneumothorax (author's transl)]. Poumon Coeur 1981; 37 (5): 317–320

Macha HN, Reichle G, von Zwehl D, Kemmer HP, Bas R, Morgan JA. The role of ultrasound assisted thoracoscopy in the diagnosis of pleural disease. Clinical experience in 687 cases. Eur J Cardiothorac Surg 1993; 7 (1): 19–22

Mack MJ, Shennib H, Landreneau RJ, Hazelrigg SR. Techniques for localization of pulmonary nodules for thoracoscopic resection. J Thorac Cardiovasc Surg 1993; 106 (3): 550–553

Mackey VS, Wheat JD. Endoscopic examination of the equine thorax. Equine Vet J 1985; 17 (2): 140–142

Mahtabifard A, Fuller CB, McKenna RJ Jr. Video-assisted thoracic surgery sleeve lobectomy: a case series. Ann Thorac Surg 2008; 85 (2): S729–S732

Mai J, Loddenkemper R, Brandt HJ. [Diagnostic thoracoscopy in mediastinal space-occupying lesions]. Pneumologie 1989; 43 (2): 122–125

Maiwand MO. Video-assisted thoracoscopic surgery: Current applications, advantages, and limitations. [Review]. J Bronchol Intervent Pulmonol 1997; 4: 321–328

Marchandise FX, Vandenplas O, Wallon J, Francis C. Thoracoscopic lung biopsy in interstitial lung disease. Acta Clin Belg 1992; 47 (3): 165–169

Marchi E, Vargas FS, Madaloso BA, et al. Pleurodesis practice in South and Central American Countries (letter to the editor). Chest 2010; 137: 739–740

Marel M, Zrůstová M, Stasný B, Light RW. The incidence of pleural effusion in a well-defined region. Epidemiologic study in central Bohemia. Chest 1993; 104 (5): 1486–1489

Marel M. Epidemiology of pleural effusion. In: Loddenkemper R, Antony VB, eds. Pleural diseases. Eur Respir Mon 2002; 7: 146–156

Mares DC, Mathur PN. Medical thoracoscopic talc pleurodesis for chylothorax due to lymphoma: a case series. Chest 1998; 114: 731–735

Marhold F, Izay B, Zacherl J, Tschabitscher M, Neumayer C. Thoracoscopic and anatomic landmarks of Kuntz's nerve: implications for sympathetic surgery. Ann Thorac Surg 2008; 86 (5): 1653–1658

Marom EM, Patz EF Jr, Erasmus JJ, McAdams HP, Goodman PC, Herndon JE. Malignant pleural effusions: treatment with small-bore-catheter thoracostomy and talc pleurodesis. Radiology 1999; 210 (1): 277–281

Marquette CH, Marx A, Leroy S, et al; Pneumothorax Study Group. Simplified stepwise management of primary spontaneous pneumothorax: a pilot study. Eur Respir J 2006; 27 (3): 470–476

Martensson G, Pettersson K, Thiringer G. Differentiation between malignant and non-malignant pleural effusion. Eur J Respir Dis 1985; 67 (5): 326–334

Martínez-Moragón E, Aparicio J, Sanchis J, Menéndez R, Cruz Rogado M, Sanchis F. Malignant pleural effusion: prognostic factors for survival and response to chemical pleurodesis in a series of 120 cases. Respiration 1998; 65 (2): 108–113

Martins Rua JF, Jatene FB, de Campos JR, et al. Robotic versus human camera holding in video-assisted thoracic sympathectomy: a single blind randomized trial of efficacy and safety. Interact Cardiovasc Thorac Surg 2009; 8 (2): 195–199

Maskell NA, Butland RJ; Pleural Diseases Group, Standards of Care Committee, British Thoracic Society. BTS guidelines for the investigation of a unilateral pleural effusion in adults. Thorax 2003; 58 (Suppl 2): ii8–ii17

Maskell NA, Gleeson FV, Davies RJ. Standard pleural biopsy versus CT-guided cutting-needle biopsy for diagnosis of malignant disease in pleural effusions: a randomised controlled trial. Lancet 2003; 361 (9366): 1326–1330

Maskell NA, Lee YC, Gleeson FV, Hedley EL, Pengelly G, Davies RJ. Randomized trials describing lung inflammation after pleurodesis with talc of varying particle size. Am J Respir Crit Care Med 2004; 170 (4): 377–382

Maskell NA. Undiagnosed pleural effusions. In: Light RW, Lee YCG, eds. Textbook of pleural diseases. 2nd ed. London: Arnold; 2008: 491–498

Mason AC, Miller BH, Krasna MJ, White CS. Accuracy of CT for the detection of pleural adhesions: correlation with video-assisted thoracoscopic surgery. Chest 1999; 115 (2): 423–427

Masood I, Ahmad Z, Pandey DK, Singh SK. Role of simple needle aspiration in the management of spontaneous pneumothorax. J Assoc Physicians India 2007; 55: 628–629

Masshoff W, Höfer W. [Pathology of so-called idiopathic spontaneous pneumothorax]. Dtsch Med Wochenschr 1973; 98 (16): 801–805

Mathlouthi A, Chabchoub A, Labbene N, et al. [An experimental anatomopathological study of pleural talcosis]. Rev Mal Respir 1992; 9 (6): 617–621

Mathur PN. How I do it. 'Medical' thoracoscopy. J Bronchol 1994; 2: 144–151

Mathur PN, Boutin C, Loddenkemper R. 'Medical' thoracoscopy: Technique and indications in pulmonary medicine [Editorial]. J Bronchol Intervent Pulmonol 1994; 1: 228–239

Mathur PN, Loddenkemper R. Medical thoracoscopy. Role in pleural and lung diseases. Clin Chest Med 1995; 16 (3): 487–496

Mathur PN, Astoul P, Boutin C. Medical thoracoscopy. Technical details. Clin Chest Med 1995; 16 (3): 479–486

Mathur PN, Loddenkemper R. Biopsy techniques in the diagnosis of pleural diseases. In: Loddenkemper R, Antony VB, eds. Pleural diseases. Eur Respir Mon 2002; 7: 120–130.

Mathur PN. Pleuroscopy: a window to the pleura. J Bronchol. 2004a; 11: 147–149

Mathur PN. Review: thoracoscopic pleurodesis with talc may be the optimal technique in patients with malignant pleural effusions. ACP J Club 2004b; 141 (2): 43

Matson RC. The role of thoracoscopy in the diagnosis and management of lung tumors. Surg Gynecol Obstet 1936; 63: 617–624

Mattison LM, Steed LL, Sahn SA. More on talc sterilization. Chest 1996; 109 (6): 1667–1668

McCarthy TC, McDermaid SL. Thoracoscopy. Vet Clin North Am Small Anim Pract 1990; 20 (5): 1341–1352

McGahren ED, Teague WG Jr, Flanagan T, White B, Rodgers BM. The effects of talc pleurodesis on growing swine. J Pediatr Surg 1990; 25 (11): 1147–1151

McKenna RJ Jr. Lobectomy by video-assisted thoracic surgery with mediastinal node sampling for lung cancer. J Thorac Cardiovasc Surg 1994; 107 (3): 879–881, discussion 881–882

McKenna RJ Jr. The current status of video-assisted thoracic surgery lobectomy. Chest Surg Clin N Am 1998; 8: 775–785, viii; discussion 787–788

McKenna RJ Jr. Thoracoscopic evaluation and treatment of pulmonary disease. Surg Clin North Am 2000; 80: 1543–1553

McKenna RJ Jr, Mahtabifard A, Pickens A, Kusuanco D, Fuller CB. Fast-tracking after video-assisted thoracoscopic surgery lobectomy, segmentectomy, and pneumonectomy. Ann Thorac Surg 2007; 84 (5): 1663–1667, discussion 1667–1668

McKneally MF, Lewis RJ, Anderson RJ, et al. Statement of the AATS/STS Joint Committee on Thoracoscopy and Video Assisted Thoracic Surgery. J Thorac Cardiovasc Surg 1992; 104 (1): 1

McLean AN, Bicknell SR, McAlpine LG, Peacock AJ. Investigation of pleural effusion: an evaluation of the new Olympus LTF semiflexible thoracofiberscope and comparison with Abram's needle biopsy. Chest 1998; 114 (1): 150–153

Medford AR. Theoretical cost benefits of medical thoracoscopy (MT). Respir Med 2010 (epub ahead of print)

Medford AR, Awan YM, Marchbank A, Rahamim J, Unsworth-White J, Pearson PJ. Diagnostic and therapeutic performance of video-assisted thoracoscopic surgery (VATS) in investigation and management of pleural exudates. Ann R Coll Surg Engl 2008; 90 (7): 597–600

Medford AR, Bennett JA, Free CM, et al. Current status of medical pleuroscopy. Clin Chest Med 2010; 31: 165–172

Melton LJ III, Hepper NG, Offord KP. Incidence of spontaneous pneumothorax in Olmsted County, Minnesota: 1950 to 1974. Am Rev Respir Dis 1979; 120 (6): 1379–1382

Mengeot P-M, Gailly C. Spontaneous detachment of benign mesothelioma into the pleural space and removal during pleuroscopy. Eur J Respir Dis 1986; 68 (2): 141–145

Menzies R, Charbonneau M. Thoracoscopy for the diagnosis of pleural disease. Ann Intern Med 1991; 114 (4): 271–276

Metintas M, Ak G, Yildirim H, et al. Medical thoracoscopy versus computed tomography guided Abrams pleural needle biopsy for diagnosis of patients with pleural effusions: a randomized controlled trial. Chest 2010; 137: 1362–1368

Migliore M, Giuliano R, Aziz T, Saad RA, Sgalambro F. Four-step local anesthesia and sedation for thoracoscopic diagnosis and management of pleural diseases. Chest 2002; 121 (6): 2032–2035

Milanez de Campos JR, Kauffman P, Werebe EdeC, et al. Quality of life, before and after thoracic sympathectomy: report on 378 operated patients. Ann Thorac Surg 2003; 76 (3): 886–891

Miller AC, Harvey YE. Guidelines for the management of spontaneous pneumothorax. Standards of Care Committee. British Thoracic Society. BMJ 1993; 307: 114–116

Miller DL, Allen MS, Deschamps C, Trastek VF, Pairolero PC. Video-assisted thoracic surgical procedure: management of a solitary pulmonary nodule. Mayo Clin Proc 1992; 67 (5): 462–464

Miller JI, Hatcher CR Jr. Thoracoscopy: a useful tool in the diagnosis of thoracic disease. Ann Thorac Surg 1978; 26 (1): 68–72

Miller JI Jr. Therapeutic thoracoscopy: new horizons for an established procedure. (Editorial) Ann Thorac Surg 1991; 52 (5): 1036–1037

Mistal OM. Endoscopie et pleurolyse. Paris: Masson; 1935

Moisiuc FV, Colt HG. Thoracoscopy: origins revisited. Respiration 2007; 74 (3): 344–355

Molin LJ, Steinberg JB, Lanza LA. VATS increases costs in patients undergoing lung biopsy for interstitial lung disease. Ann Thorac Surg 1994; 58 (6): 1595–1598

Molins L, Fibla JJ, Pérez J, Sierra A, Vidal G, Simón C. Outpatient thoracic surgical programme in 300 patients: clinical results and economic impact. Eur J Cardiothorac Surg 2006; 29 (3): 271–275

Molins L, Fibla JJ, Mier JM, Sierra A. Outpatient thoracic surgery. Thorac Surg Clin 2008; 18 (3): 321–327

Munavvar M, Khan MA, Edwards J, Waqaruddin Z, Mills J. The autoclavable semirigid thoracoscope: the way forward in pleural disease? Eur Respir J 2007; 29 (3): 571–574

Munnell ER. Thoracic drainage. Ann Thorac Surg 1997; 63 (5): 1497–1502

Mutsaerts EL, Zoetmulder FA, Meijer S, Baas P, Hart AA, Rutgers EJ. Long term survival of thoracoscopic metastasectomy vs metastasectomy by thoracotomy in patients with a solitary pulmonary lesion. Eur J Surg Oncol 2002; 28 (8): 864–868

Naito T, Satoh H, Ishikawa H, et al. Pleural effusion as a significant prognostic factor in non-small cell lung cancer. Anticancer Res 1997; 17 (6D): 4743–4746

Nakajima J, Takamoto S, Kohno T, Ohtsuka T. Costs of video-thoracoscopic surgery versus open resection for patients with lung carcinoma. Cancer 2000; 89 (11, Suppl): 2497–2501

Nasreen N, Mohammed KA, Dowling PA, Ward MJ, Galffy G, Antony VB. Talc induces apoptosis in human malignant mesothelioma cells in vitro. Am J Respir Crit Care Med 2000; 161 (2 Pt 1): 595–600

Nasreen N, Najmunnisa N, Mohammed KA, et al. Talc mediates angiostasis in malignant pleural effusions via endostatin induction. Eur Respir J 2007; 29 (4): 761–769

Newhouse MT. Thoracoscopy: diagnostic and therapeutic indications. Pneumologie 1989; 43 (2): 48–52

Nezu K, Kushibe K, Tojo T, Takahama M, Kitamura S. Thoracoscopic wedge resection of blebs under local anesthesia with sedation for treatment of a spontaneous pneumothorax. Chest 1997; 111 (1): 230–235

Nitze M. Eine neue Beleuchtungs- und Untersuchungsmethode für Harnröhre, Harnblase und Rektum. Wien Med Wochenschr 1879; 29: 713–716

Nomori H, Ohtsuka T, Horio H, Naruke T, Suemasu K. Thoracoscopic lobectomy for lung cancer with a largely fused fissure. Chest 2003; 123 (2): 619–622

Noppen M, Dhondt E, Mahler T, Malfroot A, Dab I, Vincken W. Successful management of recurrent pneumothorax in cystic fibrosis by localized apical thoracoscopic talc poudrage. Chest 1994; 106 (1): 262–264

Noppen M, Dendale P, Hagers Y. Thoracoscopic sympathicotomy. Lancet 1995; 345 (8952): 803–804

Noppen M, Vincken W. Thoracoscopic sympathicolysis for essential hyperhidrosis: effects on pulmonary function. Eur Respir J 1996; 9 (8): 1660–1664

Noppen M, Vincken W, Dhaese J, Herregodts P, D'Haese J. Thoracoscopic sympathicolysis for essential hyperhidrosis: immediate and one year follow-up results in 35 patients and review of the literature. Acta Clin Belg 1996; 51 (4): 244–253

Noppen M, Degreve J, Mignolet M, Vincken W. A prospective, randomised study comparing the efficacy of talc slurry and bleomycin in the treatment of malignant pleural effusions. Acta Clin Belg 1997; 52 (5): 258–262

Noppen M, Dab I, D'Haese J, Meysman M, Vincken W. Thoracoscopic T2-T3 sympathicolysis for essential hyperhidrosis in childhood: effects on pulmonary function. Pediatr Pulmonol 1998a; 26 (4): 262–264

Noppen M, Meysman M, D'Haese J, Vincken W. Thoracoscopic splanchnicolysis for the relief of chronic pancreatitis pain: experience of a group of pneumologists. Chest 1998b; 113 (2): 528–531

Noppen M, De Waele M, Li R, et al. Volume and cellular content of normal pleural fluid in humans examined by pleural lavage. Am J Respir Crit Care Med 2000; 162 (3 Pt 1): 1023–1026

Noppen M, Alexander P, Driesen P, Slabbynck H, Verstraeten A. Manual aspiration versus chest tube drainage in first episodes of primary spontaneous pneumothorax: a multicenter, prospective, randomized pilot study. Am J Respir Crit Care Med 2002; 165 (9): 1240–1244

Noppen M, Schramel F. Pneumothorax. In: Loddenkemper R, Antony VB, eds. Pleural diseases. Eur Respir Mon 2002; 22: 279–296

Noppen M. Management of primary spontaneous pneumothorax. Curr Opin Pulm Med 2003a; 9 (4): 272–275

Noppen M. Chest ultrasound is o.k. for mountaineers and astronauts… and for pulmonologists? [Editorial] Respiration 2003b; 70 (3): 240–241

Noppen M, Baumann MH. Pathogenesis and treatment of primary spontaneous pneumothorax: an overview. Respiration 2003; 70 (4): 431–438

Noppen M. Normal volume and cellular contents of pleural fluid. Paediatr Respir Rev 2004a; 5 (Suppl A): S201–S203

Noppen M. Medical thoracoscopy. Techniques for thoracic sympathectomy. In: Beamis JF, Mathur PN, Mehta AC, eds. Interventional pulmonary medicine. Lung biology in health and disease. Vol. 189. New York: Marcel Dekker; 2004b: 483–502

Noppen M, Dekeukeleire T, Hanon S, et al. Fluorescein-enhanced autofluorescence thoracoscopy in patients with primary spontaneous pneumothorax and normal subjects. Am J Respir Crit Care Med 2006; 174 (1): 26–30

Noppen M. Who's (still) afraid of talc? Eur Respir J 2007; 29 (4): 619–621

Noppen M, De Keukeleire T. Pneumothorax. Respiration 2008; 76 (2): 121–127

Nowak AK, Lake RA, Kindler HL, Robinson BW. New approaches for mesothelioma: biologics, vaccines, gene therapy, and other novel agents. Semin Oncol 2002; 29 (1): 82–96

O'Brien PK, Kucharczuk JC, Marshall MB, et al. Comparative study of subxiphoid versus video-thoracoscopic pericardial "window". Ann Thorac Surg 2005; 80 (6): 2013–2019

Ohata M, Suzuki H. Pathogenesis of spontaneous pneumothorax. With special reference to the ultrastructure of emphysematous bullae. Chest 1980; 77 (6): 771–776

Ojimba TA, Cameron AE. Drawbacks of endoscopic thoracic sympathectomy. Br J Surg 2004; 91 (3): 264–269

Oldenburg FA Jr, Newhouse MT. Thoracoscopy. A safe, accurate diagnostic procedure using the rigid thoracoscope and local anesthesia. Chest 1979; 75 (1): 45–50

O'Rourke N, Garcia JC, Paul J, Lawless C, McMenemin R, Hill J. A randomised controlled trial of intervention site radiotherapy in malignant pleural mesothelioma. Radiother Oncol 2007; 84 (1): 18–22

Osugi H, Takemura M, Higashino M, Takada N, Lee S, Kinoshita H. A comparison of video-assisted thoracoscopic oesophagectomy and radical lymph node dissection for squamous cell cancer of the oesophagus with open operation. Br J Surg 2003; 90 (1): 108–113

Ozkara SK, Turan G, Başyiğit I. Clinicopathologic significance of eosinophilic pleural effusions in a population with a high prevalence of tuberculosis and cancer. Acta Cytol 2007; 51 (5): 773–781

Park BJ, Flores RM. Cost comparison of robotic, video-assisted thoracic surgery and thoracotomy approaches to pulmonary lobectomy. Thorac Surg Clin 2008; 18 (3): 297–300, vii

Passlick B, Born C, Sienel W, Thetter O. Incidence of chronic pain after minimal-invasive surgery for spontaneous pneumothorax. Eur J Cardiothorac Surg 2001; 19: 355–358

Pastis NJ, Nietert PJ, Silvestri GA; American College of Chest Physicians Interventional Chest/Diagnostic Procedures Network Steering Committee. Variation in training for interventional pulmonary procedures among US pulmonary/critical care fellowships: a survey of fellowship directors. Chest 2005; 127 (5): 1614–1621

Patz EF Jr, McAdams HP, Erasmus JJ, et al. Sclerotherapy for malignant pleural effusions: a prospective randomized trial of bleomycin vs doxycycline with small-bore catheter drainage. Chest 1998; 113 (5): 1305–1311

Peroni JF, Robinson NE, Stick JA, Derksen FJ. Pleuropulmonary and cardiovascular consequences of thoracoscopy performed in healthy standing horses. Equine Vet J 2000; 32 (4): 280–286

Perry Y, Fernando HC, Buenaventura PO, Christie NA, Luketich JD. Minimally invasive esophagectomy in the elderly. JSLS 2002; 6 (4): 299–304

Petrou M, Kaplan D, Goldstraw P. Management of recurrent malignant pleural effusions. The complementary role talc pleurodesis and pleuroperitoneal shunting. Cancer 1995; 75 (3): 801–805

Pien GW, Gant MJ, Washam CL, Sterman DH. Use of an implantable pleural catheter for trapped lung syndrome in patients with malignant pleural effusion. Chest 2001; 119 (6): 1641–1646

Pierce GF, Mustoe TA, Lingelbach J, et al. Platelet-derived growth factor and transforming growth factor-beta enhance tissue repair activities by unique mechanisms. J Cell Biol 1989; 109 (1): 429–440

Piguet A, Giraud A. La pleuroscopie et la section des adhérences intrapleural au cours du pneumothorax thérapeutique. La presse médicale, No 23, 1923

Pittet O, Christodoulou M, Pezzetta E, Schmidt S, Schnyder P, Ris HB. Video-assisted thoracoscopic resection of a small pulmonary nodule after computed tomography-guided localization with a hook-wire system. Experience in 45 consecutive patients. World J Surg 2007; 31 (3): 575–578

Pompeo E, Tacconi F, Mineo D, Mineo TC. The role of awake video-assisted thoracoscopic surgery in spontaneous pneumothorax. J Thorac Cardiovasc Surg 2007; 133 (3): 786–790

Putnam JB Jr, Light RW, Rodriguez RM, et al. A randomized comparison of indwelling pleural catheter and doxycycline pleurodesis in the management of malignant pleural effusions. Cancer 1999; 86 (10): 1992–1999

Putnam JB Jr, Walsh GL, Swisher SG, et al. Outpatient management of malignant pleural effusion by a chronic indwelling pleural catheter. Ann Thorac Surg 2000; 69 (2): 369–375

Quetglas FS, Velasquez AS, Pujol JL. La toracoscopia. Madrid: Jarpyo; 1985

Qureshi RA, Stamenkovic SA, Carnochan FM, Walker WS. Video-assisted thoracoscopic lung biopsy in patients with interstitial lung disease. Ann Thorac Surg 2007; 84 (6): 2136–2137

Raffenberg M, Mai J, Loddenkemper R. [Results of thoracoscopy in localized lung and chest wall diseases]. Pneumologie 1990; 44 (Suppl 1): 182–183

Raffenberg M, Schaberg T, Loddenkemper R. Thorakoskopische Diagnostik pleuranaher Herdbefunde. Pneumologie 1992; 46: 298–299

Radomsky J, Becker HP, Hartel W. [Pleural porosity in idiopathic spontaneous pneumothorax]. Pneumologie 1989; 43 (5): 250–253

Reed DN Jr, Vyskocil JJ, Rao V. Subcutaneous access ports with fenestrated catheters for improved management of recurrent pleural effusions. Am J Surg 1999; 177 (2): 145–146

Reed MF, Lucia MW, Starnes SL, Merrill WH, Howington JA. Thoracoscopic lobectomy: introduction of a new technique into a thoracic surgery training program. J Thorac Cardiovasc Surg 2008; 136 (2): 376–381

Rehse DH, Aye RW, Florence MG. Respiratory failure following talc pleurodesis. Am J Surg 1999; 177 (5): 437–440

Robinson GR II, Gleeson K. Diagnostic flexible fiberoptic pleuroscopy in suspected malignant pleural effusions. Chest 1995; 107 (2): 424–429

Rocco G, La Rocca A, La Manna C, et al. Uniportal video-assisted thoracoscopic surgery pericardial window. J Thorac Cardiovasc Surg 2006; 131 (4): 921–922

Rocco G, Internullo E, Cassivi SD, Van Raemdonck D, Ferguson MG. The variability of practice in minimally invasive thoracic surgery for pulmonary resections. Thorac Surg Clin 2008; 18: 235–247

Roche G, Delanoe Y, Moayer N. Talcage de la plèvre sous pleuroscopie. Résultats, indications, technique (A propos de 14 observations). J Fr Med Chir Thorac 1963; 21: 177–195

Rodgers BM, Talbert JL. Thoracoscopy for diagnosis of intrathoracic lesions in children. J Pediatr Surg 1976; 11 (5): 703–708

Rodgers BM, Moazam F, Talbert JL. Thoracoscopy. Early diagnosis of interstitial pneumonitis in the immunologically suppressed child. Chest 1979a; 75 (2): 126–130

Rodgers BM, Moulder PV, DeLaney A. Thoracoscopy: new method of early diagnosis of cardiac herniation. J Thorac Cardiovasc Surg 1979b; 78 (4): 623–625

Rodgers BM, Talbert JL, Moazam F. Thoracic endoscopy in children. J Fla Med Assoc 1979c; 66 (10): 1013–1015

Rodgers BM. Thoracoscopy in children. Poumon Coeur 1981; 37 (5): 301–306

Rodgers BM. The role of thoracoscopy in pediatric surgical practice. Semin Pediatr Surg 2003; 12 (1): 62–70

Rodriguez-Panadero F, Lopez-Mejias J. Survival time of patients with pleural metastatic carcinoma predicted by glucose and pH studies. Chest 1989a; 95 (2): 320–324

Rodríguez-Panadero F, López Mejías J. Low glucose and pH levels in malignant pleural effusions. Diagnostic significance and prognostic value in respect to pleurodesis. Am Rev Respir Dis 1989b; 139 (3): 663–667

Rodriguez-Panadero F. Talc pleurodesis for treating malignant pleural effusions. Chest 1995; 108 (4): 1178–1179

Rodriguez-Panadero F, Antony VB. Pleurodesis: state of the art. Eur Respir J 1997; 10 (7): 1648–1654

Rodriguez-Panadero F, Janssen JP, Astoul P. Thoracoscopy: general overview and place in the diagnosis and management of pleural effusion. Eur Respir J 2006; 28 (2): 409–422

Rodríguez-Panadero F. Medical thoracoscopy. Respiration 2008; 76 (4): 363–372

Roe BB. Physiologic principles of drainage of the pleural space. Am J Surg 1958; 96 (2): 246–253

Rusch VW; From the International Mesothelioma Interest Group. A proposed new international TNM staging system for malignant pleural mesothelioma. Chest 1995; 108 (4): 1122–1128

Ryan CJ, Rodgers RF, Unni KK, Hepper NG. The outcome of patients with pleural effusion of indeterminate cause at thoracotomy. Mayo Clin Proc 1981; 56 (3): 145–149

Ryckman FC, Rodgers BM. Thoracoscopy for intrathoracic neoplasia in children. J Pediatr Surg 1982; 17 (5): 521–524

Sahn SA. Malignant pleural effusions. Clin Chest Med 1985; 6: 113–125

Sahn SA. Talc should be used for pleurodesis. Am J Respir Crit Care Med 2000; 162 (6): 2023–2024, discussion 2026

Sahn SA, Heffner JE. Spontaneous pneumothorax. N Engl J Med 2000; 342 (12): 868–874

Sahn SA. Pleural thickening, trapped lung, and chronic empyema as sequelae of tuberculous pleural effusion: don't sweat the pleural thickening. Int J Tuberc Lung Dis 2002; 6 (6): 461–464

Sakuraba M, Masuda K, Hebisawa A, Sagara Y, Komatsu H. Thoracoscopic pleural biopsy for tuberculous pleurisy under local anesthesia. Ann Thorac Cardiovasc Surg 2006a; 12 (4): 245–248

Sakuraba M, Masuda K, Hebisawa A, Sagara Y, Komatsu H. Diagnostic value of thoracoscopic pleural biopsy for pleurisy under local anaesthesia. ANZ J Surg 2006b; 76 (8): 722–724

Sakuraba M, Masuda K, Hebisawa A, et al. Pleural effusion adenosine deaminase (ADA) level and occult tuberculous pleurisy. Ann Thorac Cardiovasc Surg 2009; 15: 294–296

Salati M, Brunelli A, Xiumè F, et al. Uniportal video-assisted thoracic surgery for primary spontaneous pneumothorax: clinical and economic analysis in comparison to the traditional approach. Interact Cardiovasc Thorac Surg 2008a; 7 (1): 63–66

Salati M, Brunelli A, Rocco G. Uniportal video-assisted thoracic surgery for diagnosis and treatment of intrathoracic conditions. Thorac Surg Clin 2008b; 18 (3): 305–310, vii.

Salyer WR, Eggleston JC, Erozan YS. Efficacy of pleural needle biopsy and pleural fluid cytopathology in the diagnosis of malignant neoplasm involving the pleura. Chest 1975; 67 (5): 536–539

Sanchez-Armengol A, Rodriguez-Panadero F. Survival and talc pleurodesis in metastatic pleural carcinoma, revisited. Report of 125 cases. Chest 1993; 104 (5): 1482–1485

Sartori S, Tombesi P, Tassinari D, et al. Sonographically guided small-bore chest tubes and sonographic monitoring for rapid sclerotherapy of recurrent malignant pleural effusions. J Ultrasound Med 2004; 23 (9): 1171–1176

Sasaki M, Kawabe M, Hirai S, et al. Preoperative detection of pleural adhesions by chest ultrasonography. Ann Thorac Surg 2005; 80 (2): 439–442

Sattler A. Zur Behandlung des Spontanpneumothorax mit besonderer Berücksichtigung der Thorakoskopie. Beitr Klin Tuberk 1937a; 89: 395–408

Sattler A. Zur Pathogenese und Therapie des idiopathischen Spontanpneumothorax. Wien Arch Inn Med 1937; 30: 77–96

Sattler A. Der idiopathische Spontanpneumothorax und ähnliche Krankheitsbilder. Ergeb Inn Med Kinderheilkd 1940; 59: 213–283

Sattler A. Biopsie zur ätiologischen Diagnose pleuraler Ergüsse. Wien Med Wochenschr 1956; 106: 620–622

Sattler A. La thoracoscopie: intérêt thérapeutique dans les syndromes pleuro-pulmonaires d'urgence et intérêt diagnostique. Poumon Coeur (Paris) 1981; 37: 265–267

Savcenko M, Wendt GK, Prince SL, Mack MJ. Video-assisted thymectomy for myasthenia gravis: an update of a single institution experience. Eur J Cardiothorac Surg 2002; 22 (6): 978–983

Schaberg T, Süttmann-Bayerl A, Loddenkemper R. [Thoracoscopy in diffuse lung diseases]. Pneumologie 1989; 43 (2): 112–115

Scherpereel A, Astoul P, Baas P, et al. Guidelines of the European Respiratory Society and the European Society of Thoracic Surgeons for the management of malignant pleural mesothelioma. Eur Respir J 2010; 35: 479–495

Schmidt W. Der künstliche Pneumothorax. In: Hein, Kremer, Schmidt. Kollapstherapie der Lungentuberkulose. Leipzig: Thieme; 1938: 269–428

Schönfeld N, Schwarz J, Kollmeier J, Blum T, Bauer TT, Ott S. Narrow band imaging (NBI) during medical thoracoscopy: first impressions. J Occup Med Toxicol 2009; 4: 24–28

Schramel FMNH, Postmus PE, Vanderschueren RGJRA. Current aspects of spontaneous pneumothorax. Eur Respir J 1997; 10 (6): 1372–1379

Schwarz C, Lübbert H, Rahn W, Schönfeld N, Serke M, Loddenkemper R. Medical thoracoscopy: hormone receptor content in pleural metastases due to breast cancer. Eur Respir J 2004; 24 (5): 728–730

Schwarz C, Bittner R, Kirsch A, et al. A 62-year-old woman with bilateral pleural effusions and pulmonary infiltrates caused by extramedullary hematopoiesis. Respiration 2009; 78 (1): 110–113

Sears D, Hajdu SI. The cytologic diagnosis of malignant neoplasms in pleural and peritoneal effusions. Acta Cytol 1987; 31 (2): 85–97

Seijo LM, Sterman DH. Interventional pulmonology. N Engl J Med 2001; 344 (10): 740–749

Seitz B, Delpierre S, Choux R, Lama A, Boutin C. [Experimental study of the pleural effects of the pulverization, under thoracoscopic control, of a fibrin glue (Tissucol)]. Rev Mal Respir 1989; 6 (6): 537–542

Semm K. Tissue-puncher and loop-ligation—new aids for surgical-therapeutic pelviscopy (laparoscopy) = endoscopic intra-abdominal surgery. Endoscopy 1978; 10 (2): 119–124

Semm K. Endoscopic appendectomy. Endoscopy 1993; 15: 59–64

Shaw P, Agarwal R. Pleurodesis for malignant pleural effusions. Cochrane Database Syst Rev 2004; (1): CD002916

Shichinohe T, Hirano S, Kondo S. Video-assisted esophagectomy for esophageal cancer. Surg Today 2008; 38 (3): 206–213

Shigemura N, Akashi A, Funaki S, et al. Long-term outcomes after a variety of video-assisted thoracoscopic lobectomy approaches for clinical stage IA lung cancer: a multi-institutional study. J Thorac Cardiovasc Surg 2006; 132 (3): 507–512

Shigemura N, Yim AP. Variation in the approach to VATS lobectomy: effect on the evaluation of surgical morbidity following VATS lobectomy for the treatment of stage I non-small cell lung cancer. Thorac Surg Clin 2007; 17 (2): 233–239, ix

Siebert WW. Endothorakale Kinematographie. Dtsch Med Wochenschr 1930; 1: 1003–1006

Singer JJ. The thoracoscope in pulmonary diagnosis. Am Rev Tuberc 1924; 10: 67–71

Society of Thoracic Surgeons. Practice guidelines—video-assisted thoracic surgery. Ann Thorac Surg 1994; 58: 596–602

Solaini L, Prusciano F, Bagioni P, di Francesco F, Solaini L, Poddie DB. Video-assisted thoracic surgery (VATS) of the lung: analysis of intraoperative and postoperative complications over 15 years and review of the literature. Surg Endosc 2008; 22 (2): 298–310

Solèr M, Wyser C, Bolliger CT, Perruchoud AP. Treatment of early parapneumonic empyema by "medical" thoracoscopy. Schweiz Med Wochenschr 1997; 127 (42): 1748–1753

Spiegler PA, Hurewitz AN, Groth ML. Rapid pleurodesis for malignant pleural effusions. Chest 2003; 123 (6): 1895–1898

Stefani A, Natali P, Casali C, Morandi U. Talc poudrage versus talc slurry in the treatment of malignant pleural effusion. A prospective comparative study. Eur J Cardiothorac Surg 2006; 30 (6): 827–832

Steiropoulos P, Kouliatsis G, Karpathiou G, Popidou M, Froudarakis ME. Rare cases of primary pleural Hodgkin and non-Hodgkin lymphomas. Respiration 2009; 77 (4): 459–463

Sterman DH. Gene therapy for malignant pleural mesothelioma. Hematol Oncol Clin North Am 2005; 19 (6): 1147–1173, viii

Stewart DJ, Edwards JG, Smythe WR, Waller DA, O'Byrne KJ. Malignant pleural mesothelioma—an update. Int J Occup Environ Health 2004; 10 (1): 26–39

Stolz D, Chhajed PN, Leuppi JD, Brutsche M, Pflimlin E, Tamm M. Cough suppression during flexible bronchoscopy using combined sedation with midazolam and hydrocodone: a randomised, double blind, placebo controlled trial. Thorax 2004; 59 (9): 773–776

Storey CF. Thoracoscopy. Surg Clin North Am 1957; 37 (5): 1327–1336

Storey DD, Dines DE, Coles DT. Pleural effusion. A diagnostic dilemma. JAMA 1976; 236 (19): 2183–2186

Stovroff M, Teague G, Heiss KF, Parker P, Ricketts RR. Thoracoscopy in the management of pediatric empyema. J Pediatr Surg 1995; 30 (8): 1211–1215

Sudduth CD, Sahn SA. Pleurodesis for nonmalignant pleural effusions. Recommendations. Chest 1992; 102 (6): 1855–1860

Sugarbaker DJ, Jaklitsch MT, Bueno R, et al. Prevention, early detection, and management of complications after 328 consecutive extrapleural pneumonectomies. J Thorac Cardiovasc Surg 2004; 128 (1): 138–146

Sugiura S, Ando Y, Minami H, Ando M, Sakai S, Shimokata K. Prognostic value of pleural effusion in patients with non-small cell lung cancer. Clin Cancer Res 1997; 3 (1): 47–50

Swanson SJ, Herndon JE II, D'Amico TA, et al. Video-assisted thoracic surgery lobectomy: report of CALGB 39802—a prospective, multi-institution feasibility study. J Clin Oncol 2007; 25 (31): 4993–4997

Swierenga J, Wagenaar JPM, Bergstein PGM. The value of thoracoscopy in the diagnosis and treatment of diseases affecting the pleura and lung. Pneumonologie 1974; 151 (1): 11–18

Swierenga J. Atlas of Thoracoscopy. Ingelheim/Rhein: Boehringer, 1978

Takeno Y. Thoracoscopic treatment of spontaneous pneumothorax. Ann Thorac Surg 1993; 56 (3): 688–690

Tamura M, Ohta Y, Sato H. Thoracoscopic appearance of bilateral spontaneous pneumothorax. Chest 2003; 124 (6): 2368–2371

Tan C, Sedrakyan A, Browne J, Swift S, Treasure T. The evidence on the effectiveness of management for malignant pleural effusion: a systematic review. Eur J Cardiothorac Surg 2006a; 29 (5): 829–838

Tan C, Treasure T, Browne J, Utley M, Davies CW, Hemingway H. Appropriateness of VATS and bedside thoracostomy talc pleurodesis as judged by a panel using the RAND/UCLA appropriateness method (RAM). Interact Cardiovasc Thorac Surg 2006b; 5 (3): 311–316

Tape TG, Blank LL, Wigton RS. Procedural skills of practicing pulmonologists. A national survey of 1,000 members of the American College of Physicians. Am J Respir Crit Care Med 1995; 151 (2 Pt 1): 282–287

Tassi G, Marchetti G. Minithoracoscopy: a less invasive approach to thoracoscopy. Chest 2003; 124 (5): 1975–1977

Tassi GF, Davies RJ, Noppen M. Advanced techniques in medical thoracoscopy. Eur Respir J 2006; 28 (5): 1051–1059

Terashima H, Sugawara F, Hirayama K. [The optimal procedure for chylothorax after operation for thoracic esophageal cancer; reasonable approaches to the thoracic duct from the point of view of routes for esophageal replacement]. Kyobu Geka 2003; 56 (6): 465–468

Thiberville L, Salaün M, Lachkar S, et al. Human in vivo fluorescence microimaging of the alveolar ducts and sacs during bronchoscopy. Eur Respir J 2009; 33 (5): 974–985

Thompson RL, Yau JC, Donnelly RF, Gowan DJ, Matzinger FR. Pleurodesis with iodized talc for malignant effusions using pigtail catheters. Ann Pharmacother 1998; 32 (7–8): 739–742

Trajman A, Pai M, Dheda K, et al. Novel tests for diagnosing tuberculous pleural effusion: what works and what does not? Eur Respir J 2008; 31 (5): 1098–1106

Treasure T. Minimally invasive surgery for pneumothorax: the evidence, changing practice and current opinion. J R Soc Med 2007a; 100 (9): 419–422

Treasure T. Minimal access surgery for pneumothorax. Lancet 2007b; 370 (9584): 294–295

Treasure T, Internullo E, Utley M. Resection of pulmonary metastases: a growth industry. Cancer Imaging 2008; 8: 121–124

Tremblay A, Michaud G. Single-center experience with 250 tunnelled pleural catheter insertions for malignant pleural effusion. Chest 2006; 129 (2): 362–368

Tremblay A, Mason C, Michaud G. Use of tunnelled catheters for malignant pleural effusions in patients fit for pleurodesis. Eur Respir J 2007; 30 (4): 759–762

Tribble CG, Selden RF, Rodgers BM. Talc poudrage in the treatment of spontaneous pneumothoraces in patients with cystic fibrosis. Ann Surg 1986; 204 (6): 677–680

Tschopp JM, Bolliger CT, Boutin C. Treatment of spontaneous pneumothorax: why not simple talc pleurodesis by medical thoracoscopy? Respiration 2000; 67 (1): 108–111

Tschopp JM, Boutin C, Astoul P, et al; ESMEVAT team. (European Study on Medical Video-Assisted Thoracoscopy). Talcage by medical thoracoscopy for primary spontaneous pneumothorax is more cost-effective than drainage: a randomised study. Eur Respir J 2002; 20 (4): 1003–1009

Tschopp JM, Rami-Porta R, Noppen M, Astoul P. Management of spontaneous pneumothorax: state of the art. Eur Respir J 2006; 28 (3): 637–650

Tschopp JM, Schnyder JM, Astoul P, et al. Pleurodesis by talc poudrage under simple medical thoracoscopy: an international opinion. Thorax 2009; 64 (3): 273–274, author reply 274

UEMS Charter on training of medical specialists in the EU—Requirements for the specialty Pneumology. Union Européenne de Médecins Spécialistes, European Board of Pneumology, 1995

Unverricht W. Weitere Erfahrungen mit der Kaustik im Pleuraraum und der Thorako- und Laparoskopie. Beitr Klin Tuberk 1923; 55: 296–307

Unverricht W. Thorakoskopie, ihre Technik und Ergebnisse. 2nd ed. Leipzig: Barth; 1931

Vachon AM, Fischer AT. Thoracoscopy in the horse: diagnostic and therapeutic indications in 28 cases. Equine Vet J 1998; 30 (6): 467–475

Valdés L, Alvarez D, Valle JM, Pose A, San José E. The etiology of pleural effusions in an area with high incidence of tuberculosis. Chest 1996; 109 (1): 158–162

Valdés L, Alvarez D, San José E, et al. Tuberculous pleurisy: a study of 254 patients. Arch Intern Med 1998; 158 (18): 2017–2021

van de Brekel JA, Duurkens VAM, Vanderschueren RGJRA. Pneumothorax. Results of thoracoscopy and pleurodesis with talc poudrage and thoracotomy. Chest 1993; 103 (2): 345–347

Vanderschueren RG. [Pleural talcage in patients with spontaneous pneumothorax (author's transl)]. Poumon Coeur 1981; 37 (4): 273–276

Van Schil P. Cost analysis of video-assisted thoracic surgery versus thoracotomy: critical review. Eur Respir J 2003; 22 (5): 735–738

Vansteenkiste J, Verbeken E, Thomeer M, Van Haecke P, Eeckhout AV, Demedts M. Medical thoracoscopic lung biopsy in interstitial lung disease: a prospective study of biopsy quality. Eur Respir J 1999; 14 (3): 585–590

Vargas FS, Milanez JR, Filomeno LT, Fernandez A, Jatene A, Light RW. Intrapleural talc for the prevention of recurrence in benign or undiagnosed pleural effusions. Chest 1994; 106 (6): 1771–1775

Venekamp LN, Velkeniers B, Noppen M. Does 'idiopathic pleuritis' exist? Natural history of non-specific pleuritis diagnosed after thoracoscopy. Respiration 2005; 72 (1): 74–78

Verfaillie G, Herreweghe RV, Lamote J, Noppen M, Sacre R. Use of a Port-a-Cath system in the home setting for the treatment of symptomatic recurrent malignant pleural effusion. Eur J Cancer Care (Engl) 2005; 14 (2): 182–184

Viallat JR, Rey F, Convert G, et al. [Yield of the thoracoscopic biopsy in experimental pulmonary infections in the immunosuppressed rabbit]. Rev Mal Respir 1985; 2 (3): 161–166

Viallat JR, Tubiana N, Boutin C, Farisse P, Lejeune C, Carcassonne Y. [Pleurisy in blood diseases: value of thoracoscopic poudrage]. Rev Pneumol Clin 1986; 42 (6): 274–278

Viallat JR, Rey F, Astoul P, Boutin C. Thoracoscopic talc poudrage pleurodesis for malignant effusions. A review of 360 cases. Chest 1996; 110 (6): 1387–1393

Villanueva AG, Gray AW Jr, Shahian DM, Williamson WA, Beamis JF Jr. Efficacy of short term versus long term tube thoracostomy drainage before tetracycline pleurodesis in the treatment of malignant pleural effusions. Thorax 1994; 49 (1): 23–25

Viskum K, Enk B. Complications of thoracoscopy. Poumon Coeur 1981; 37 (1): 25–28

Viskum K. Contraindications and complications to thoracoscopy. Pneumologie 1989; 43 (2): 55–57

Vlug MS, Wind J, Eshuis JH, Lindeboom R, van Berge Henegouwen MI, Bemelman WA. Feasibility of laparoscopic Nissen fundoplication as a day-case procedure. Surg Endosc 2009; 23 (8): 1839–1844

Voellmy W. [Results of thoracoscopies in the diagnosis of diseases of the lungs and of the pleura (author's transl)]. Poumon Coeur 1981; 37 (1): 67–73

Vogel B, Mall W. [Thoracoscopic pericardial fenestration—diagnostic and therapeutic aspects]. Pneumologie 1990; 44 (Suppl 1): 184–185

Vogelzang NJ, Rusthoven JJ, Symanowski J, et al. Phase III study of pemetrexed in combination with cisplatin versus cisplatin alone in patients with malignant pleural mesothelioma. J Clin Oncol 2003; 21 (14): 2636–2644

Vohra HA, Adamson L, Weeden DF. Does video-assisted thoracoscopic pleurectomy result in better outcomes than open pleurectomy for primary spontaneous pneumothorax? Interact Cardiovasc Thorac Surg 2008; 7 (4): 673–677

Wakabayashi A. Expanded applications of diagnostic and therapeutic thoracoscopy. J Thorac Cardiovasc Surg 1991; 102 (5): 721–723

Wakai A, O'Sullivan RG, McCabe G. Simple aspiration versus intercostal tube drainage for primary spontaneous pneumothorax in adults. Cochrane Database Syst Rev 2007 Jan 24; (1): CD004479

Walker-Renard PB, Vaughan LM, Sahn SA. Chemical pleurodesis for malignant pleural effusions. Ann Intern Med 1994; 120 (1): 56–64

Wall CP, Gaensler EA, Carrington CB, Hayes JA. Comparison of transbronchial and open biopsies in chronic infiltrative lung diseases. Am Rev Respir Dis 1981; 123 (3): 280–285

Waller DA, Martin-Ucar AE. Surgery of the pleural cavity. In: Light RW, Lee YCG, eds. Textbook of pleural diseases. 2nd ed. London: Arnold; 2008: 599–611

Walzl G, Wyser C, Smedema J, et al. Comparing the diagnostic yield of Abrams needle pleural biopsy and thoracoscopy. Am J Respir Crit Care Med 1996; 153: A460

Wang Z, Tong ZH, Li HJ, et al. Semi-rigid thoracoscopy for undiagnosed exudative pleural effusions: a comparative study. Chin Med J (Engl) 2008; 121 (15): 1384–1389

Warren WH, Kalimi R, Khodadadian LM, Kim AW. Management of malignant pleural effusions using the Pleur(x) catheter. Ann Thorac Surg 2008; 85 (3): 1049–1055

Weiss LD, Generalovich T, Heller MB, et al. Methemoglobin levels following intravenous lidocaine administration. Ann Emerg Med 1987; 16 (3): 323–325

Weissberg D. Pleuroscopy in empyema: is it ever necessary? Poumon Coeur 1981; 37 (4): 269–272

Weissberg D, Kaufman M, Schwecher I. Pleuroscopy in clinical evaluation and staging of lung cancer. Poumon Coeur 1981; 37 (4): 241–243

Weissberg D. Handbook of practical pleuroscopy. Mount Kisko, NY: Futura; 1991

Weissberg D, Ben-Zeev I. Talc pleurodesis. Experience with 360 patients. J Thorac Cardiovasc Surg 1993; 106 (4): 689–695

Wetzer K, Schilling W, Wenzel D, et al. Die thorakoskopische Lungenbiopsie. Erkrank Atem-Org 1980; 155: 82–88

Whitlow CB, Craig R, Brady K, Hetz SP. Thoracoscopic pleurodesis with minocycline vs talc in the porcine model. Surg Endosc 1996; 10 (11): 1057–1059

Whitson BA, Andrade RS, Boettcher A, et al. Video-assisted thoracoscopic surgery is more favorable than thoracotomy for resection of clinical stage I non-small cell lung cancer. Ann Thorac Surg 2007; 83: 1965–1970

Wilkinson HA. Radiofrequency percutaneous upper-thoracic sympathectomy. Technique and review of indications. N Engl J Med 1984; 311 (1): 34–36

Wittmoser R. Thoracoscopic sympathectomy and vagotomy. In: Cuschieri A, Buess G, Perissat J, eds. Operative manual of endoscopic surgery. Berlin: Springer; 1992

Wittmoser R. Surgical thoracoscopy. Langenbecks Arch Chir Suppl II Verh Deutsch Ges Chir. 1990: 1325–1331

World Health Organization. Global tuberculosis control: epidemiology, strategy, financing: Report WHO. Geneva: World Health Organization 2009: 49–54

Wright GM, Barnett S, Clarke CP. Video-assisted thoracoscopic thymectomy for myasthenia gravis. Intern Med J 2002; 32 (8): 367–371

Wyser C, Walzl G, Smedema JP, et al. Corticosteroids in the treatment of tuberculous pleurisy. A double-blind, placebo-controlled randomized study. Chest 1996; 111: 333–338

Yildirim E, Dural K, Yazkan R, et al. Rapid pleurodesis in symptomatic malignant pleural effusion. Eur J Cardiothorac Surg 2005; 27 (1): 19–22

Yim AP, Chan AT, Lee TW, Wan IY, Ho JK. Thoracoscopic talc insufflation versus talc slurry for symptomatic malignant pleural effusion. Ann Thorac Surg 1996; 62 (6): 1655–1658

Yim AP, Lee TW, Izzat MB, Wan S. Place of video-thoracoscopy in thoracic surgical practice. World J Surg 2001; 25 (2): 157–161

Yoneda KY, Mathur PN, Gasparini S. The evolving role of interventional pulmonary in the interdisciplinary approach to the staging and management of lung cancer. Part III: diagnosis and management of malignant pleural effusions. Clin Lung Cancer 2007; 8 (9): 535–547

Young O, Neary P, Keaveny TV, Mehigan D, Sheehan S. Evaluation of the impact of transthoracic endoscopic sympathectomy on patients with palmar hyperhydrosis. Eur J Vasc Endovasc Surg 2003; 26 (6): 673–676

Zarić B, Kuruc V, Milovancev A, et al. Differential diagnosis of tuberculous and malignant pleural effusions: what is the role of adenosine deaminase? Lung 2008; 186 (4): 233–240

Zehtabchi S, Rios CL. Management of emergency department patients with primary spontaneous pneumothorax: needle aspiration or tube thoracostomy? Ann Emerg Med 2008; 51 (1): 91–100, 100, e1

Zgoda MA, Lunn W, Ashiku S, Ernst A, Feller-Kopman D. Direct visual guidance for chest tube placement through a single-port thoracoscopy: a novel technique. Chest 2005; 127 (5): 1805–1807

Zocchi L. Physiology and pathophysiology of pleural fluid turnover. Eur Respir J 2002; 20 (6): 1545–1558

# Subject Index

Note: Page numbers in *italics* refer to illustrations; page numbers in **bold** refer to tables.

Abbreviations: MT/P – medical thoracoscopy/pleuroscopy; VATS – video-assisted thoracic surgery